Neuro-oncology

NEUROLOGY IN PRACTICE

SERIES EDITORS: ROBERT A. GROSS, DEPARTMENT OF NEUROLOGY, UNIVERSITY OF ROCHESTER MEDICAL CENTER, ROCHESTER, NY, USA

JONATHAN W. MINK, DEPARTMENT OF NEUROLOGY, UNIVERSITY OF ROCHESTER MEDICAL CENTER, ROCHESTER, NY, USA

Neuro-oncology

First Edition

EDITED BY

Roger J. Packer, MD
Center for Neuroscience and Behavioral Medicine
Brain Tumor Institute
Gilbert Neurofibromatosis Institute
Children's National
Washington, DC, USA

David Schiff, MD
Departments of Neurology, Neurological Surgery, and Medicine (Hematology-Oncology)
University of Virginia Health Science Center
Charlottesville, VA, USA

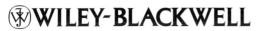

A John Wiley & Sons, Ltd., Publication

This edition first published 2012 © 2012 by John Wiley & Sons, Ltd

Wiley-Blackwell is an imprint of John Wiley & Sons, formed by the merger of Wiley's global Scientific, Technical and Medical business with Blackwell Publishing.

Registered office: John Wiley & Sons, Ltd, The Atrium, Southern Gate, Chichester, West Sussex, PO19 8SQ, UK

Editorial offices: 9600 Garsington Road, Oxford, OX4 2DQ, UK
The Atrium, Southern Gate, Chichester, West Sussex, PO19 8SQ, UK
111 River Street, Hoboken, NJ 07030-5774, USA

For details of our global editorial offices, for customer services and for information about how to apply for permission to reuse the copyright material in this book please see our website at www.wiley.com/wiley-blackwell

Library of Congress Cataloging-in-Publication Data
Neuro-oncology / edited by Roger J. Packer, David Schiff. – 1st ed.
    p. ; cm.
  Includes bibliographical references and index.
  ISBN 978-0-470-65575-7 (pbk. : alk. paper)
  I. Packer, Roger J., 1951–   II. Schiff, David, 1959–
  [DNLM: 1. Central Nervous System Neoplasms.   WL 358]
  616.99'481–dc23

                          2011044220

A catalogue record for this book is available from the British Library.

Wiley also publishes its books in a variety of electronic formats. Some content that appears in print may not be available in electronic books.

Set in 8.75/11.75 pt Utopia by Toppan Best-set Premedia Limited
Printed in Singapore by Ho Printing Singapore Pte Ltd

1   2012

Contents

Contributors

Jeffrey C. Allen, MD
Departments of Pediatrics and Neurology
NYU Langone Medical Center
New York, NY, USA

Isabel C. Arrillaga-Romany, MD, PhD
Center for Neuro-Oncology
Dana-Farber/Brigham and Women's Cancer
Center
Boston, MA, USA

Melissa L. Bondy, PhD
Department of Pediatrics
Dan L. Duncan Cancer Center
Baylor College of Medicine
Houston, TX, USA

Marc Chamberlain, MD
Department of Neurology and Neurological
Surgery
Fred Hutchinson Cancer Research Center
University of Washington;
Division of Neuro-Oncology
Seattle Cancer Care Alliance
Seattle, WA, USA

Jennifer L. Clarke, MD, MPH
Departments of Neurology and Neurological
Surgery
Division of Neuro-Oncology
University of California, San Francisco
San Francisco, CA, USA

Bruce H. Cohen, MD, FAAN
Department of Neurology
Children's Hospital Medical Center of Akron;
Department of Pediatrics
Northeast Ohio Medical University
Akron, OH, USA

Shlomi Constantini, MD, MSc
Department of Pediatric Neurosurgery
The Gilbert Israeli Neurofibromatosis Center
(GINFC)
Dana Children's Hospital
Tel Aviv Medical Center
Tel Aviv, Israel

Robert Dallapiazza, MD, PhD
Department of Neurological Surgery
University of Virginia Health System
Charlottesville, VA, USA

Josep Dalmau, MD, PhD
Department of Neurology
Hospital Clinic/Institute of Biomedical Investi-
gation (IDIBAPS)
University of Barcelona
Barcelona, Spain

Mark R. Gilbert, MD
Department of Neuro-Oncology
The University of Texas MD Anderson
Cancer Center
Houston, TX, USA

Jerome J. Graber, MD, MPH
Department of Neurology and Oncology
Montefiore Medical Center of the Albert
Einstein College of Medicine
New York, NY, USA

Sean Grimm, MD
Northwestern University
Chicago, IL, USA

Daphne A. Haas-Kogan, MD
Departments of Radiation Oncology and
Neurological Surgery
University of California, San Francisco
San Francisco, CA, USA

Jethro Hu, MD
Johnnie L. Cochran Jr. Brain Tumor Center
Departments of Neurology and Neurosurgery
Cedars-Sinai Medical Center
Los Angeles, CA, USA

Michael Ivan, MD
Department of Neurological Surgery
University of California, San Francisco
San Francisco, CA, USA

Kurt A. Jaeckle, MD
Departments of Neurology and Oncology
Mayo Clinic
Jacksonville, FL, USA

John A. Jane Jr., MD
Department of Neurological Surgery
University of Virginia Health System
Charlottesville, VA, USA

Derek R. Johnson, MD
Department of Neurology
Mayo Clinic
Rochester, MN, USA

Thomas J. Kaley, MD
Department of Neurology
Memorial Sloan-Kettering Cancer Center
New York, NY, USA

Santosh Kesari, MD, PhD
Department of Neurosciences
Moores UCSD Cancer Center
University of California San Diego
Health System
La Jolla, CA, USA

Akiva Korn, MMedSci
Department of Pediatric Neurosurgery
Dana Children's Hospital
Tel Aviv Medical Center
Tel Aviv, Israel

Eudocia Quant Lee, MD, MPH
Center for Neuro-Oncology
Dana-Farber/Brigham and Women's
Cancer Center
Boston, MA, USA

Geneviève Legault, MD
Departments of Pediatrics and Neurology
NYU Langone Medical Center
New York, NY, USA

Zvi Lidar, MD
Spine Unit, Department of Neurosurgery
Tel Aviv Medical Center
Tel Aviv, Israel

Yanhong Liu, PhD
Department of Pediatrics
Dan L. Duncan Cancer Center
Baylor College of Medicine
Houston, TX, USA

Robert G. Louis, MD
Department of Neurological Surgery
University of Virginia Health System
Charlottesville, VA, USA

Melike Mut, MD, PhD
Department of Neurosurgery
Hacettepe University
Ankara, Turkey

Antonio M.P. Omuro, MD
Department of Neurology
Memorial Sloan-Kettering Cancer Center
New York, NY, USA

Roger J. Packer, MD
Center for Neuroscience and Behavioral
Medicine
Brain Tumor Institute
Gilbert Neurofibromatosis Institute
Children's National
Washington, DC, USA

Kanwal P. S. Raghav, MD
Department of Medical Oncology
The University of Texas MD Anderson
Cancer Center
Houston, TX, USA

Jeffrey Raizer, MD
Department of Neurology
Northwestern University
Chicago, IL, USA

Alyssa T. Reddy, MD
University of Alabama at Birmingham
Departments of Pediatrics, Neurology
and Surgery
Children's of Alabama
Birmingham, AL, USA

Myrna R. Rosenfeld, MD, PhD
Department of Neurology
Hospital Clinic/Institute of Biomedical
Investigation (IDIBAPS)
University of Barcelona
Barcelona, Spain

Michael E. Scheurer, PhD, MPH
Department of Pediatrics
Dan L. Duncan Cancer Center
Baylor College of Medicine
Houston, TX, USA

Mark E. Shaffrey, MD
Department of Neurological Surgery
University of Virginia Health System
Charlottesville, VA, USA

Wendy J. Sherman Sojka, MD
Department of Neurology
Northwestern University
Chicago, IL, USA

Ben Shofty, BMedSci
Department of Pediatric Neurosurgery
The Gilbert Israeli
Neurofibromatosis Center (GINFC)
Dana Children's Hospital
Tel Aviv Medical Center
Tel Aviv, Israel

Matthew Tate, MD, PhD
Department of Neurological Surgery
University of California, San Francisco
San Francisco, CA, USA

Mary R. Welch, MD
Department of Neurology
Memorial Sloan-Kettering Cancer
Center
New York, NY, USA

Patrick Y. Wen, MD
Center for Neuro-Oncology
Dana-Farber/Brigham and Women's Cancer
Center
Boston, MA, USA

Brian J. Williams, MD
Department of Neurological Surgery
University of Virginia Health System
Charlottesville, VA, USA

Jennifer S. Yu, MD, PhD
Department of Radiation Oncology
Department of Stem Cell Biology and
Regenerative Medicine
Cleveland Clinic
Cleveland, OH, USA

Series Foreword

The genesis for this book series started with the proposition that, increasingly, physicians want direct, useful information to help them in clinical care. Textbooks, while comprehensive, are useful primarily as detailed reference works but pose challenges for uses at point of care. By contrast, more outline-type references often leave out the "how's and why's" – pathophysiology, pharmacology – that form the basis of management decisions. Our goal for this series is to present books, covering most areas of neurology, that provide enough background information for the reader to feel comfortable, but not so much to be overwhelming; and to combine that with practical advice from experts about care, combining the growing evidence base with best practices.

Our series will encompass various aspects of neurology, the topics and specific content chosen to be accessible and useful. *Neuro-oncology*, by Roger J. Packer and David Schiff, covers the field broadly, with detail when needed and helpful pointers along the way. Overview chapters cover etiology, epidemiology, and diagnosis, followed by treatment overviews concerning surgery, radiation therapy, and chemotherapy and biologic agents. Chapters on specific topics follow, covering the major areas of neuro-oncology encountered in pediatric and adult practice. We hope this approach will appeal to students, trainees, experts, and practicing neurologists alike. The editors are expert in their field and have recruited superb contributors to share their views on best treatment and management options.

Chapters cover critical information that will inform the reader of the disease processes and mechanisms as a prelude to treatment planning.

Algorithms and guidelines are presented, when appropriate. "Tips and Tricks" boxes provide expert suggestions. Other boxes present cautions and warnings to avoid pitfalls. Finally, we provide "Science Revisited" sections which review the most important and relevant science background material. Bibliographies guide the reader to additional material.

We welcome feedback. As additional volumes are added to the series, we hope to refine the content and format so that our readers will be best served.

Our thanks, appreciation, and respect goes out to our editors and their contributors, who conceived and refined the content for each volume, assuring a high quality, practical approach to neurologic conditions and their treatment.

And our thanks also go to our mentors and students (past, present, and future), who have challenged and delighted us; to our book editors and their contributors, who were willing to take on additional work for an educational goal; and to our publisher, Martin Sugden, for his ideas and support, for wonderful discussions, and for commiseration over baseball and soccer teams that might not quite have lived up to expectations. We would like to dedicate the series to Marsha, Jake, and Dan; and to Janet, Laura, and David. And to Steven R. Schwid, MD, our friend and colleague, whose ideas helped shape this project and whose humor brightened our lives, but who could not complete this goal with us.

Robert A. Gross
Jonathan W. Mink
Rochester, MN, USA

Preface

Neuro-oncology is a broad, ever-changing discipline, involving the specialties of neurology, neurosurgery, medical and pediatric oncology, radiation oncology, neuroradiology, and neuropathology, among others. Under its purview are the management of primary central nervous system tumors, the effects of systemic cancer on the nervous system, oncologic-related autoimmune conditions causing significant neurologic compromise, and the acute and long-term sequelae of oncologic treatment. For decades, the care of patients with primary central nervous system tumors was frustrating, with little progress being made. Recently there have been remarkable advances in the understanding of the molecular pathogenesis of cancer, the biology of neurodevelopment, basic mechanisms of cellular signaling, and how these all have a role in brain tumor development. Furthermore, there have been advances in the understanding of the mechanisms involved in paraneoplastic conditions and factors that predispose to treatment-related untoward effects on the adult and immature nervous systems. There has also been confirmation that tumors arising in children are molecularly different from those occurring in adults, and because of these molecular differences and the increased susceptibility of the developing nervous system to treatment-related injury, pediatric brain tumors require different management from those with similar histologies arising in adulthood.

While tremendous gains in molecular understanding of cancer in developing nervous system have not yet been widely translated into improved outcomes, innovative, biologically based approaches to treatment are rapidly being incorporated into management schema with the promise of better, less toxic therapy. This has given rise to the hope that "personalized" approaches to the treatment of brain tumors is within reach.

It is with this rapidly changing and maturing landscape that this volume in the series of Neurology in Practice has been developed. The textbook is not intended as an all-encompassing detailed reference, but rather as an easy-to-read, comprehensive text that covers the general aspects of therapy of adult and pediatric brain tumors, present concepts of the pathogenesis and management of the most common types of primary central nervous system tumors, and the effects of systemic cancer on the nervous system. Aspects of present management are emphasized while attempting to integrate newer concepts, especially biologic, which will soon have a direct impact on management and outcome of these lesions. Realizing the dynamic nature of the field, there was an attempt to move this text rapidly into press, so as not to be outdated at the time of publication. The neuro-oncology contribution to this series is designed to update both the academic and practicing neurologist and neurosurgeon, as well as physicians in practice and others caring for patients with brain tumors and cancers affecting the nervous system, with a readable review of all of the major types of tumors and a framework to understand new therapies, as they are being introduced. There is a purposeful emphasis on unique management approaches for adult and pediatric tumors where such distinctions are driven by the biology of the tumor or the effects of the required therapy on the developing nervous system. Although biases are unavoidable in such a complex field, there is every attempt, in this volume, to focus on evidence-based best practices.

Roger J. Packer, MD
Washington, DC, USA

David Schiff, MD
Charlottesville, VA, USA

Acknowledgments

I would like to thank David Schiff for his willingness to work with me on this text (I could not have had a better co-editor) and all of the authors for giving of their time and expertise. I want to thank the superb neuro-oncology team at Children's National, including Brian Rood, Lindsay Kilburn, Eugene Hwang, Gilbert Vezina, and Elizabeth Wells, for their support. Over the years, Betsy Schaefer has provided tremendous editorial help and expertise, allowing me to complete this and other works. Lastly, and most importantly, I want to thank my family: Bashi, Michael, Zavi, Rachael, Ophir, and Anabel for their love and encouragement.

Roger J. Packer

I would like to thank Roger J. Packer for the opportunity to participate in this worthwhile endeavor and the individual chapter authors for their top-notch and timely contributions. The incredible neuro-oncology team at UVA, including B.J. Purow, Jennie Friend, Marcia Molnar, Gina Petersen, Jim Finn, Stacy Smith, Kristie Coles, and most importantly Bruce Leffler, helped me carve out the time to complete this project. Over many years, the love and support from Julie and Dick Leerburger, Evie Joss, and Datsie Adams among others has been invaluable. Last and most of all, thanks to Tanya, Jasper, and Gracie, who keep me smiling.

David Schiff

Part I

Overview and General Aspects of Therapy

Diagnosis of Brain Tumors: Clinical and Radiographic

Isabel C. Arrillaga-Romany, Eudocia Quant Lee and Patrick Y. Wen

Center for Neuro-Oncology, Dana-Farber/Brigham and Women's Cancer Center, Boston, MA, USA

Introduction

Recent epidemiologic studies by the Central Brain Tumor Registry of the United States report the rate of symptomatic brain tumors at 19 per 100,000 person-years. An estimated 64,500 new cases of primary central nervous system (CNS) tumors and 150,000 cases of brain metastases are expected to be diagnosed in the United States in 2011. Surgery, chemotherapy, and radiation are the mainstays of therapy, and early diagnosis may produce better outcomes.

This chapter focuses on the diagnosis of tumors of the CNS and reviews both presenting clinical and neuroimaging features. Clinical recognition and imaging are essential early steps in identification of CNS tumors, although pathologic evaluation of tissue samples remains the gold standard for diagnosis. Rarely, when a biopsy is not feasible (for example with pediatric brainstem tumors), imaging has an even more valuable role. Our goal is to familiarize clinicians with general principles that are useful in the clinical recognition of potential brain tumors and to review imaging modalities that help differentiate brain tumors from other mass lesions.

Clinical diagnosis of brain tumors

History

Diagnosis of CNS neoplasms begins with a good clinical history and examination. Both nonspecific and focal neurologic complaints and symptoms can alert the primary care physician or neurologist to the possibility of an underlying mass lesion and indicate the need for further work-up. Key aspects of the history that help differentiate neoplastic lesions from other diagnoses include timing of symptom onset, tempo of progression, and severity of symptoms. Systemic symptoms and the presence of other diseases or hereditary syndromes are additional valuable pieces of information that can help narrow the diagnosis by their association with specific CNS tumors.

Symptoms produced by brain tumors may be either nonspecific or focal, and in general tend to be subacute in onset. The presentation varies widely and neither a normal neurologic exam nor presentation with acute onset of symptoms rules out a brain tumor. At the outset many brain tumors produce minimal or no symptoms. In

Neuro-oncology, First Edition. Edited by Roger J. Packer, David Schiff.

contrast, brain tumors can also present with acute onset stroke-like symptoms. This type of acute presentation is usually the result of a focal seizure or hemorrhage into the tumor bed. Less common causes include infarction or intraparenchymal hemorrhage resulting from stroke or venous sinus thrombosis, two conditions to which brain tumor patients are predisposed given their inherent hypercoagulable state.

The rate of progression of symptoms is also quite variable but tends to be gradual over weeks to months, helping to differentiate neoplasms from other more static disorders such as degenerative disease or more rapidly progressing infectious conditions. By paralleling the growth and spread of CNS neoplasms, the rate of symptomatic progression can serve as a rough clinical estimate to tumor grade. Typically, benign tumors such as meningiomas, or low-grade neoplasms such as oligodendrogliomas, will have a slower progression of symptoms than more malignant tumors such as glioblastomas.

Various other historical factors associated with brain tumors that can be elicited in the history are helpful in the formulation of a differential diagnosis. A careful review of systems, for instance, should identify symptoms such as weight loss, lethargy, and night sweats that are nonspecific but can be associated with many types of cancers. When combined with neurologic symptoms, these symptoms should raise suspicion of primary or metastatic CNS neoplasms, though should not rule out subacute infectious, inflammatory, or autoimmune CNS processes. Likewise, a detailed review of past medical history may identify genetic syndromes or other conditions with a higher than normal incidence of CNS neoplasms. Li–Fraumeni syndrome, resulting from germline mutations in the p53 tumor suppressor gene, is associated with a strong family history of multiple cancers including breast cancer, sarcoma, and leukemia, and associated with glioblastomas. Neurofibromatosis type 1 is associated with gliomas and cutaneous manifestations, neurofibromatosis type 2 is associated with vestibular schwannomas and meningiomas, while von Hippel–Lindau syndrome is associated with hemangioblastomas. Other systemic illnesses increase the risk for specific CNS neoplasm; one of the best examples

of this is the human immunodeficiency virus/acquired immunodeficiency syndrome (HIV/AIDS). Neurologic symptoms in immunocompromised patients, and in particular those with HIV/AIDS, should raise concern for primary CNS lymphoma (PCNSL). Likewise, focal neurologic symptoms in patients with a prior history of systemic cancers or lymphoma raises suspicion for brain metastases or CNS lymphoma. Lastly, knowledge of prior exposure to ionizing radiation can be helpful. Irradiation of the cranium is the only environmental exposure or behavior that is known unequivocally to increase the risk for intracranial tumors, specifically meningiomas, glial tumors, and schwannomas.

Clinical presentation and symptoms

Though classically patients with mass lesions are thought to present with focal or lateralizing symptoms, the reality is that many patients present with impairments reflecting multifocal, global, or nonspecific cerebral dysfunctions. The variety of symptoms and symptom subtypes reflect the diverse actions of tumors, either directly or indirectly, on brain function. Tumors such as gliomas or lymphomas can directly invade and destroy brain parenchyma. Others, such as meningiomas, directly compress and distort brain tissue. Such direct effects can result in a disruption of brain functioning at the cellular or circuit level resulting in focal neurologic signs. Alternatively, compression or invasion of other intracranial structures such as blood vessels, leptomeninges, and CSF outflow tracts is possible, and could lead to infarctions, venous sinus thromboses, elevated intracranial pressure, and hydrocephalus. Disruption of the blood–brain barrier (BBB) is another frequent occurrence that leads to vasogenic edema and thus increases the territory of brain parenchyma that becomes affected. Importantly, other factors inherent to the tumor itself, including location, size, and growth rate, impact the clinical presentation. Tumor size will determine how much of the brain is affected, which can correlate with both the number and severity of symptoms. The rate of tumor growth impacts the brain's ability to adapt to pathologic changes, and slower growing tumors often produce milder symptoms.

Generalized non-focal symptoms

Generalized tumor-associated symptoms are global and nonlocalizable. Often, patients with intracranial neoplasms have generalized impairments of cerebral function and present with vague complaints, making accurate diagnosis difficult. Headaches, nausea, vomiting, and changes in mental status, cognition, and level of consciousness usually reflect raised intracranial pressure from mass effect or hydrocephalus. Other symptoms and signs, such as global mental status changes, are quite pervasive and include apathy, change in personality, irritability, psychomotor retardation, lethargy, and forgetfulness. Such nonspecific impairments in mental function have been linked to lesions in the frontal and temporal lobes, corpus callosum, thalamocortical fibers, and reticular formation, among others. Occasionally, increased intracranial pressure can present in a similar fashion though usually alongside other indicative signs such as papilledema or with progressive altered levels of consciousness. Still other nonlocalizable presentations are the result of multifocal tumors, often seen in metastatic disease, presenting with a mixture of focal signs and symptoms that can be confused for generalized clinical manifestations.

Headache is one of the most pervasive symptoms in neuro-oncology, occurring in over 50% of this patient population. Pre-existing headache conditions appear to predispose patients to tumor-related headaches, making it difficult to distinguish between tumor and nontumor-related complaints. Some clues, such as change in headache character and increasing frequency or severity of headache, can help with diagnosis and point to the need for further work-up. Importantly, most tumor-related headaches do not appear in isolation. Recent estimates indicate that just 2% of brain tumor patients present with headache as their only clinical manifestation. The association of focal neurologic signs or symptoms with headache is another indication for prompt work-up.

Unfortunately, the character of the headache is not especially helpful in diagnosis. The classical teaching is that headache attributable to an intracranial neoplasm will be progressive, worse in the morning, or wake the patient from sleep, and may be aggravated by coughing, straining, or bending forward. These characteristics were thought to reflect raised intracranial pressures and theoretically to help identify tumor-related headaches. Recent reviews, however, have not corroborated an association between intracranial tumors and headache that is worse in the morning or with cough. Instead, tension-type headaches that are dull, moderate in intensity, and not particularly localizable are found to be the most common headache type in patients with intracranial tumors.

⚠ CAUTION!

Patients with headaches that wake them at night or are worse in the morning, or who have focal neurologic deficits, require urgent neuroimaging. However, many patients with brain tumors present with headaches that are indistinguishable from tension headaches.

Nausea and vomiting occur most frequently in association with severe tumor headache, but can also be present in isolation. These symptoms typically manifest first thing in the morning and are only rarely associated with food intake. Usually, tumor-associated vomiting reflects an increase in intracranial pressure or compression of the area postrema, a chemoreceptive trigger zone for vomiting, located in the inferolateral portion of the fourth ventricle. Specific tumor types with a predilection for the fourth ventricle and thus for inducing nausea and vomiting include medulloblastomas and ependymomas. Projectile vomiting without preceding nausea is fairly specific to posterior fossa childhood tumors and is rarely seen in adults. Tumors of the brainstem can also lead to similar symptoms via their effect on the nucleus solitarius.

Dizziness is another frequent complaint in brain tumor patients which can be either vague and ill-described or consistent with frank vertigo. A complaint of classic vertigo should raise suspicion of a tumor in the cerebellopontine angle such as a schwannoma, meningioma, or metastasis, or tumors in the pons or posterior fossa. Posterior fossa tumors sometimes present with vertigo and concomitant headache or dizziness.

Concomitant signs of incoordination such as dysmetria or ataxia are highly suggestive of a cerebellar or pontine lesion. Tumors that are supratentorial may at times also present with dizziness, though this is usually of the vague, ill-defined type that is more consistent with a sensation of lightheadedness and can be related to elevations in intracranial pressure.

Seizures are another common clinical manifestation of intracranial tumors. Although they are the result of a focal lesion, their frequent secondary generalization often prevents accurate localization. There may be post-ictal clues, such as Todd paralysis or post-ictal aphasia, which aid in localization of the lesion. If secondary generalization does not occur, or if the seizure semiology prior to generalization is clear, localization may be possible. The frequency of seizures in patients with brain tumors is around 30%, with significant variability by tumor type. Typically, slow-growing low-grade tumors are most epileptogenic and cause seizures that are often difficult to manage clinically. As an example, low-grade gliomas have a seizure frequency of 65–85% whereas the incidence of seizures in glioblastoma is 30–50%, closer to the average across all tumor types. The reason for the higher frequency in lower grade tumors remains elusive but may simply be related to the longer survival times of these patients. About 10–25% of patients with meningiomas or metastasis also develop seizures, with some variation by location. High convexity meningiomas and cortical metastasis are associated with higher seizure frequencies. Seizure frequencies for other specific tumor types have been less well defined, though brain lesions in close proximity to the cortex will be more epileptogenic than lesions deeper in the brain parenchyma.

Focal symptoms

Focal signs and symptoms may not be present initially in brain tumor patients but almost always develop as the disease progresses. There is great variety in symptom type based on location of the lesion (Table 1.1), and we describe some of the more typical signs and symptoms.

Supratentorial lesions frequently result in motor, sensory, language, or visual impairments. Hemiparesis, for instance, can occur in up to 50%

of patients with brain metastasis and 36% of patients with glioblastoma. Of course, the severity and side of the paresis, as well as the presence of concomitant signs and symptoms, depends on both the location and size of the tumor. Gross sensory disturbances are typical of tumors in the sensory cortex or thalamus, whereas higher level impairment in sensory discrimination or processing are typical of tumors in the parietal lobes. Diverse aphasias are possible when tumors affect the dominant postero-inferior frontal lobe or superior, perinsular, or insular regions of the dominant temporal lobe. When the aphasia presents in isolation of other symptoms it should raise concern for seizure and be further evaluated with an electroencephalogram (EEG). Visual impairments such as hemianopsias can be caused by lesions in the occipital lobes or parieto-temporal regions where the optic radiations may be impacted. Tumors of the hypothalamic or pituitary regions can compress the optic chiasm, producing bitemporal hemianopsia. Double vision can result from involvement of cranial nerves III, IV, and VI, usually with tumor invasion of the cavernous sinus, but also with tumors in the brainstem. Notably, double vision can present as a false localizing sign from VIth nerve palsy when increased intracranial pressure is the culprit.

Several tumor types frequently occur in specific locations and tend to produce a characteristic constellation of associated localizing symptoms. Their symptom pattern makes them readily recognizable. For example, craniopharyngiomas, slow-growing suprasellar tumors, can damage the pituitary and hypothalamus and compress the nearby optic chiasm, producing hormone imbalances manifesting with excessive thirst and urination or stunted growth, along with the classic bitemporal hemianopsia. Pituitary tumors can have a similar presentation though often the hormone imbalance is brought about by an overproduction of the hormone corresponding to the specific tumor cell type. Schwannomas are benign nerve sheath tumors that have a predilection for cranial nerve VIII, often causing hearing loss, tinnitus, and vertigo. Pineal gland region tumors, including pineal parenchymal tumors and germ cell tumors, present with symptoms of obstructive hydro-

Table 1.1. Symptom type based on location of lesion.

Frontal lobe	Seizures
	Headaches, nausea, vomiting
	Abulia
	Personality and behavioral changes
	Hemiparesis
	Aphasia (Broca [inferior frontal gyrus], conduction, or transcortical)
Temporal lobe	Seizures
	Headaches, nausea, vomiting
	Aphasia (Wernicke [superior temporal gyrus]; conduction
	Memory loss
	Visual field loss (superior quadrantinopsia)
Parietal lobe	Headaches, nausea, vomiting
	Sensory loss
	Seizures
	Visual field loss (inferior quadrantinopsia or homonymous hemianopsia)
	Visual spatial problems; problems with directions, dressing apraxia
Occipital lobe	Visual field loss (homonymous hemianopsia)
	Headaches, nausea, vomiting
	Seizures
Cerebellum	Ataxia
	Headaches, nausea, vomiting
Brainstem	Dizziness
	Diplopia
	Dysarthria
	Weakness
	Numbness
	Ataxia
Pineal region	Headaches, nausea, vomiting (from tumor and hydrocephalus)
	Visual problems
Pituitary/ hypothalamic region	Headaches
	Visual field loss (bitemporal hemianopsia)
	Hormonal disturbance (overproduction or underproduction of hormones)

cephalus including headache, nausea and vomiting, and lethargy. These tumors frequently compress the midbrain, potentially resulting in Parinaud (dorsal midbrain) syndrome, characterized by a group of specific eye and pupil abnormalities including impaired upgaze, light-near dissociation, convergence nystagmus, and eyelid retraction.

Radiographic diagnosis of brain tumors

Clinical clues can help formulate a differential diagnosis that includes intracranial neoplasms, but the differential remains vast and other tools are required to help narrow the diagnosis. Imaging with computerized tomography (CT) and/or magnetic resonance imaging (MRI) should be the next step in the confirmatory process of a suspected intracranial mass lesion. To date, MRI with gadolinium represents the best noninvasive and sensitive tool in the evaluation and characterization of intracranial neoplasms. Several specific MRI characteristics, along with more advanced imaging techniques, which are discussed below, are especially useful in differentiating among various types of intracranial masses such as brain tumors, demyelinating or inflammatory lesions, abscesses, and other infections. They do so by approximating lesion cellularity, invasiveness, metabolic rate, and vascularity. Many of these imaging characteristics can also be used to differentiate between specific tumor types and grades, and are helpful for preoperative planning, monitoring of treatment effect, and assessment of tumor recurrence.

Computer tomography imaging

Despite the many advantages of MRI, CT remains the most commonly used imaging modality in the initial evaluation of patients suspected of having a brain tumor. The reasoning behind this includes the speed and ease of CT scanning, the availability of scanners across emergency departments and hospitals, and the relatively low cost of CT compared with MRI. Occasionally, when an MRI is contraindicated such as when a patient has a pacemaker or metallic foreign body or implanted device, CT may be the only imaging modality available for use. CT scans can identify enhancing brain lesions that are larger than 5 mm. Lesions that are small or located in the posterior fossa can often be missed. CT scan can also readily identify tumors that are calcified such as oligodendrogliomas and craniopharyngiomas and can detect bony abnormalities-associated skull-based tumors. In the acute setting this imaging modality is essential for the rapid identification of mass effect, midline shift, vasogenic edema, hemorrhage, herniation, and hydrocephalus. The speedy identification of these complications is crucial to providing patients with appropriate and sometimes life-saving treatments.

Brain magnetic resonance imaging

MRI with gadolinium provides a great deal of information about intracranial tumors and their effects on surrounding brain parenchyma. Basic MRI sequences, such as T1, T2, and fluid attenuated inversion recovery (FLAIR), can identify the number, location, and size of lesions, the amount of associated vasogenic edema, and the presence of mass effect, midline shift, and hydrocephalus. T1 post-gadolinium sequences and more advanced sequences can provide detailed information that help differentiate among diverse types of mass lesions and intracranial tumors.

Contrast enhancement

The evaluation of an intracranial lesion with MRI should be performed with and without contrast, unless contraindicated. Gadolinium, a chelated rare earth element, is the contrast material of choice for MRI. The BBB acts as a first line of defense by impeding entrance of toxic substances, including gadolinium, into brain. Contrast enhancement of brain parenchyma thus reflects a breakdown in the BBB leading to increased permeability. The degree of enhancement should parallel the amount of BBB permeability, though imaging technique and contrast dose result in significant variability.

Neoplastic lesions, and in particular higher grade tumors, increase permeability and cerebral capillary blood volume via the cooption of existing capillaries and the formation of new distorted blood vessels with abnormal endothelium and incomplete basement membranes. This results in a leaky BBB that is permeable to gadolinium, making high-grade neoplastic lesions more apt to enhance on T1 post-gadolinium sequences. Theoretically, higher grade tumors with increased angiogenesis should result in higher degrees of contrast enhancement than lower grade lesions. In practice, however, the correlation between the degree of enhancement (aside from present or absent) and grade of glial tumors can be variable. Some low-grade tumors, such as pilocytic astrocytomas, gangliogliomas, and hemangioblastomas, enhance with contrast while a very small minority of glioblastomas do not.

Various other pathologic states increase BBB permeability including active inflammation from infectious and noninfectious causes, cerebral ischemia, and increased pressure states. Specific tumor types, however, tend to possess unique patterns of enhancement that can differ from patterns in these other disease states (Table 1.2). Extra-axial tumors, for instance, can produce pachymeningeal enhancement through a reactive process that results in increased dural thickness. Meningiomas, one type of extra-axial tumor with a broad-based dural attachment, are often identifiable by their characteristic "enhancing dural tail" on MRI. Leptomeningeal enhancement is another pattern of enhancement seen when neoplasms spread into the subarachnoid space, a process often referred to as "leptomeningeal metastases or neoplastic meningitis." Occasionally, this type of enhancement will be more nodular, helping to differentiate it from the

Table 1.2. Differential diagnosis of brain tumors.

SINGLE BRAIN LESION	
Tumors	Brain metastases
Primary brain tumor (including primary CNS lymphoma)	Primary CNS lymphoma
	Intravascular lymphoma
	Lymphomatoid granulomatosis
Metastatic brain tumor	Multifocal glioma
Hamartoma	Leptomeningeal metastases
Vascular	**Vascular**
Cerebral hemorrhage	Multiple cerebral infarction
Cerebral infarction	Small vessel disease
Aneurysm	Cavernous angiomas
Arteriovenous malformation	Multiple hemorrhages (amyloid angiopathy, blood dyscrasias, anticoagulation)
Cavernous angioma	
Infection	**Inflammatory**
Abscess	Systemic lupus erythematosus
Progressive multifocal leukoencephalopathy (PML)	Vasculitis
	Demyelination
Lyme disease	Multiple sclerosis
Syphilis	Acute disseminated encephalomyelitis
Viral encephalitis (e.g. herpes simplex encephalitis)	Behçet
	Sarcoidosis
Inflammation	**Infections**
Multiple sclerosis	Abscesses
Post-infectious encephalomyelitis	Bacterial
Systemic lupus erythematosus (SLE)	Tuberculosis
	Syphilis
Sarcoidosis	Fungal
Vasculitis	*Toxoplasma*
	Cysticercosis
Degenerative disorders	Progressive multifocal leukoencephalopathy (PML)
Trauma	
Benign cyst	**Developmental**
MULTIPLE BRAIN LESIONS	Heterotopia
Tumor	**Trauma**

smooth leptomeningeal enhancement caused by infectious forms of meningitis. The presence of small nodular cortical and subcortical enhancing lesions at the brain gray–white junction is typically seen in parenchymal brain metastasis. The gray–white matter junction is usually a transition zone between abundant and sparse vasculature creating a filtration zone for intravascular particulate matter in the region, including hematogenously spread neoplasms. However, brain metastases may occur anywhere in the brain parenchyma.

Another classic pattern of enhancement is ring enhancement, which can be associated with numerous types of benign and malignant intraparenchymal brain lesions. Ring enhancing lesions can be both superficial or deep and can represent high-grade gliomas, metastasis, abscesses, and other infections as well as demyelinating diseases, usually in that order of frequency. Both metastases and glioblastomas may appear initially as nodular and solidly enhancing lesions which become ring-enhancing with further growth as a result of central necrosis. Glioblastomas are usually single lesions, while metastases, demyelinating disease, and infections more frequently present as multiple lesions.

Patterns of ring enhancement can also vary, providing another clue in diagnosis. A smooth thin ring of enhancement is typically seen with abscesses and other infectious lesions. An open ring pattern can be quite characteristic of tumefactive demyelinating lesions. Thick irregular and nodular rings are usually seen in high-grade gliomas. Both glioblastoma and primary CNS lymphoma can present as expansile masses involving the corpus callosum, making it sometimes difficult to distinguish the two entities.

Diffusion MRI

Diffusivity measures the anisotropic movement of water molecules through tissues and is greater in extracellular than intracellular compartments. Lower diffusivity, which on MRI corresponds to a dark area on the apparent diffusion coefficient (ADC) sequence and a bright area on diffusion-weighted imaging (DWI) sequence, can thus serve as an approximation for higher cellularity and help to distinguish neoplastic lesions from non-neoplastic ones. It is particularly useful when attempting to distinguish hypercellular neoplasms, such as lymphomas and some high-grade gliomas, from less cellular lesions such as tumefactive demyelinating lesions. Diffusivity can also be used to differentiate solid viable tumors from tumors with necrotic centers. Importantly, abscesses are hypercellular lesions and will exhibit restricted diffusion on MRI. Low diffusivity will be seen both at the periphery and core of the abscess, helping to distinguish it from high-grade gliomas, which can have a similar ring enhancement pattern but a necrotic high-diffusivity core. Acute strokes also presents with restricted diffusion secondary to cytotoxic injury and may be difficult to differentiate from tumor, though the vascular distribution of the former is an important clue. Information from patterns of enhancement described above, diffusivity and appearance of lesions in other MRI sequences and other advanced imaging techniques must be taken into account in the radiographic diagnosis of intracranial lesions.

Identification of postoperative injury by noting new areas of restricted diffusion in the tumor resection cavity is also valuable to the clinician. Intraoperative injury can occur for numerous reasons, and areas of injury will subsequently evolve both physiologically and radiographically. Specifically, an area of injury with low diffusivity can evolve to become contrast enhancing. Without knowledge of prior tissue injury to the area it would be almost impossible to distinguish the lesion from tumor recurrence.

Perfusion MRI (dynamic susceptibility MRI)

Perfusion MRI techniques help identify the degree of tumor angiogenesis and capillary permeability by approximating cerebral blood volume and flow. Because increased tumor vascularity (with some notable exceptions especially among extra-axial tumors such as meningiomas) correlates with malignancy, this imaging technique provides additional hemodynamic information that can help distinguish neoplastic from benign lesions. Perfusion imaging also provides valuable information for preoperative tumor grading and planning, with more accurate estimates of the degree of vascularity than contrast enhancement provides. Biopsies can be obtained from regions of high perfusion, increasing the likelihood of obtaining tissue from regions corresponding to the highest grades. The technique has also been used with some success to differentiate tumor recurrence from radiation effect, including "pseudoprogression," and to measure response to antiangiogenic therapies.

Dynamic contrast-enhanced MRI

Although not routinely used in the diagnosis of brain tumors, dynamic contrast-enhanced (DCE) MRI provides useful information on tumor vascular permeability and is occasionally used to follow the effects of antiangiogenic therapies.

Magnetic resonance spectroscopy

Magnetic resonance spectroscopy is a noninvasive MRI technique that measures freely mobile metabolites within a specific area of interest in the brain, thereby relaying information about the regional biochemical milieu. The major metabolites of interest in the study of brain tumors include N-acetyl aspartate (NAA), choline, creatine, and lactate. Each of these provides unique biochemical information of the area of interest. Specifically, NAA, which is high in normal brain tissue, is a marker of neuronal integrity and will be decreased in regions corresponding to brain tumors. Creatine levels correspond to energy stores. Malignant tumors with high metabolic activity will usually have decreased levels of this metabolite. Choline is a marker of membrane turnover that is low in normal parenchymal tissue and will increases within brain tumors. Lactate and lipid levels vary in the typical spectra of malignant gliomas, with lactate representing the presence of anaerobic glycolysis and lipids reflecting any type of tissue necrosis.

Magnetic resonance spectroscopy may occasionally be useful in the radiographic diagnosis of brain tumors but generally has only limited value in the differentiation of intracranial masses. This is because spectroscopic patterns may be similar for gliomas, demyelinating disease, ischemia, and infection. Some niche applications of this technique include the differentiation of meningiomas, dural-based metastasis, and high-grade gliomas. More common clinical applications have included tumor grading, assessment of tumor recurrence, and preoperative planning.

Elevation of lipid within a malignant lesion corresponds to tissue necrosis suggesting a high grade. Information about metabolite levels in regions of T2 hyperintensity just beyond areas of contrast enhancement is also helpful in differentiating between tumor infiltration and vasogenic edema. The same pattern of low NAA and creatine with high choline characteristic of a neoplastic lesion will correspond to tumor infiltration, a mechanism of tumor spread characteristic of high grade but not low grade or metastatic lesions. Metabolite analysis can further help to differentiate areas of radiation necrosis from areas of tumor recurrence, a common clinical diagnostic dilemma. Radiation changes will typically exhibit low NAA and creatine similar to tumors, but will also have low choline levels in contradistinction to neoplasms. Lastly, magnetic resonance spectroscopy can be clinically useful in preoperative planning, where regions that appear most metabolically active can be identified for brain biopsy thereby decreasing the likelihood of false negatives based on sampling error.

Positron emission tomography

Positron emission tomography (PET) is a functional nuclear medicine imaging modality that can provide information about glucose metabolic activity, blood flow, and oxygen consumption. ^{18}Fluorodeoxyglucose (FDG) is the most available and commonly used tracer. It concentrates in regions of high glucose metabolism, thus highlighting lesions with high metabolic activity such as malignant neoplasms. Importantly, inflammatory lesions may also display increased FDG uptake, which can complicate the diagnosis of brain tumors. Amino acid tracers such as ^{11}C-methionine (MET) and ^{18}F-fluoroihydroxyphenylalanine (DOPA) are being developed as alternative tracers. As with FDG, increased concentrations of these tracers can be seen in neoplastic lesions known to upregulate carrier-mediated transport of amino acids.

In addition to its utility in the diagnosis of intracranial neoplasms, PET can be used to distinguish between radiation necrosis and tumor recurrence, and in monitoring response to treatment, although its sensitivity and specificity are limited. PET is also used occasionally in preoperative planning by highlighting regions of high metabolic activity, which can be targeted for biopsy.

Conclusions

Accurate diagnosis of intracranial tumors is challenging and usually requires histopathologic evaluation of sampled tissue. The process of diagnosis begins with a detailed clinical evaluation and continues with imaging. Both of these steps are crucial to the identification of intracranial lesions and provide significant information that helps formulate a differential diagnosis, sometimes narrowing the possibilities to one or two entities. The clinical history provides information regarding symptoms, their onset and progression that can begin to point in the direction of an intracranial neoplasm. The exam then provides direct observation of neurologic deficits and impairments, which allows for corroboration of the history and localization of potential brain lesions. Imaging confirms the presence of intracranial pathology. The use of a combination of standard and advanced imaging modalities provides anatomic, metabolic, functional, and physiologic information about intracranial pathologies that is frequently necessary to make an accurate diagnosis.

Selected bibliography

Cha S. (2006) Update on brain tumor imaging: from anatomy to physiology. *Am J Neuroradiol* **27**, 475–85.

Cha S. (2008) Physiological imaging. In: Bernstein M, Berger MS (eds) *Neuro-oncology: The Essentials*, 2nd edn. Thieme, New York, pp. 79–90.

Kracht LW, Jacobs AH, Heiss W. (2008) Metabolic imaging. In: Bernstein M, Berger MS (eds) *Neuro-oncology: The Essentials*, 2nd edn. Thieme, New York, pp. 71–8.

Nyak L, DeAngelis LM. (2010) Clinical features of brain tumors. In: Reese J, Wen PY (eds) *Neuro-Oncology: Blue Books of Neurology Series*. Saunders Elsevier, Philadelphia, pp. 54–70.

O'Neill AM. (2005) Clinical presentation of patients with brain tumors. In: Black PM, Loeffler JS (eds) *Cancer of the Nervous System*. Lippincott Williams & Wilkins, Philadelphia, pp. 47–52.

Schankin CJ, Ferrari U, Reinisch VM, Birnbaum T, Goldbrunner R, Straube A. (2007) Characteristics of brain tumour-associated headache. *Cephalgia* **27**, 904–11.

Smirniotopoulos JG, Murphy FM, Rushing EJ, Rees JH, Schroeder JW. (2007) Patterns of contrast enhancement in the brain and meninges. *Radiographics* **27**, 521–55.

van Breemen MS, Wilms EB, Vecht CJ. (2007) Epilepsy in patients with brain tumours: epidemiology, mechanisms, and management. *Lancet Neurol* **6**, 421–30.

Yamada K, Sorensen AG. (2008). Anatomic imaging. In: Bernstein M, Berger MS (eds) *Neuro-oncology: The Essentials*, 2nd edn. Thieme, New York, pp. 47–69.

Young GS, Stauss J, Mukundan S. (2010) Advanced imaging of adult brain tumors with MRI and PET. In: Reese J, Wen PY (eds.) *Neuro-Oncology: Blue Books of Neurology Series*. Saunders Elsevier, Philadelphia, pp. 71–98.

2

Epidemiology and Etiology

Melissa L. Bondy, Yanhong Liu and Michael E. Scheurer

Department of Pediatrics, Dan L. Duncan Cancer Center, Baylor College of Medicine, Houston, Texas, USA

Introduction

Brain tumors account for a small proportion of all cancers (1.4%) and cancer-related deaths (2.4%). However, most of these tumors are rapidly fatal, and even benign brain tumors can interfere with essential brain functions. An estimated 64,530 new cases of primary nonmalignant and malignant brain and central nervous system (CNS) tumors are expected to be diagnosed in the United States in 2011. Because of the extremely high mortality – especially among patients diagnosed with glioblastoma – and significant morbidity from brain tumors, there is ever-intensifying interest in understanding their etiology. The etiology of brain tumors remains largely unknown, and the relationship between and the contribution of heritable conditions and environmental exposures are unclear. Epidemiologic studies enhance this understanding in two ways. First, descriptive epidemiology studies characterize the incidence of brain tumors and the mortality and survival rates associated with them with respect to histologic tumor type and demographic characteristics. Second, analytic epidemiology studies compare the risk of brain tumors in people with and without certain characteristics (cohort studies) or compare the histories of people with and without brain tumors (case–control studies) to provide information on a wide range of possible environment risk factors, including inherited and acquired alterations in genes related to carcinogenesis, exposures to ionizing or nonionizing radiation, occupation, lifestyle, medical history, and certain common infections.

Descriptive epidemiology

Data on the occurrence of brain tumors in the United States are gathered primarily by two agencies: the Surveillance, Epidemiology, and End Results (SEER) program of the National Cancer Institute (http://seer.cancer.gov) and the Central Brain Tumor Registry of the United States (CBTRUS) (www.cbtrus.org). These programs collect different types of data: the SEER program reports on malignant primary brain tumors, whereas CBTRUS reports on both malignant and nonmalignant tumors. Using data from both programs allows the estimation of the incidence and mortality of brain tumors in the United States.

Incidence

The latest statistical report (data collected 2004–2007) from CBTRUS estimates an incidence of all

Neuro-oncology, First Edition. Edited by Roger J. Packer, David Schiff.
© 2012 John Wiley & Sons, Ltd. Published 2012 by John Wiley & Sons, Ltd.

primary nonmalignant and malignant brain and CNS tumors of 19.3 cases per 100,000 person-years (7.3 per 100,000 person-years for malignant tumors and 12.1 per 100,000 person-years for nonmalignant tumors). The rate was higher in females (20.7 per 100,000 person-years) than in males (17.9 per 100,000 person-years). SEER program data (collected 2003–2007) indicates an annual incidence of primary malignant brain and CNS tumors of 6.5 per 100,000 person-years. In contrast to CBTRUS data, the rate was higher in males (7.6 per 100,000 person-years) than in females (5.5 per 100,000 person-years). The age-adjusted incidence rate was 6.5 per 100,000 men and women per year. These rates were based on cases diagnosed in 2003–2007 from 17 SEER geographic areas.

Mortality and survival

The American Cancer Society estimated that 13,140 deaths due to primary malignant brain and CNS tumors would occur in the United States in 2010. Data from the SEER program (1995–2007 data) gives an estimated overall 5-year survival rate of 35.1%. Five-year relative survival by sex was 33.8% for men and 37.5% for women. Survival rates decrease dramatically with increasing age at diagnosis for all brain tumor types. Of all the histologic types of brain cancer, glioblastoma has the lowest 2- and 5-year survival rates for all age groups. The 2-year survival rate for glioblastoma is approximately 30% for those diagnosed before 45 years of age and decreases dramatically as age increases, to less than 2% for those aged

75 years or older. The 5-year survival rate of glioblastoma and most other histologic types of brain cancer is even worse, especially for older patients.

Differences by age, sex, and ethnicity

According to CBTRUS (2007–2008), the mean age at onset for all primary brain tumors, whether they are malignant or benign, is 57 years. However, the average age at onset for glioblastoma and meningioma, the two most common types of tumors among adults, is about 62 years. More important, the age distribution varies greatly by tumor site and histologic type. For example, the incidences of glioblastoma and astrocytoma peak at ages 65–74 years and then decrease, whereas the incidence of meningioma continues to increase with increasing age. An intriguing feature of brain tumor epidemiology is the peak in incidence of medulloblastoma and other primitive neuroectodermal tumors in young children. Age-specific incidence rates for selected histologies are graphically displayed in Figure 2.1.

There are also sex differences for certain types of brain tumors. The most consistent such finding is that neuroepithelial tumors are more common among men, whereas meningeal tumors are more common among women. For example, the incidence of glioma is 40% higher among men than women, whereas the incidence of meningioma is 80% higher among women. Biologic or social factors may account for these consistently observed sex differences. Therefore, although they are not well understood, these

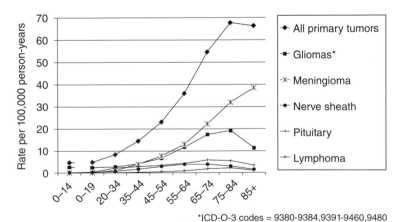

*ICD-O-3 codes = 9380-9384,9391-9460,9480

Figure 2.1. Age-specific incidence of primary brain and CNS tumors by selected histologies (CBTRUS Statistical Report: NPCR and SEER data 2004–2007).

factors must be considered in the etiology of brain tumors.

Cultural, ethnic, and geographic differences in risk factors also influence differences in tumor incidence. According to the 2011 CBTRUS data, by race and ethnicity, the overall incidence rate for primary brain tumors among African-Americans is 17.36 per 100,000, compared with 17.73 per 100,000 for Hispanic Americans and 19.13 per 100,000 for white people. The difference between these rates is statistically significant. The interpretation of ethnic variations is often confounded not only by ascertainment bias resulting from lack of access to health care by some populations, but also by inconsistencies in reporting. However, these differences cannot be attributed only to differences in access to health care or in diagnostic practices between black and white populations. There is also some evidence of ethnic variation in molecular subtypes of tumors. Although other explanations could exist, these associations justify further research into ethnic differences in molecular subtypes of gliomas.

Analytic epidemiology of risk factors

Despite the increasing number of epidemiologic studies, there is little consensus about the nature and magnitude of the risk factors for primary brain tumors. Several aspects of the epidemiologic study of these tumors hinder the comparison of studies and the formation of precise estimates of association. These factors include methodologic differences in patient recruit eligibility; the lack of representativeness of the patients studied; the use of proxies to report information about the cases; the use of inappropriate control groups; the substantial heterogeneity of primary brain tumors; inconsistencies in histologic diagnoses, definitions, and groupings; the difficulties in retrospective assessments of exposure to risk factors; and undefined latency periods.

Environmental risk factors

To date, the only established environmental risk factor for brain tumors is therapeutic ionizing radiation (IR). Some studies have investigated the role of chemical exposures (pesticides, heavy metals, and nitroso compounds), physical agents (electromagnetic fields, including mobile phones, and head trauma), biologic factors (viruses), and immunologic conditions (asthma, eczema, autoimmune diseases, and diabetes), but no definitive conclusions can be drawn.

Ionizing radiation

High-dose therapeutic IR is the only established environmental risk factor for brain tumors. Relatively low doses (1.5 Gy) used to treat ringworm of the scalp (tinea capitis) and skin hemangioma in children and infants have been associated with an increased risk for nerve sheath tumors, meningiomas, and gliomas. An increased risk of adult onset gliomas has been shown for people who received radiation treatment for acute lymphoblastic leukemia as children. In addition, an elevated risk of subsequent primary or recurrent brain tumors has been observed after radiation treatment for childhood cancer other than leukemia. Results from preliminary studies have suggested that the capability to repair DNA and the predisposition to cancer are related to differences in sensitivity to γ-radiation. Clearly, much work remains to be done to establish the importance of sensitivity to radiation exposure to the risk of developing gliomas. Other types of radiation exposures (parental exposure to IR, diagnostic radiation, or working as an airline pilot or in nuclear facilities and materials production) have also been suspected but not consistently implicated in brain tumor risk.

Cell phone use

Because the brain is the organ with the highest near-field exposure to microwaves during the use of both mobile and desktop cordless phones, an increased risk for brain tumors has been of concern. Several studies have shown an association. A meta-analysis of long-term use of mobile phones indicated that using a cell phone for >10 years approximately doubles the risk of being diagnosed with a brain tumor on the same side of the head as that preferred for cell phone use. The data achieve statistical significance for glioma and acoustic neuroma but not for meningioma. The authors stated that findings of the laterality analysis of the Hardell group are consistent with those of the Interphone group when the long-term data are specifically assessed.

Furthermore, the findings pertaining to brain tumors are strengthened by long-term data recently reported by Sadetzki *et al.* that show significantly elevated odds of developing ipsilateral parotid gland tumors among heavy cell phone users, an effect observed to be dose dependent. However, the 2010 Interphone study, which recruited participants in 13 countries, ran for a decade and included 5117 patients with brain tumors and 5634 matched control subjects. Overall, that study found little evidence of an association between brain tumors and cell phone use. However, when the two cohorts – cancer and no cancer – were subdivided according to the frequency of cell phone use, bizarre results emerged, including an apparently decreased risk of brain tumors in regular phone users, compared with rare users or nonusers. Clearly, further study is needed to establish the relationship between brain tumors and cellular phone usage on the incidence of brain tumors.

Occupational exposures

Despite the likelihood that brain tumors arise from specific workplace exposures, no definitive links have been made, even for known or strongly suspected carcinogens. In addition, there have been only small numbers of brain tumor cases even in large occupational cohort studies. The majority of studies that have examined occupational exposure to IR and the risk of brain tumors have not reported evidence of an association. Also, only very limited evidence has suggested an increased risk of brain tumors after exposure to low-level radiofrequency fields, with exposure duration of up to 10–15 years. A French population-based case–control study investigated the putative association between residential and occupational electromagnetic fields and the risk of brain tumors and found a nonsignificant increase in risk for occupational exposure to electromagnetic fields. This increase became significant for meningiomas, especially when electromagnetic field was considered separately. The risk of meningioma was also higher in subjects living in the vicinity of power lines (<100 m), but not significant. These data suggest that occupational or residential exposure to electromagnetic fields may have a role in the occurrence of meningioma.

Hormone use

Sex differences in glioma and meningioma incidence suggest that hormones could influence the development of these tumors. Increased growth rates of meningiomas have been observed during pregnancy, and a strong association exists between breast cancer and meningioma. Taken together, these observations support a role for female hormones in the etiology of meningiomas. A review of the epidemiologic literature for brain tumors and hormonal factors showed that an increased glioma risk was observed with later menarche and menopause, whereas a reduced glioma risk was observed for the use of hormone replacement therapy (HRT) and oral contraceptives, but duration of use had no effect on risk. Meningioma risk increased after menopause and with HRT use. These results are globally concordant with the biologic hypothesis assuming that female sex hormones are protective against glioma and may increase the risk of meningioma. However, more comprehensive epidemiologic studies should be conducted to confirm these associations and to refine the role of hormonal factors in brain etiology.

Diet

Dietary factors, especially those that add to the total body burden of oxidants, may be a factor in the development of cancers such as gliomas. It has been suggested that the degree of aggressiveness of the glioma can be modulated by dietary interventions and that some phytochemicals with antioxidant properties participate in that process. Epidemiologic studies of diet (particularly of *N*-nitroso compounds) have had problems obtaining accurate measurements of exposure to extremely common and widespread compounds. In addition, assessing each compound's individual effects is difficult because exposure to several compounds, especially in the diet, is unavoidable.

Tobacco and alcohol use

Although cigarette smoke is a major environmental source of carcinogens, studies of smoking have generally shown no evidence of an important association with adult or childhood brain tumors. One hypothesis that has been proposed to explain the lack of association between smoking and glioma observed in most studies is that the blood–brain barrier may limit the amount of carcinogens, such as *N*-nitroso compounds, reaching the brain tissue.

Alcohol is also an established carcinogen, and epidemiologic studies have shown that it is associated with an increased risk of several types of cancer; however, few epidemiologic studies have tested the association between alcohol consumption and risk of glioma. Epidemiologic studies have reported inconsistent results. Recently, Baglietto *et al.* provided evidence of a dose–response relationship between alcohol consumption and the risk of glioblastoma. By contrast, results for adults have suggested a decreased risk for gliomas with consumption of beer and wine.

Medical history and medication use

Serious head trauma has been suspected as a cause of some types of brain tumors, especially meningiomas and acoustic neuromas, but not gliomas. An increased risk of brain tumors has been linked to a history of seizures in several studies involving persons with epilepsy. Despite this, little is known about the effects of most medications on the risk of brain tumors. Previous studies have indicated that vitamin supplements provide a protective effect against gliomas, with increased protection resulting from increasing frequency of use. Epidemiologic studies have highlighted associations between reduced glioma risks and the use of over-the-counter medications associated with inflammation, particularly nonsteroidal anti-inflammatory drugs (NSAIDs) and antihistamines. While a reduced glioma risk associated with NSAIDs seems to span the different subtypes of glioma and is consistent with those reported for other cancers, the findings to date for antihistamine use are not as clear and suggest differing effects by glioma subtype and may act differently among those with a personal history of asthma or allergy.

Allergy, infection, and the immunologic response

Allergies and/or atopic disease have been associated with a significantly decreased risk of glioma in many but not all studies. The decreased risk associated with glioma has been hypothesized to result from an increase in immune surveillance related to atopic disease; this hyperactive immune surveillance may limit abnormal cell growth. Several types of viruses, including retroviruses, polyomaviruses, and adenoviruses, cause brain tumors in experimental animals. However, with the exception of studies of HIV-related brain lymphomas, few epidemiologic studies have addressed the potential role of viruses in causing human brain malignancies. Studies of the effects of SV40-contaminated polio vaccine on cancer incidence have found unconvincing results of an association with brain tumors. Recently, the investigation of another herpesvirus, human cytomegalovirus (HCMV), has been the topic of many reports; some supporting the role in gliomagenesis and some showing a lack of association. The debate over the role for HCMV in glioma risk continues; however, the presence of this virus in a majority of gliomas has led to the development of various immunotherapies for glioma-targeting HCMV antigens. Therefore, further study of the role of common infections and allergies in preventing brain tumors may be warranted.

⚠ CAUTION!

Although past research has elucidated environmental, genetic, and epigenetic factors in brain tumors, evidence linking a majority of brain tumors to specific genetic or environmental exposures is limited. Environmental exposure assessments (e.g. the concentration, amount, frequency, duration, setting, and route of exposure for occupation, diet, lifestyle choice) will continue to hinder progress in case–control and cohort studies, which are hampered by variability and uncertainty itself, information bias because of poor or differential recall by study subjects, and the lack of verifiable biomarkers of exposure given that information is obtained retrospectively. Additionally, the ability to measure quantitative levels of exposure at time of tumor development or predisposition to disease through molecular biomarkers has been limited.

Genetic risk factors

Cancers are believed to develop through an accumulation of genetic alterations that allow cells to grow out of the control of normal regulatory mechanisms and escape destruction by the immune system. Genetic and familial factors implicated in brain tumors have been reviewed previously. The term "genetic susceptibility" is often used to refer to relatively common genetic alterations that influence metabolism, carcinogenesis, and DNA stability and repair; these alterations are distinguished from the highly penetrant genes, which are rare alterations that lead to genetic predisposition to a disease.

✭ TIPS AND TRICKS

Recent advances in human genome studies have opened new avenues for the identification of susceptibility genes for many complex genetic disorders, especially in the field of rare brain tumors such as glioma. Our knowledge of predisposition to glioma is now developing. Improved research methods and tools, combined with larger studies involving homogenous tumor types, should help answer questions about the etiology of brain tumors. In addition to collecting data on environmental risk factors, new projects will need to consider including information on relevant genetic variants derived from ongoing whole-genome and gene pathway scans. Moreover, in addition to exploring environmental and genetic factors for brain tumor risk separately, the interaction between the two must be examined.

Family history and familial aggregation

Three to five percent of patients with CNS tumors have a first-degree family member also diagnosed with such neoplasms. A number of heritable syndromes are associated with increased incidence of brain tumors, such as Li–Fraumeni, neurofibromatosis (types 1 and 2), tuberous sclerosis, nevoid basal cell carcinoma syndrome, familial polyposis, and von Hippel–Lindau, but these syndromes explain only about 4% of the pediatric cases and even fewer of the adult cases,

approximately 1–2%. Several large studies have suggested an increased risk of primary brain tumors and other cancers for relatives of patients with glioma. These studies reported the risk of developing cancer at any site to be between 1.0 and 1.8 and the risk of developing a brain tumor to be between 1.0 and 3.0 for individuals with a family history of brain tumors. The differences in results among these studies may reflect differences in study methodologies, sample sizes, types of relatives included in the study (e.g. first- vs. second-degree), and ascertainment and validation of the family members' cancers. Although the familial aggregation studies suggest a genetic etiology for brain tumors, it is also possible that the aggregation may have resulted from shared environmental exposures. Although the data on familial risks in CNS cancer are overwhelmingly positive in showing an effect, with some exceptions, the data on childhood brain tumors have not shown strong familial effects.

Candidate gene-association studies

Candidate gene-association studies for glioma have mainly focused on four hypothesized pathways: DNA repair, cell cycle, metabolism, and inflammation (including allergies and infections). Only a few genes and single-nucleotide polymorphisms (SNPs) have been reliably associated with glioma in at least two populations from case–control studies: DNA repair genes *PRKDC* (also known as *XRCC7*) G6721T, *XRCC1* W399R, *PARP1* A762V, *MGMT* F84L, *ERCC1* A8092C, *ERCC2* Q751K; cell cycle gene *EGF* +61 A/G; and inflammation gene *IL-13* R110G. Despite much research, no definitive susceptibility alleles have been unequivocally identified through association studies. The inherent statistical uncertainty of case–control studies involving just a few hundred cases and controls seriously limits the power of such studies to reliably identify genetic determinants.

Genomewide association studies

The genomewide association study (GWAS) approach does not depend upon prior knowledge of function or presumptive involvement of any gene in disease causation. Moreover, it avoids the possibility of missing the identification of important variants in hitherto unstudied genes.

Shete *et al.* identified five risk loci for glioma: 5p15.33 *TERT*, 8q24.21 *CCDC26*, 9p21.3 *CDKN2A-CDKN2B*, 20q13.33 *RTEL1*, and 11q23.3 *PHLDB1*. Wrensch *et al.* provided further evidence to implicate the *CDKN2A-CDKN2B*, *RTEL1*, and *TERT* variants in high-grade glioma. Furthermore, a recent GWAS from France and Germany identified two additional genetic variations at 7p11.2 *EGFR* and 7q36.1 *XRCC2* and showed clear heterogeneity according to histologic subtypes of glioma *CDKN2B*, *TERT*, and *RTEL1* were found in glioblastoma, and *CCDC26* and *PHLDB1* variants most prominent in astrocytic and oligodendroglial tumors. Egan *et al.* replicated the glioma associations in *CDKN2B*, *RTEL1*, *TERT*, and *PHLDB1* in a US case–control study, and Chen *et al.* validated glioma risk at *RTEL1*, *PHLDB1*, and *TERT* in a Chinese population. It is interesting to note that the function of the seven glioma susceptibility genes identified by GWAS, four (*RTEL1*, *TERT*, *CCDC26*, and *CDKN2B*) have very close links to telomerase.

Linkage studies

Family studies have been traditionally hampered by their relatively small size and much lower marker density, unlike the newer GWAS method. However, despite their relatively low power, results of pedigree analysis can provide strong and convincing indications of genetic effects because they are based on genetic transmission of disease alleles within a family and thus do not have to make the population assumptions that association analyses do. Recently, the International Consortium GLIOGENE used a genomewide SNP approach to conduct a linkage scan in US families and identified a major disease locus on chromosome 17q12-21.32 (logarithm of the odds [LOD, to the base 10] score 3.39) and another region with evidence suggestive of linkage on 18q23 (LOD score 2.45). Thus, these two regions may harbor important genes that contribute to gliomagenesis.

Selected bibliography

Baldi I, Coureau G, Jaffré A, Gruber A, Ducamp S, Provost D, *et al.* (2011) Occupational and residential exposure to electromagnetic fields and risk of brain tumors in adults: a case–control study in Gironde, France. *Int J Cancer* **129** (6), 1477–84.

Bondy ML, Scheurer ME, Malmer B, Barnholtz-Sloan JS, Davis FG, Il'yasova D, *et al.*; Brain Tumor Epidemiology Consortium (2008) Brain tumor epidemiology: consensus from the Brain Tumor Epidemiology Consortium. *Cancer* **113** (7 Suppl), 1953–68.

Chen H, Chen Y, Zhao Y, Fan W, Zhou K, Liu Y, *et al.* (2011) Association of sequence variants on chromosomes 20, 11, and 5 (20q13.33, 11q23.3, and 5p15.33) with glioma susceptibility in a Chinese population. *Am J Epidemiol* **173** (8), 915–22.

Egan KM, Thompson RC, Nabors LB, Olson JJ, Brat DJ, Larocca RV, et al. (2011) Cancer susceptibility variants and the risk of adult glioma in a US case–control study. *J Neurooncol* **104** (2), 535–42.

Gu J, Liu Y, Kyritsis AP, Bondy ML. (2009) Molecular epidemiology of primary brain tumors. *Neurotherapeutics* **6** (3), 427–35.

Hardell L, Carlberg M, Hansson K. (2006) Mild pooled analysis of two case–control studies on the use of cellular and cordless telephones and the risk of benign brain tumours diagnosed during 1997–2003. *Int J Oncol* **28** (2), 509–18.

Interphone Study Group (2010) Brain tumour risk in relation to mobile telephone use: results of the Interphone international case–control study. *Int J Epidemiol* **39** (3), 675–94.

Khurana VG, Teo C, Kundi M, Hardell L, Carlberg M. (2009) Cell phones and brain tumors: a review including the long-term epidemiologic data. *Surg Neurol* **72** (3), 205–214; discussion 214–5.

Mitchell DA, Xie W, Schmittling R, Learn C, Friedman A, McLendon RE, *et al.* (2008) Sensitive detection of human cytomegalovirus in tumors and peripheral blood of patients diagnosed with glioblastoma. *Neuro-Oncology* **10** (1), 10–18.

Sadetzki D, Chetrit A, Jarus-Hakak A, Cardis E, Deutch Y, Duvdevani S, *et al.* (2008) Cellular phone use and risk of benign and malignant parotid gland tumors: a nationwide case–control study. *Am J Epidemiol* **167** (4), 457–67.

Scheurer ME, Bondy ML, Aldape KD, Albrecht T, El-Zein R. (2008) Detection of human cytomegalovirus in different histological types of gliomas. *Acta Neuropathol* **116** (1), 79–86.

Scheurer ME, Amirian ES, Davlin SL, Rice T, Wrensch M, Bondy ML. (2011) Effects of anti-histamine and anti-inflammatory medication use on risk of specific glioma histologies. *Int J Cancer* **129** (9), 2290–6.

Scheurer ME, El-Zein R, Thompson PA, Aldape KD, Levin VA, Gilbert MR, et al. (2008) Long-term anti-inflammatory and antihistamine medication use and adult glioma risk. *Cancer Epidemiol Biomarkers Prevent* **17** (5), 1277–81.

Shete S, Hosking FJ, Robertson LB, Dobbins SE, Sanson M, Malmer B, *et al.* (2009) Genome-wide association study identified five susceptibility loci for glioma. *Nat Genet* **41** (8), 899–904.

Wrensch M, Jenkins RB, Chang JS, Yeh RF, Xiao Y, Decker PA, *et al.* (2009) Variants in the CDKN2B and RTEL1 regions are associated with high-grade glioma susceptibility. *Nat Genet* **41** (8), 905–8.

3

General Aspects of Surgery

Robert G. Louis, Brian J. Williams and Mark E. Shaffrey

Department of Neurological Surgery, University of Virginia Health System, Charlottesville, VA, USA

Introduction

With few exceptions, operative neurosurgical intervention remains the primary method for definitive diagnosis and treatment of tumors involving the central nervous system (CNS). Even lesions for which cytoreductive surgery is not critical, such as primary CNS lymphoma (PCNSL), require stereotactic biopsy to establish a tissue diagnosis before treatment can be initiated. It has been nearly 125 years since Bennett and Godlee successfully performed the first reported resection of a cerebral tumor and concluded that "surgical intervention to the human cerebrum is indeed possible." Despite miraculous advances in surgical technique and technology, neurosurgeons of the modern era still face many of the same challenges as these early pioneers. The unique and intricate nature of the brain poses equally unique and complex challenges for those who mean to intervene upon tumors involving it. Unlike other branches of surgical oncology, where surgeons may aim to resect a malignant tumor with a clear margin of normal tissue, the very nature of neurosurgery does not allow this luxury. Rather, the neurosurgeon often faces difficult decisions on how best to maximize surgical resection, while avoiding possibly devastating and permanent neurologic complications through injury of eloquent brain tissue. In fact, often the main bulk of the tumor is managed differently from the residual margin that may exist at the interface with "normal" brain. The aim of this chapter is to introduce the principles that guide this decision-making process, provide an overview of the surgical procedures involved, and discuss surgical complications and the technologic advances that have helped to decrease their incidence.

Goals of surgery

Tissue diagnosis

At the most basic level, one of the primary goals of almost every operation in neurosurgical oncology is the sampling of tissue to establish a histopathologic diagnosis. For some tumors, such as PCNSL, this may be the extent of the neurosurgeon's involvement, whereas for the vast majority it is only the beginning. Regardless, histopathologic diagnosis has an important role in the management of almost all tumors involving the CNS. The discrepancy between clinical impression and histologic diagnosis leading to a change in patient management has been reported by Lee *et al.* as ranging from 13% to 40%. Despite significant advances in modern imaging techniques, a definitive diagnosis requires sampling of the pathologic entity in question.

Neuro-oncology, First Edition. Edited by Roger J. Packer, David Schiff.
© 2012 John Wiley & Sons, Ltd. Published 2012 by John Wiley & Sons, Ltd.

The particular approach taken by the neurosurgeon to obtain tissue for histopathologic analysis may vary according to the demographic and clinical features of the patient as well as the size, location, and imaging characteristics of the lesion. In general, a biopsy sample may be obtained in a direct, open fashion during a craniotomy for attempted resection; or it may be performed stereotactically with a thin biopsy cannula. While the tissue specimen obtained during open surgical biopsy often contains abnormal tissue, stereotactic biopsies provides a small sample of specimen which is susceptible to sampling error. Considering the treatment plan and ultimately the prognosis are heavily dependent on an accurate tissue diagnosis, it goes without saying that establishing the reliability of biopsy techniques is of paramount importance.

Stereotactic biopsy

All stereotactic procedures are based on some mathematical system of three-dimensional spatial coordinates such as Cartesian or polar coordinate systems. Once the coordinate system is established as a reference, the stereotactic apparatus allows controlled movement along a defined geometric axis. This can be accomplished either through the use of a rigid frame, which is fixed to the patient's head, or through "frameless" techniques that use optical or electromagnetic reference points to localize the instrumentation in three-dimensional space. The accuracy of frame-based stereotactic biopsy in establishing a definitive histologic diagnosis has been reported by Haines and Walters as ranging from 62% to 95%. While this seems like a broad range, many of the studies reporting lower diagnostic accuracies are those mandating accurate differentiation between anaplastic astrocytoma and glioblastoma. Most studies report sensitivities and specificities greater than 90% in diagnosing malignant glioma (inclusive of World Health Organization [WHO] grade 3 and 4 lesions). These results are true for both frame-based and frameless techniques. Inaccurate diagnosis most commonly results from sampling error in heterogeneous zones of the tumor, such as infiltrating margin or necrosis, which are not representative of the entire neoplasm. As a result, most authors recommend taking multiple biopsies from different areas of the tumor to avoid this "sampling error."

Avoidance of sampling error is one of the benefits of open resection, as the large volume of specimen provided usually allows for an accurate diagnosis. The risk of misdiagnosis from sampling error must be weighed against the risk of open surgical resection in the case of a tumor that might not benefit from such a procedure. In cases where the diagnosis is questionable, stereotactic biopsy should be performed. If, based upon the biopsy, the histopathologic diagnosis is uncertain or is one that would benefit from cytoreduction, open surgical sampling and resection can be performed at a later date. Proposed indications for stereotactic biopsy are listed in the Tips and Tricks box.

☆ TIPS AND TRICKS

INDICATIONS FOR STEREOTACTIC BRAIN BIOPSY

- Tumors in eloquent or inaccessible areas of the brain in which open surgical intervention has a high risk of neurologic deficit, such as the brainstem or thalamus
- Small tumors with minimal deficit
- Lesions in which the imaging diagnosis is uncertain and those in which management plan may include further surgical or medical treatment based on the histologic diagnosis (e.g. sarcoid, primary CNS lymphoma)
- Patients in poor medical condition, precluding anesthesia

A highly vascular lesion or one in close proximity to a major vascular structure are contraindications to stereotactic biopsy. In these cases, open biopsy offers the safest method for obtaining tissue for histopathologic analysis.

The complications associated with stereotactic biopsy include hemorrhage, new neurologic deficit, seizures, and infection. The overall complication rate associated with stereotactic biopsy is less than 5%. While it bears mentioning that the reported rate of hemorrhage after stereotactic biopsy is as high as 60%, the vast majority of these are small, asymptomatic bleeds without clinical consequences. In a series of 500 consecutive patients undergoing stereotactic biopsy, 8% were found to have hemorrhage on postoperative computer tomography (CT) scan. Of these, neurologic deficit developed in six patients (1.2%) and one patient (0.2%) died. There is also a small risk of delayed hemorrhage and neurologic deficit, even in patients with a negative postoperative CT scan. According to Field *et al.*, this risk justifies overnight hospitalization in all patients undergoing stereotactic brain biopsy. Despite the low risk (0.2–0.8%) of infection after stereotactic biopsy, perioperative antibiotics (1 g cefazolin IV prior to incision and every 8 hours for 24 hours) are recommended. In addition, dexamethasone and antiepileptics are frequently given to prevent postoperative edema and seizures, respectively, although the clinical necessity is not proven.

Cytoreduction vs. surgical cure

At the most elementary level, the surgical approach to tumors can be distinguished by whether the tumor is intra-axial or extra-axial (Figure 3.1). Although trends exist for each tumor type, intra-axial tumors including gliomas, gli-

oneuronal tumors, PCNSL, primitive neuro-ectodermal tumors (PNETs), and metastases can occur anywhere within the brain parenchyma, including the cerebellum or brainstem. With the exception of PCNSL and some metastases (e.g. small cell lung cancer), the optimal initial treatment modality for these tumors is surgical resection. Although gross total resection determined by magnetic resonance imaging (MRI) may be curative in some cases, this is often not the case, particularly in cases of infiltrating gliomas. Even though surgical cure may not be possible, resection can be beneficial in both providing histopathologic diagnosis, reducing both mass effect and overall tumor burden, and improving outcome.

Although a subject of much controversy, there is a growing body of literature to suggest that cytoreductive surgery for low-grade and malignant gliomas improves survival. Several studies have also demonstrated survival benefits for the resection of single and multiple brain metastases. Extent of resection (EOR) may be significant in determining survival for both low-grade and high-grade gliomas. After adjusting for other factors known to influence survival (age, Karnofsky performance status [KPS], tumor location, and tumor subtype), improvements in both

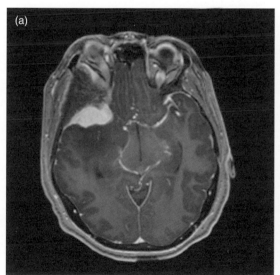 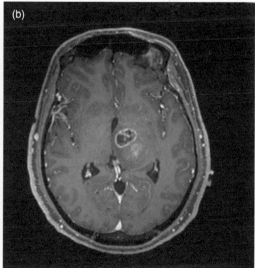

Figure 3.1. (a) Right medial sphenoid wing meningioma, a classic extra-axial tumor. (b) An example of a left-sided glioblastoma based in the thalamus, an intra-axial tumor.

overall survival (OS) and progression free survival (PFS) have been demonstrated in patients with low-grade gliomas whose EOR was ≥90%. The utility of aggressive surgery has also been demonstrated with anaplastic astrocytoma and glioblastoma. Neurosurgeons agree that every attempt should be made to perform as complete a resection as possible while, if possible, avoiding resections that can damage normal brain tissue.

✋ CAUTION!

EXTENT OF RESECTION AND SURVIVAL IN MALIGNANT GLIOMA

- No class I evidence exists to either support or refute the benefit of extent of resection (EOR) on survival.
- McGirt *et al.* retrospectively reviewed 949 patients and demonstrated improved overall survival in patients with both anaplastic astrocytoma and glioblastoma who underwent gross total resection compared with those who received near-total or subtotal resection.
- Sanai *et al.* retrospectively reported on a series of 500 patients with newly diagnosed glioblastoma and found that a significant survival advantage was seen with as little as 78% EOR and stepwise improvement in survival was evident even in the 95–100% EOR range.
- Hart *et al.* Cochrane Review in 2003 with a meta-analysis of 2100 articles addressing the EOR in malignant glioma excluded all studies as being unable to identify appropriate randomized data for inclusion.
- Lacroix *et al.* retrospectively reviewed EOR in 416 patients with glioblastoma, and reported that a significant survival advantage was associated with resection of 98% or more of the tumor volume (median survival 13 months, 95% confidence interval [CI] 11.4–14.6 months), compared with 8.8 months (95% CI 7.4–10.2 months; $P < 0.0001$) for resections of less than 98%.

- Six of the eight available prospective studies report that EOR is an important indicator of postoperative survival.

In contrast to many glial and metastatic intraparenchymal tumors, in which complete resection is often not feasible, many extra-axial tumors and some intra-axial tumors afford the neurosurgeon the opportunity for gross total resection and surgical cure. Benign tumors such as meningiomas, pituitary adenomas, cranial nerve schwannomas, chordomas, dermoids and epidermoids, choroid plexus papillomas, pilocytic astrocytomas, and hemangioblastomas may, in many cases, be cured with complete surgical resection. In these cases, gross total resection may offer significant advantages in both OS and PFS over subtotal or partial resection. Meningiomas have a 10-year recurrence rate of only 9% with complete tumor resection including overlying dura and bone (Simpson Grade 1) compared with 40% recurrence with subtotal resection. While more recent reports have called into question the need for resection of underlying bone and dura, most agree that gross total resection of the tumor provides the best opportunity for long-term cure. However, in a series of 373 patients with WHO Grade 1 meningiomas, no significant difference in PFS were found in patients who received Simpson Grade 1–4 resections, arguing that removing the entire tumor or even leaving small amounts of tumor attached to critical structures was an acceptable alternative to potentially neuro-damaging surgery.

While they may not always directly involve cortical or subcortical structures, extra-axial tumors often exert significant mass effect upon the brain and may become adherent and even infiltrative, making safe resection a challenge. Because of their location, often near the skull base, many of these tumors can often be intimately involved with vital cerebrovascular structures, cranial nerves, and the brainstem itself. Patients and surgeons must recognize and discuss the risk–benefit profile for attempting complete removal of tumors involving these critical structures.

Alleviation of mass effect

Even in cases where surgical cure is not possible and cytoreduction is of limited or questionable survival benefit, surgical debulking may still be indicated as a palliative measure. This is true for both intraparenchymal and extra-axial tumors. Even a modest reduction in tumor volume can accomplish enough of a decrease in intracranial pressure (ICP) to provide significant relief of the headaches, nausea, and vomiting associated with increased ICP. Similarly, obstructive hydrocephalus may often be relieved by debulking the inciting tumor; although often these patients require permanent cerebrospinal fluid (CSF) diversion. Fixed neurologic deficits from intra-axial tumors such as gliomas and metastases can arise either from compression or direct invasion of eloquent brain regions. Cytoreductive surgery can often result in improvement of those focal neurologic symptoms caused by compression, while those caused by direct invasion will often be worse after surgery if tumor is removed from eloquent areas. Reduction in tumor volume may also lead to decreases in local edema, which can also help to alleviate both neurologic symptoms and those related to increased ICP. In addition, patients developing seizures as a result of a mass lesion may benefit significantly from epilepsy surgery. The neurosurgeon, in combination with a multidisciplinary epilepsy team, must decide whether the seizures are more likely to be controlled purely by removal of the tumor (lesionectomy) or a more extensive operation which could include a seizure focus remotely located from the tumor itself. Intraoperative electrocorticography can often help to make this distinction.

Craniotomy

Just as the spectrum of tumors affecting the CNS is broad, so too is the armamentarium of surgical procedures to address them. Any attempt at surgical intervention for an intracranial tumor must be preceded by a frank and detailed discussion of the possible outcomes and complications. Patients must be counseled about the undesirable but often expected complications of the particular procedure they are to undergo. Perhaps in no other field of medicine is the consent process so necessary and involved. Because of the poten-

tial for neurologic devastation, a patient's condition must be considered in the context of familial, social, cultural, religious, and economic circumstances, some of which may be in conflict with each other.

While numerous variations in positioning, approach, and technique exist, the fundamental operation in neurosurgical oncology is the craniotomy. With the possible exception of intrasellar tumors, craniotomy or craniectomy in some form is required as the initial step of every attempted resection of both intra-axial and extra-axial tumors. Routine medical and laboratory screening must be performed in order to assess suitability for surgery. To prevent excessive bleeding, platelet count should be >100,000 and international normalized ratio (INR) <1.4 before initiating any elective craniotomy. At least two units of blood should be typed and held for surgery. Patients should be risk stratified according to their medical comorbidities to assess for the suitability of a prolonged anesthetic and surgical procedure.

All patients are given preoperative antibiotics (e.g. 1–2 g cefazolin IV) and dexamethasone and most patients are given either phenytoin or levetiracetam as seizure prophylaxis. After induction of anesthesia, the patient's head is placed in Mayfield pins in order to allow for rigid fixation to the operating table. The head is then positioned so the tumor is the most elevated site of the body. The head is generally elevated at 30 degrees to facilitate venous drainage and decrease ICP. Gentle hyperventilation by the neuroanesthesiologist with a target PCO_2 of 25–30 mmHg will also help to accomplish this goal. In select cases, mannitol or lumbar drainage may also be used to further decrease ICP and prevent trans-cranial herniation through the craniotomy defect. The neurosurgeon then localizes the site of the tumor using surface landmarks, often employing neuronavigation to improve accuracy. The site for the incision is then marked, clipped, and prepped in a sterile fashion. Local anesthetic with epinephrine is employed for local hemostasis and to help prevent postoperative pain. The incision generally involves creation of a galeocutaneous flap, which is elevated, exposing the skull. The pericranium may be kept intact and harvested separately as a dural substitute for dural repair at the completion of the case. A pneumatic drill is then used to place burr holes through the skull as entry points for the craniotomy. These are generally placed in strategic locations, away from critical structures, and allow dissection of the underlying dura away from the deep surface of the calvarium. Once the dura has been separated, a high-speed saw is used to create a bone flap which is then carefully elevated, removed, and placed aside until the completion of the case. The dura is then carefully incised, creating a dural flap which can be reflected.

With the brain exposed, the next step depends upon the nature, location, and depth of the tumor. Tumors that are superficial can be easily visualized at the cortical surface, while deeper lesions may appear to cause localized swelling or may be invisible at the surface. Adequate visualization of the tumor and its interface with the surrounding brain is of paramount importance in maximizing the EOR and preventing neurologic complications. There are several mechanisms by which brain tumor patients can sustain neurologic deterioration during neurosurgical resection. Deficits from direct cortical injury usually appear immediately postoperatively and are not progressive in nature. Often, this may include completion or worsening of a pre-existing deficit as a result of tumor proximity to eloquent brain structures. These issues are further complicated by the very nature of certain intrinsic brain tumors. Specifically, gliomas are typified by their infiltrative nature, often making it impossible to visualize the demarcation between tumor and surrounding normal brain. Detailed knowledge of neuroanatomy and intraoperative mapping can allow the surgeon to predict and sometimes prevent these complications.

Intraoperative localization of subcortical and deep tumors can be accomplished with the help of neuronavigation or ultrasound. Once the tumor has been localized, a small corticotomy is performed, taking care to avoid major surface arteries and veins. The approach taken to gain access to a particular tumor is beyond the scope of this chapter, but both trans-gyral and trans-sulcal routes have been advocated. Upon identification of the tumor, a biopsy is sent for intraoperative consultation. The intraoperative diagnosis will often dictate how aggressive a resection the surgeon will attempt. Those lesions that may be cured surgically are often targeted for more aggressive resection, while debulking may suffice for higher grade lesions that involve critical structures. Resection of a tumor with a defined border generally involves identification and dissection of the superficial aspects of the tumor–brain interface, followed by internal debulking in order to allow the tumor to collapse upon itself. This alternating technique of external dissection and internal debulking allows for safe resection of the tumor while minimizing retraction of surrounding brain structures. Depending on the consistency, the tumor may be evacuated using a combination of techniques, including cautery, suction, and ultrasonic aspiration. Throughout the resection, it remains critical to visualize the tumor margin clearly in order to prevent accidental transgression into the surrounding brain.

After the resection is complete, meticulous hemostasis must be accomplished within the tumor cavity. This often involves the use of multiple hemostatic agents including peroxide, thrombin-soaked gel foam, or foam-like hemostatic agents. After gentle irrigation of the brain surface, the dural flap is returned to place and closed primarily if possible. In cases where insufficient dura exists to repair the defect, pericranium may be used as a substitute or synthetic dural substitutes are available. Although not always possible, the goal is to obtain a watertight dural closure to prevent postoperative CSF leakage. This is primarily a concern in cases involving the posterior fossa or skull base including trans-sphenoidal approaches. Hemostasis must again be achieved at the dural and bone edges. The craniotomy flap is then replaced and secured to the skull with titanium plates and screws that are MRI compatible. A drain may be introduced to prevent formation of a sub-galeal hematoma. The galea and skin are closed in two separate layers. Finally, a sterile head wrap is applied to both protect the wound and provide some degree of compression for hemostasis.

Postoperative care

The potential for neurologic decline, postoperative hemorrhage, increased ICP, and seizures dictates mandatory postoperative placement within an intensive care unit (ICU), preferably one with experience in the care of neurologic and neurosurgical patients. Serial exams are performed in order to ensure that the patient returns to the baseline level of consciousness (LOC) and neurologic functioning. After emergence from anesthesia, most patients return to their neurologic baseline. Patients must be monitored closely for seizures, and hypertension must be avoided. Maintenance fluid should be isotonic (normal saline or lactated Ringer solution). Hypotonic solutions should be avoided as hyponatremia will increase cerebral edema. Dexamethasone is generally continued at high doses in the initial postoperative period and may be tapered slowly or rapidly, depending on the nature of the tumor and degree of edema. Antibiotics are continued for 24 hours or until all drains have been removed. Based upon the American Academy of Neurology recommendations, seizure prophylaxis is not mandated except in patients with a history of seizures. Postoperative imaging is performed on the evening of postoperative day zero and usually includes a CT scan with and without contrast. The noncontrast CT allows for evaluation of postoperative hematomas, hydrocephalus, pneumocephalus, edema, mass-effect, and herniation, while the addition of contrast will allow for visualization of any residual enhancing tumor.

If the postoperative CT scan is negative for complicating factors and the patient is neurologically stable, s/he is transitioned from the ICU to the neurosurgical floor. The typical hospital course is uncomplicated and lasts for 3–5 days. Surgical sutures or staples are typically removed at 7–10 days postoperatively. Most surgeons perform routine postoperative MRI 6 weeks after surgery, although many perform "early" MRI within 72 hours to evaluate the extent of resection. The final surgical pathology results are typically available 5–7 days after surgery, at which time a multidisciplinary treatment plan involving the neurosurgeon, the neuro-oncologist, and the radiation oncologist should be formulated and discussed with the patient.

Technologic advances in brain tumor surgery

In addition to the advancement of anatomic knowledge and surgical technique, several modern technologies have been developed that allow neurosurgeons to maximize the extent of resection while minimizing risk to normal brain structure and function. The advent of neuronavigation, cortical mapping and monitoring, and intraoperative MRI have played a significant part in allowing neurosurgeons to continue to evolve their surgical skills and thus effect better outcomes for patients.

Awake craniotomy

Awake craniotomy is considered the gold standard for neurophysiologic monitoring during glioma surgery. The surgery is performed under local anesthesia with some mild sedation during the initial positioning, incision, craniotomy, and approach. Once the tumor is visualized, the patient is aroused and the cortical surface is directly stimulated with an electric current. Motor and language testing is performed while stimulating at various sites. If cortical stimulation causes movement of the contralateral limb, those areas are considered as primary motor cortex and avoided during resection. Language is most commonly tested by naming, and language areas are identified when cortical stimulation leads to speech arrest. The cortical map created by this process can be effectively used to determine which areas are safe for resection, thus significantly decreasing the risk of new neurologic deficit. Awake craniotomy has been routinely performed with improved outcomes for patients with tumors involving or in proximity to eloquent cortex. Many advocate expanding the use of awake craniotomy to improve safety and decrease risk of neurologic complications in all patients with intra-axial tumors. While negative mapping of eloquent areas may provide a safe margin for surgical resection, in some studies identification of eloquent areas increased the risk of postoperative deficits, likely indicating close proximity of functional cortex to tumor. If speech mapping is not necessary, the patient can be anesthetized and cortical evoked electromyography (EMG) can be performed as described below.

Intraoperative neurophysiology

Intraoperative neurophysiology has evolved over the last 20 years as a method of delineating functional areas of the brain and monitoring their status during surgery. These techniques can be broadly classified into two groups: mapping and monitoring. Neurophysiologic mapping is a technique that allows identification of certain cortical and subcortical structures based on their function. This includes mapping of the sensory and motor cortex with phase reversal, mapping of cranial nerve nuclei at the floor of the fourth ventricle, and mapping the corticospinal tract at the cerebral peduncle or in the spinal cord. One of the simplest applications of cortical mapping is the identification of the central sulcus by somatosensory evoked potential (SEP) phase reversal. This technique is based on the observation that the morphology of cortical SEP recordings at the precentral and postcentral gyri are mirror images. Phase reversal can accurately localize the central sulcus in up to 97% of cases and can be performed without the need to keep the patient "awake." Accurate localization of primary motor and sensory cortex based on surface landmarks can be inaccurate and is invaluable in preventing inadvertent neurologic injury during tumor resection. Once the precentral gyrus has been identified using phase reversal, direct cortical stimulation can be used to confirm localization of the motor cortex. With this technique, electrical current is applied directly to cortical or subcortical areas and the corresponding muscle group is monitored for activity, either through direct visualization or through EMG. If established stimulation thresholds are reached without motor response, the area can be considered functionally silent and thus most likely safe for resection. These techniques have been modified over the past several years to increase sensitivity and decrease the incidence of seizures. Many cranial nerves (e.g. facial nerve) can be stimulated for identification and determination of their integrity during skull base surgical procedures. While mapping techniques are useful to delineate eloquent areas of cortex, they do not help to detect injury as they do not allow continuous assessment of the functional integrity of neural pathways.

Intraoperative neurophysiologic monitoring allows constant feedback for several functional pathways and can detect injury to cortical and subcortical structures. This includes real-time monitoring of SEPs, motor evoked potentials (MEPs), and brainstem auditory evoked responses (BAERs). With SEPs, stimulating needle electrodes are placed in various muscle groups and electrical current applied. Recording electrodes are placed either at the scalp (trans-cranial) or directly on the brain (cortical). Changes from baseline in the signals reflect disruption of the physiologic pathway and may be indicative of injury to the involved structures. MEPs monitor the integrity of the corticospinal tract and can be elicited either through trans-cranial or direct cortical stimulation. A persistent increase in the threshold to elicit muscle MEPs or a persistent drop in MEP amplitude represents a warning sign. Once systemic (mean arterial pressure, temperature), technical and anesthetic causes have been ruled out, injury to the functional pathway must be considered. While some debate exists for the threshold criteria, most agree that 10–15% increase in latency or greater than 50% decrease in amplitude correlates with some degree of postoperative motor deficit.

Neuronavigation

Prior to the development of modern neuroimaging techniques, craniotomy flaps for resection of brain tumors were necessarily large in order to ensure adequate exposure of the lesion. Tumor localization was based on surface landmarks, was often imprecise, and not infrequently led to injury of normal structures. The development of neuronavigation and frameless stereotaxy has also allowed us to maximize surgical resection while minimizing risk. The enhanced ability afforded by neuronavigation to localize tumors has allowed surgeons to minimize the use of large craniotomy flaps in favor of more precise "keyhole" approaches. The advantage is that minimally invasive approaches still allow the surgeon to identify the tumor and key anatomic structures, while minimizing the risk of injury and the risks and discomforts of larger approaches. As a result, neuronavigation based on CT and MRI has become the standard for tumor resection. MRI guided stereotactic resection is particularly useful for intra-axial tumors if precise location is not immediately obvious on visual inspection and the interface between tumor and normal brain is indistinct.

Many authors have reported improved results when comparing stereotactic resection with traditional resection techniques. In one series of 76 patients with malignant astrocytomas, the percentage of a gross total resection was significantly higher in the neuronavigation group than that in the no-navigation group (64.3% vs. 38.2%; $P < 0.05$). In addition, neurologic deterioration occurred in 9.5% of patients after surgery with neuronavigation and in 17.6 % after surgery without neuronavigation.

Intraoperative MRI

One of the known disadvantages of stereotactic techniques is that the accuracy of the system decreases as an open surgical resection progresses. The reason for this is that the stereotactic images are based on a fixed set of reference points. However, during the course of the approach and resection, as a result of tumor debulking and CSF egress, some "shift" occurs. As a result, while the navigation system may indicate that the resection has reached the limits of the tumor or that the resection margin is safely away from eloquent brain tissue, this may not actually be the case. This presents a particular challenge with intra-axial tumors where the difference between normal brain and tumor is not always clear. As a result, intraoperative imaging technology has been developed in order to allow the surgeon to reimage the lesion to determine the volume and precise location of any residual tumor. Real-time magnetic resonance images of the tumor cavity and residual tumor may then be used to further the operation, often allowing more complete resection.

In a study comparing traditional image-guided resection with image-guided resection with the addition of intraoperative MRI (iMRI), Bohinski et al. demonstrated that 53% of patients have some demonstrable residual after traditional image-guided surgery. Their conclusion was that iMRI can help to identify residual tumor even after maximal resection was thought to be achieved through both conventional and image-guided techniques. Senft et al. compared outcomes in patients who underwent standard surgical resection with neuronavigation in those who underwent resection with iMRI and found a significantly higher rate of gross total resection in the iMRI group. On multivariate analysis, increased extent of resection was associated with improved prognosis, leading to the conclusion that iMRI assisted resection can improve outcomes in glioma surgery. Modern techniques allow for the addition of functional sequences to iMRI, thus combining the benefits of image guidance with functional mapping. While intraoperative mapping, monitoring, and image guidance may help to increase both the safety and efficacy of our resection, fundamentals of anatomic awareness and meticulous surgical technique remain as the cornerstone of preventing direct neurologic complications in surgical neuro-oncology.

Complications

Neurologic decline

The overall rate of neurologic complications for surgery for intra-axial tumors ranges 7–32%. These rates vary widely based upon several factors including patient age, KPS, tumor location, histology, use of intraoperative mapping, the number of previous operations, proximity to eloquent brain, skill and experience of surgeon, and differences in reporting. In a prospectively collected series of 408 patients enrolled in the Glioma Outcome Project who underwent craniotomy for resection of malignant glioma, the overall incidence of neurologic worsening was 9.8%. The same study reported neurologic improvement in 53% and that KPS, but not patient age, tumor size, or location were important in predicting neurologic outcome. Although some of these factors are controversial, it is important to consider all aspects of the patient's preoperative condition when attempting to assess risk for neurologic deterioration.

✋ CAUTION!

POSTOPERATIVE DECLINE IN LEVEL OF CONSCIOUSNESS

- Diminished level of consciousness (LOC) is uncommon after most tumor resections and often indicates a complication.
- Failure of emergence from anesthesia or delayed decline in LOC should prompt urgent investigation.

- Common causes include seizures, infarction, increased intracranial pressure (ICP), hydrocephalus, hematoma, and sedating medications.
- Sedative medications and narcotics should be minimized or avoided entirely in all postoperative craniotomy patients in order to avoid confounding the neurologic exam.
- Emergency evaluation with CT scan is indicated for all patients who have an alteration in LOC to evaluate for hematoma, infarction, herniation, and hydrocephalus.
- Seizures must be treated promptly in order to avoid severe elevations in ICP and blood pressure.

While direct injury most often leads to immediate and predictable neurologic deficits, many patients will experience delayed or extended deterioration that stretches beyond the boundaries of the local anatomic function. In such cases where the pattern of deficit exceeds or differs from that expected within the area of resection, the surgeon must consider injury to vascular structures as a possible cause. Neurologic deficits from arterial injury and infarct are usually present immediately upon awakening and encompass a larger area of cortical structures than would be included within the immediate surgical vicinity. In contrast, venous injury and infarction often present in a delayed manner. Intraoperative sacrifice or injury to a draining vein from retractor placement can be initially clinically silent. However, as venous congestion ensues, a hemorrhagic infarct may develop more than 24–48 hours after surgery. As with arterial injuries, these deficits often present as more extensive than would be expected from direct surgical trauma and have a characteristic appearance of hemorrhage and edema on noncontrast CT scan. Fortunately, unlike arterial injuries, neurologic deficits suffered from venous congestion and infarction can be recoverable.

Hematoma

The incidence of hematoma after craniotomy for intra-axial lesions is approximately 1.4–2.0%. Predictive factors include older age and more eloquent lesion. The clinical presentation of a postoperative hematoma varies widely upon the size and location, however typically includes new neurologic deficit including weakness, numbness, aphasia/dysphasia, or decreased level of consciousness after reversal of anesthesia. Noncontrast CT is sufficient to confirm this suspicion. In general, if the patient is symptomatic and a hematoma is present, then the treatment is operative evacuation. If the bleed is small and found on routine postoperative CT, then the management is strict blood pressure control and maintenance of normal coagulation parameters.

Infection

The incidence of infectious complications after craniotomy ranges 1.75–3.4%. The most common causative pathogens are typical skin flora including *Staphylococcus aureus* and coagulase-negative staphylococcus. Factors contributing to postoperative wound infections include prolonged use of corticosteroids or immunosuppression in general, nutritional status, operative factors (entrance into a sinus cavity, e.g. frontal sinus or mastoid air cells), and mechanical factors (e.g. pressure on the wound or CSF leak). A postoperative wound infection manifests with the classic findings of erythema, edema, induration, and purulent drainage. Other infectious complications include subdural empyema, abscess, meningitis, and encephalitis. Wound infections are typically managed with antibiotics and wound care. Occasionally, surgical débridement and reclosure are required. Meningitis is treated with intravenous antibiotics with a regimen focusing on broad-spectrum coverage initially then more specific treatment tailored to culture results. Subdural empyema and abscess require surgical evacuation as well as intravenous antibiotics.

Hydrocephalus

Hydrocephalus occurs in 0.25–1.4% of cases of intraparenchymal tumor resections; however, important factors associated with risk of postoperative hydrocephalus are location and violation of the ependymal surface during resection. Tumors that are located in the pineal region, posterior fossa, and near the ventricular system can cause obstructive hydrocephalus. Postoperative hematomas can lead to ventricular obstruction, depending upon location. Signs and symptoms of hydrocephalus include depressed level of consciousness, herniation syndromes, sun-setting sign (paresis of upgaze), nausea, and vomiting. The diagnosis is confirmed with postoperative imaging demonstrating ventriculomegaly of an obstructed aspect of the ventricular system. The treatment includes diversion of CSF and/or relief of the obstructing lesion with surgical decompression.

Selected bibliography

Bohinski RJ, Kokkino AK, Warnick RE, Gaskill-Shipley MF, Kormos DW, Lukin RR, et al. (2001) Glioma resection in a shared-resource magnetic resonance operating room after optimal image-guided frameless stereotactic resection. Neurosurgery 48 (4), 731–42; discussion 742–4.

Chang SM, Parney IF, McDermott M, Barker FG 2nd, Schmidt MH, Huang W, et al. (2003) Perioperative complications and neurological outcomes of first and second craniotomies among patients enrolled in the Glioma Outcome Project. J Neurosurg 98 (6), 1175–81.

Delctis, V, Sala F. (2006) Intraoperative neurophysiology: a tool to prevent and/or document intraoperative injury to the nervous system. In: Schmidek HH, Roberts DW (eds) Schmidek and Sweet Operative Neurosurgical Techniques, 5th edn. Elsevier, Philadelphia, pp. 596–610.

Field M, Witham TF, Flickinger JC, Kondziolka D, Lunsford LD. (2001) Comprehensive assessment of hemorrhage risks and outcomes after stereotactic brain biopsy. J Neurosurg 94, 545–51.

Haines SJ, Walters BC. (2006) Establishing the diagnosis and evaluating the intervention. In: Haines SJ, Walters BC (eds) Evidence Based Neurosurgery: An Introduction. Thieme, New York, pp. 37–103.

Hart MG, Grant R, Metcalfe SE. Biopsy versus resection for high grade glioma. Cochrane Database of Systematic Reviews 2000, Issue 2.

Art. No.: CD002034. DOI: 10.1002/14651858.CD002034.

Kurimoto M, Hayashi N, Kamiyama H, Nagai S, Shibata T, Asahi T, et al. (2004) Impact of neuronavigation and image-guided extensive resection for adult patients with supratentorial malignant astrocytomas: a single-institution retrospective study. Minim Invasive Neurosurg 47 (5), 278–83.

Lacroix M, Abi-Said D, Fourney DR, Gokaslan ZL, Shi W, DeMonte F, et al. (2001) A multivariate analysis of 416 patients with glioblastoma multiforme: prognosis, extent of resection, and survival. J Neurosurg 95, 190–8.

Lee KH, Harris BT, Roberts DW. (2006) Frame based stereotactic brain biopsy. In: Schmidek HH, Roberts DW (eds) Schmidek and Sweet Operative Neurosurgical Techniques, 5th edn. Elsevier, Philadelphia, pp. 625–36.

McGirt MJ, Chaichana KL, Gathinji M, Attenello FJ, Than K, Olivi A, et al. (2009) Independent association of extent of resection with survival in patients with malignant brain astrocytoma. J Neurosurg 110 (1), 156–62.

Patchell RA, Tibbs PA, Walsh JW, Dempsey RJ, Maruyama Y, Kryscio RJ, et al. (1990) A randomized trial of surgery in treatment of single metastases to the brain. N Engl J Med 322 (8), 494–500.

Ryken TC, Frankel B, Bernstein M. (2006) Neuro-oncology: the role of surgery in the management of malignant glioma. In: Haines SJ, Walters BC (eds) Evidence Based Neurosurgery. Thieme Publishers, New York, pp. 37–99.

Ryken TC, Frankel B, Julien T, Olson JJ. (2008) Surgical management of newly diagnosed glioblastoma in adults: role of cytoreductive surgery. J Neurooncol 89 (3), 271–86.

Sanai N, Polley MY, McDermott MW, Parsa AT, Berger MS. (2011) An extent of resection threshold for newly diagnosed glioblastomas. J Neurosurg 115 (1), 3–8.

Sawaya R, Hammoud M, Schoppa D, Hess KR, Wu SZ, Shi WM, et al. (1998) Neurosurgical outcomes in a modern series of 400 craniotomies for treatment of parenchymal tumors. Neurosurgery 42 (5), 1044–55.

Senft C, Franz K, Blasel S, Oszvald A, Rathert J, Seifert V, et al. (2010) Influence of iMRI-guidance on the extent of resection and survival of patients with glioblastoma multi-forme. *Technol Cancer Res Treat* **9**, 339–46.

Simpson D. (1957) The recurrence of intracranial meningiomas after surgical treatment. *J Neurol Neurosurg Psychiatry* **20**, 22–39.

Smith JS, Chang EF, Lamborn KR, Chang SM, Prados MD, Cha S, *et al.* (2008) Role of extent of resection in the long-term outcome of low-grade hemispheric gliomas. *J Clin Oncol* **26** (8), 1338–45.

Stummer W, Pichlmier U, Meinel T, Wiestler OD, Zanella F, Reulen HJ; ALA-Glioma Group. (2006) Flourescence-guided surgery with 5-aminolevulinic acid for resection of malig-nant glioma: a randomized controlled multi-centre phase III trial. *Lancet Oncol* **7** (5), 392–401.

Sughrue ME, Kane AJ, Shangari G, Rutkowski MJ, McDermott MW, Berger MS, *et al.* (2010) The relevance of Simpson Grade I and II resection in modern neurosurgical treatment of World Health Organization Grade I meningiomas. *J Neurosurg* **113**, 1029–35.

Taylor MD, Bernstein M. (2005) Surgical manage-ment. In: Schiff D, O'Neill BP (eds) *Principles of Neuro-oncology*. McGraw Hill, New York, pp. 121–42.

4

General Approach to Radiation Oncology

Jennifer S. Yu[1] and Daphne A. Haas-Kogan[2]

[1]Department of Radiation Oncology, Department of Stem Cell Biology and Regenerative Medicine, Cleveland Clinic, Cleveland, OH, USA
[2]Departments of Radiation Oncology and Neurological Surgery, University of California, San Francisco, CA, USA

Introduction

Radiation is often used in the treatment of central nervous system (CNS) malignancies. This chapter reviews the fundamental elements of therapeutic radiation biology and physics, and discusses the radiobiologic and clinical rationales behind selection of different dose fractionation schemes. The different types of radiation used in clinical practice are highlighted, including three-dimensional conformal, intensity modulated radiation therapy, and stereotactic radiotherapy/radiosurgery. Therapeutic approaches to commonly encountered adult and pediatric malignancies are also discussed.

Radiation biology and physics

Ionizing radiation

The major sources of radiation used in therapy are X-rays, gamma-rays, electrons, and, more recently, protons. These sources of radiation are ionizing; that is, they eject electrons from atoms. These ejected electrons can amplify the energy deposited by causing secondary ionizations. Resulting free radicals can directly damage cellular macromolecules such as DNA. Because of the high water content in tissues, however, they more commonly damage DNA indirectly by forming hydroxyl radicals.

> **⚛ SCIENCE REVISITED**
>
> The distinction between X-rays and gamma-rays lies in their origins. Whereas X-rays are produced in linear accelerators, gamma-rays are derived from atomic nuclei.

Both X-rays and gamma-rays may be considered photons, which have no mass. Electrons and protons are charged, fundamental particles that have a mass. Their interaction with matter is therefore different from that of X-rays and gamma-rays.

Photons deposit energy throughout their tracks. Depending upon their energy, photons may travel over 1 cm before the maximum dose is achieved. For example, the maximum dose for a 6-MV photon is at 1.5 cm. The dose fall-off beyond the depth of maximum energy deposition is gradual. Therefore, photons are skin-sparing and are useful for treating deep-seated tumors.

Neuro-oncology, First Edition. Edited by Roger J. Packer, David Schiff.
© 2012 John Wiley & Sons, Ltd. Published 2012 by John Wiley & Sons, Ltd.

Electrons are charged and light; they scatter readily and dissipate energy quickly when they hit their target. Consequently, electrons have high surface doses compared to photons. Electrons deposit their energy over a known pathlength that varies as a function of their energy. The dose fall-off at the end of this path is steep and accounts for only 5% of the maximum dose. Because of their high surface dose and shallow tissue penetration, electrons are useful for treating superficial tumors such as skin cancers or rib metastases.

Protons are charged and have a greater mass than electrons. At the end of the proton's pathlength, dose is deposited in a sharp peak, termed the Bragg peak. Protons are useful for restricting the high dose area to a tumor target volume while sparing critical structures. Protons may be most beneficial in pediatric patients or patients with base of skull, spinal cord, or eye tumors. Their utility in other types of cancer treatment is actively under investigation.

Radiation sensitizers

Significant efforts have been underway to enhance the effects of radiation. The most common and arguably the most effective radiosensitizer is oxygen. Under normoxic conditions, oxygen can "fix" radiation damage by free radicals. The efficiency of most therapeutic forms of radiation is threefold greater under normoxic than hypoxic conditions. Thus, tumors that are well perfused and normoxic are more responsive to radiation than hypoxic tumors.

Traditional chemotherapy and biologic agents have also been used concurrently with radiation to enhance cell kill. Some commonly used drugs include 5-fluorouracil, cisplatin, mitomycin C, temozolomide, and the epidermal growth factor receptor (EGFR) inhibitor cetuximab. Novel drugs and biologic agents, and their various combinations, are currently under investigation as potential radiosensitizers.

Radiation fractionation

Radiation doses for CNS malignancies are typically in the range 50.4–54 Gy for benign tumors, and 60 Gy for malignant tumors. These total doses are given in daily fractions of 1.8–2 Gy, so-called "conventional fractionation." The purpose of this fractionation is to exploit the differences in the response of normal cells and tumor cells to ionizing radiation.

Both normal and tumor cells may be stimulated to repopulate to maintain tissue homeostasis, reassort to specific phases of the cell cycle, repair DNA damage, and reoxygenate as tumors shrink and remodel. With 1.8–2 Gy fractions, normal cells but not tumor cells can efficiently repair DNA damage, allowing physicians to deliver high total doses of radiation with acceptable toxicity.

The radiation dose needed to control a tumor must be tempered by the dose that critical structures in the tumor vicinity can tolerate. In some cases, delivering high doses of radiation may be preferred, but because of the location of the tumor, such high doses may not be feasible because of normal tissue tolerances. For example, radiation treatment for optic gliomas is limited by the dose tolerance of the optic nerve and chiasm.

In some cases, altered fractionation schedules may be entertained. Hypofractionation, the use of large daily fractions in few sessions, may be preferred in the setting of palliative care. A sufficient dose of radiation is delivered over a short period of time to improve symptoms.

Common fractionation schemes used in the treatment of bone metastases include 8 Gy in 1 fraction, 30 Gy in 10 fractions, and 20 Gy in 5 fractions. These fractionation schemes have been shown to have similar efficacies in onset of pain relief, although the duration of relief may be shorter with 8 Gy in 1 fraction.

Altered fractionation may be considered for patients with poor prognosis and poor performance status. The morbidity of standard fractionation may be too excessive for these patients. For example, standard radiation treatment of glioblastoma patients entails concurrent chemoradiation for 6 weeks, followed by adjuvant chemotherapy. Some patients may be unable to tolerate this prolonged and intense treatment. They may instead be considered for hypofractionated radiation over 2–3 weeks.

Hypofractionation may also be used to treat cancers that are traditionally thought to be "radioresistant," such as melanoma or renal cell cancers. The mechanism behind this improved sensitivity to high dose radiation is currently under investigation.

The radiation oncologist's toolbox

Contemporary radiation is typically based on three-dimensional planning. The radiation oncologist can make use of many imaging techniques including computer tomography (CT) scans, magnetic resonance imaging (MRI) scans, positron emission tomography (PET) scans, ultrasound, and nuclear imaging to aid in treatment planning. These images may be fused with a treatment planning CT scan to help define tumor volumes and critical structures. The radiation oncologist prescribes radiation to areas at risk for disease and limits dose to critical structures. Physicians work with a team of physicists or dosimetrists to develop a unique radiation plan for each individual patient.

Whole brain radiation is typically delivered using opposed lateral beams. A CT scan may be performed to help delineate critical structures. Plate 4.1 (see plate section opposite p. 52) shows a beam's eye view of a whole brain radiation field. Three-dimensional conformal plans often involve 3–5 beam arrangements. Intensity-modulated radiation therapy (IMRT) plans are very conformal and may use more than 5 beams. The intensity of the radiation beam is modulated throughout treatment so that the radiation dose can be sculpted around critical structures. IMRT may permit simultaneous integrated boost, such that different targets can receive different daily doses of radiation in a dose-painting technique. Both three-dimensional conformal and IMRT plans are useful when treating large fields with a high degree of accuracy. An example of an IMRT plan is shown in Plate 4.2 (see plate section opposite p. 52). In this case, a radiation treatment plan for an anaplastic astrocytoma is shown; the radiation conforms to the target volume and spares the optic chiasm.

Stereotactic radiosurgery (SRS) and stereotactic body radiotherapy (SBRT) can deliver highly conformal radiation with accuracy within 1–2 mm. SRS refers to treatment in 1 fraction, whereas stereotactic radiotherapy refers to treatment in 2 or more fractions. These modalities are useful for treating small targets to high doses. This is possible because of numerous sources or beamlets that converge upon the target, as shown in Plates 4.3–4.5 (see plate section opposite p. 52). SRS may be performed with a Gamma Knife®, which utilizes cobalt-60 sources, or with linear accelerators. SBRT can be performed with linear accelerators.

Management

Adult CNS tumors

Gliomas

Low grade gliomas

Surgery with maximal safe resection remains the mainstay of treatment. Postoperative radiation for low grade gliomas is often deferred until disease progression.

EVIDENCE AT A GLANCE

The EORTC 22845 study randomized patients with grade 2 gliomas to adjuvant radiation to 54 Gy or observation. There was no difference in overall survival between the two arms (7.4 years for the radiation arm vs. 7.2 years for the observation arm), but adjuvant radiation improved progression free survival (PFS) (5.3 vs. 3.4 years). Within the observation arm, 65% of patients went on to salvage radiation.

Subset analysis of patients <40 years old with gross total resection in the radiation only arm of RTOG 9802 (which randomized patients to adjuvant radiation to 54 Gy with or without PCV chemotherapy × 6 cycles) had an overall survival of 94% and PFS of 50% at 5 years, suggesting that these low-risk patients may be considered for observation. Together, these data suggest that radiation may be delayed in patients with low grade gliomas without impacting overall survival.

Two randomized trials studied whether outcomes could be improved with dose escalation. In the EORTC 22844 trial, patients were randomized to adjuvant radiation of 45 vs. 59.4 Gy. Both overall survival (58% vs. 59%) and progression free survival (PFS) (47% vs. 50%) were similar between the treatment arms. An Intergroup trial randomized patients to 50.4 vs. 64.8 Gy. Similar to the EORTC 22844 trial, 5-year overall survival was comparable between the low dose and high dose arms (64% vs. 72%). Interestingly, 92%

of failures occurred within the irradiated field, suggesting that a subset of tumor cells may be radioresistant.

A subset of high risk, low grade glioma patients may be considered for upfront adjuvant radiation. These include patients who are symptomatic with residual disease, and those with three or more adverse features, based on the EORTC trials. These risk factors include age ≥40 years old, astrocytoma histology, tumors ≥6 cm, tumors crossing the midline, and presence of neurologic deficits before surgery. The ongoing RTOG 0424 study asks whether high risk, low grade glioma patients, defined as those patients with three or more adverse features, may benefit from adjuvant radiation to 54 Gy with concurrent temozolomide. The EORTC 22033 trial randomizes high risk patients (three or more adverse features) to adjuvant radiation to 50.4 Gy or temozolomide.

High grade gliomas

The treatment paradigm for these tumors is maximum safe resection followed by adjuvant chemoradiation and additional chemotherapy. Because of the infiltrative nature of many of these tumors, complete resection of the tumor may not be possible.

While early trials have shown improved survival with adjuvant radiation, prognosis remains dismal. Radiation dose-escalation trials that utilized altered fractionation, brachytherapy boost, and radiosurgery boost have not proven to be advantageous. Moreover, early trials of adjuvant concurrent radiation and nitrogen mustard-based chemotherapy failed to improve survival compared with radiation alone. It was not until 2005 when chemoradiation with temozolomide demonstrated an improvement in survival.

⚠ CAUTION!

The EORTC/NCIC study randomized patients with glioblastomas to radiation with or without concurrent and adjuvant temozolomide. Patients received radiation to 60 Gy with daily temozolomide, followed by six cycles of adjuvant temozolomide. Median survival was 14.6 months in the chemoradiation arm compared to 12.1 months in the control radiation alone arm.

While only patients with glioblastoma were eligible for this trial, these results have been extrapolated to patients with grade 3 gliomas. Prior to this, the EORTC 26951 trial showed no survival advantage to induction chemotherapy with procarbazine, CCNU, vincristine (PCV) compared with radiation alone.

★ TIPS AND TRICKS

For patients with advanced age and poor performance status, alternative fractionation schemes may be considered. Radiation alone to 30–35 Gy in 10 fractions or 40 Gy in 15 fractions may be prescribed.

Meningiomas

Depending on the size and location of the meningioma, presence or absence of symptoms, and performance status of the patient, therapeutic options include observation, surgery, or radiation. In general, low grade meningiomas grow slowly, at about 1 mm per year and, if small and asymptomatic, observation may be appropriate. Higher grade tumors, however, have higher proliferation indices and may invade brain parenchyma and bone. In suspected high grade meningiomas, overlying osteostosis should be considered as osseous involvement.

Surgical resection remains the cornerstone of meningioma treatment and can relieve symptoms because of mass effect and provide histologic diagnosis. Local control rates vary with completeness of resection and are typically in the range of 80–90% for gross total resections and approximately 60% for subtotal resection. Adjuvant radiation may be considered when grade 1 meningiomas are subtotally resected, or if histology reveals a higher grade meningioma. For grade 1 meningiomas, local control after subtotal resection and adjuvant radiation is comparable with that achieved with gross total resection alone. Five-year overall survival is 85% for benign lesions and 58% for malignant meningiomas.

Definitive radiation may be considered an alternative to resection. Control rates rival those of gross total resection, with local control in the 80–90% range. Because of the slow proliferation rates of most meningiomas, radiation treatment more often stabilizes growth of meningiomas rather than producing rapid shrinkage. Meningiomas treated with radiation may take several years to reduce in size.

Grade 1 meningiomas are typically treated to 54 Gy, while grade 3 meningiomas to 60–63 Gy, and grade 2 meningiomas to 54–60 Gy. In the current RTOG 0539 phase II trial, patients with grade 1 meningiomas undergo observation regardless of extent of resection, those with grade 2 meningiomas or recurrent grade 1 meningiomas receive 54 Gy, and grade 3 meningiomas or recurrent grade 2–3 meningiomas receive 60 Gy.

For small meningiomas not involving the optic apparatus or brainstem, stereotactic radiosurgery may be considered. A median dose of 16 Gy in 1 fraction offers local control rates over 90%.

Pituitary adenomas

The mainstay of treatment is surgical resection, which provides local control rates >90%, and for functional tumors hormone normalization rates of 70–80%. Medical management of secretory tumors may help to restore proper hormone levels. Radiation is reserved for patients with residual or recurrent disease, disease refractory to surgical or medical management, and inoperable patients. Local control with radiation is comparable to that following surgery. Normalization of hormones varies by subtype: 80% for growth hormone-secreting tumors, 50–80% for adenocorticotropic hormone (ACTH) secreting tumors, and 30–40% for prolactin-secreting tumors. Radiation doses range 45–50.4 Gy for non-secreting tumors and 50.4–54 Gy for secreting tumors. For select tumors, radiosurgery may be considered. Doses range 12–20 Gy for non-secreting tumors, and 15–30 Gy for secreting tumors. Optic chiasm dose is limited to <8 Gy and pituitary stalk to <5.5 Gy. Radiosurgery may improve hormone levels faster than conventional radiation. Radiation for hypersecreting tumors may be more efficacious when patients are off medical management.

♨ CAUTION!

Long-term side effects of treatment include loss of vision and hypopituitarism. Therefore these patients need formal visual field testing and endocrine follow-up.

Vestibular schwannomas

Similar to low grade meningiomas, these tumors grow slowly at a rate of 1–2 mm per year. If asymptomatic, observation with serial imaging may be an option. Treatment approaches include microsurgical resection, fractionated radiation therapy, and stereotactic radiosurgery. Local control rates of >90% are similar among these approaches, but complications appear to be reduced with radiosurgery compared with microsurgery: preservation of useful hearing is about 75% with SRS and external beam radiation therapy versus 30–50% with surgery, and facial nerve function is >90% with SRS and external beam radiation therapy versus >60% with surgery. Typical external beam doses are 50–60 Gy and radiosurgery doses are 12–13 Gy in 1 fraction. Patients should undergo formal audiometry prior to and after treatment.

Primary CNS lymphomas

Primary CNS lymphomas are rare forms of non-Hodgkin lymphoma, predominantly associated with immunocompromised patients. The most common histology is diffuse large B-cell lymphoma. These tumors may involve the entire neuraxis and eyes. Therefore, CSF studies, brain and spine MRIs, and formal ophthalmologic examination with slit-lamp examination should be performed. These tumors are responsive to steroids and chemotherapy, which remain first line treatment. Despite excellent response rates, these tumors are incurable, and patients have poor prognoses, with median survival of 12 months. Radiation may cause remission, but results are short-lived. For patients with good performance, adjuvant radiation is given after high dose methotrexate-based chemotherapy. For elderly patients, radiation may be reserved for recurrence after chemotherapy. Because of the infiltrative nature of primary CNS lymphomas, the whole brain is treated to 45 Gy. Patients with leptomeningeal disease may have intrathecal methotrexate-based chemotherapy or craniospinal irradiation to 39.6 Gy with a boost to 45–50.4 Gy to areas of gross disease.

Pediatric CNS tumors

Treatment of pediatric primary CNS tumors involves multidisciplinary teams of medical oncologist, neurosurgeon, and radiation oncologist. Side effects of treatment may be more pronounced in children than adults, and must be minimized while maintaining tumor control. Radiation therapy to the brain may result in neurocognitive sequelae manifest as a decline in intelligence and behavioral changes. The degree of neurocognitive decline is a function of the volume of the brain treated and radiation dose. It is estimated that children younger than 7 years undergoing craniospinal irradiation for medulloblastomas can lose 2.4–3.7 IQ points per year. Radiation to the growth plate in bones may retard growth. For example, treatment of one orbit may result in hypoplasia in the treated area, while the contralateral orbit grows normally, resulting in facial asymmetry as the child grows. Depending on the area treated, radiation treatment may also cause hormonal dysfunction, which may affect puberty and fertility, and may cause cataracts, hearing loss, and vascular damage. Moreover, children, some of whom may have germline mutations that predispose them to malignancy, may be at increased risk of developing radiation-induced cancers, particularly because many patients have long life expectancies. It is estimated that approximately 4% of patients who undergo brain radiation will develop a radiation-induced malignancy. In addition to the side effects of radiation, young children may also require general anesthesia if they are unable to hold still during their radiation treatment. Daily anesthesia for radiation treatments up to 6 weeks long may also add to the morbidity.

Because of the many long-term side effects of radiation, efforts have been made to limit the radiation field to spare normal tissues. Highly conformal radiation techniques with three-dimensional conformal or IMRT planning may be utilized to minimize normal tissue toxicity. Proton therapy, which may better be able to spare normal tissues, may prove to be safer for pediatric patients.

✋ CAUTION!

For infants and toddlers less than 3 years old with malignant brain tumors, the "Baby POG" study demonstrated that radiation may be postponed without decrement in progression free survival (33–39%) or overall survival (53–55%). Patients instead received chemotherapy until age 3 or disease progression.

★ TIPS AND TRICKS

Because of the rarity of pediatric tumors, all patients should be enrolled in protocols and preferably be treated in pediatric oncology specialty centers.

Gliomas

In contrast to adults, pediatric patients more often present with low grade rather than high grade gliomas. The most common types are pilocytic astrocytomas (PA) and World Health Organization (WHO) grade 2 gliomas. PAs may have solid nodular and cystic components and may arise in the cortex or brainstem. Less frequently, these tumors may be diffuse and present as gliomatosis cerebri. Because of the indolent nature and well-circumscribed nature of many PAs and low grade gliomas, patients with these tumors undergo maximal safe resection followed by observation. Adjuvant chemotherapy with carboplatin and vincristine can improve 3-year PFS to 68% and delay radiation treatment to allow the child's brain to develop. Patients younger than 5 years stand to benefit more than those older than 5 years, with 3-year PFS of 74% vs. 39%.

High grade gliomas are less common in children. Anaplastic gliomas are more common than glioblastomas. Similar to their adult counterparts, children undergo maximal safe resection followed by radiation with concurrent and adjuvant temozolomide-based chemotherapy. The current Children's Oncology Group (COG) protocol, ACNS 0423, tests radiation with concurrent temozolomide and adjuvant temozolomide and lomustine. Patients receive 54 Gy to the involved field with a boost to 59.4 Gy to areas of residual disease.

Diffuse intrinsic pontine gliomas (DIPGs) are more common in children than adults. Tumors arising in the midbrain and thalamus are frequently focal and low grade lesions, whereas tumors in the pons are more often diffuse and of high grade. Radiation dose is limited by brainstem tolerance of 54 Gy. Median survival for patients with DIPGs is poor at 11 months, and for those with focal gliomas is excellent with 4-year PFS of 94% and overall survival of 100%.

★ TIPS AND TRICKS

Because of the possible morbidity of biopsy, patients with diffuse intrinsic pontine gliomas may be diagnosed based on their clinical presentation and radiographic imaging.

Medulloblastomas

Patients are treated in a multidisciplinary approach with a combination of surgical resection, chemotherapy, and radiation therapy. Because of the propensity for these tumors to spread throughout the neuraxis, patients need craniospinal irradiation. Standard risk patients receive 23.4 Gy craniospinal irradiation, whereas high risk patients receive 36 Gy. Both receive a boost to the posterior fossa to 54 Gy. The current COG protocol for standard risk patients, ACNS 0331, examines whether reduced craniospinal dose and a smaller boost volume will offer comparable control rates while limiting toxicity. One randomization compares craniospinal dose of 18 Gy versus standard 23.4 Gy in children age 3–7 years; the other randomization compares involved field boost versus posterior fossa boost. Patients over age 3 years with supratentorial primitive neuroectodermal tumors (PNET) and pineoblastomas are treated like high risk medulloblastoma patients and have 5-year survivals of 50–70%.

Ependymomas

Ependymomas arise in the posterior fossa, supratentorium, or spinal cord. The treatment paradigm is maximal safe resection with postoperative radiation. Adjuvant radiation therapy improves local control compared to surgery alone (100% with radiation therapy vs. 50% with observation). The current COG protocol

studies whether a subset of patients with completely resected grade 2 supratentorial ependymomas may forgo postoperative radiation therapy.

Intracranial ependymomas are typically treated to the involved field to 54–59.4 Gy. Patients with spinal involvement as evidenced by cerebrospinal fluid (CSF) analysis or spine imaging should receive craniospinal irradiation to 36–39.6 Gy followed by a boost to the primary tumor to 54–59.4 Gy and spinal disease to 45 Gy. For patients with spinal ependymomas, myxopapillary ependymomas that arise in the conus or filum terminale should receive 45 Gy to the tumor bed with a boost to 50.4–59.4 Gy.

Craniopharyngiomas

Craniopharyngiomas derive from the Rathke pouch or pituitary stalk. They frequently have solid and cystic components. Treatment options include cystic decompression, surgical resection, or radiation therapy. Cystic and surgical resection may offer immediate relief of symptoms, but often radical surgery is highly morbid and not possible because of involvement of the pituitary stalk, hypothalamus, and optic nerves and chiasm.

Conservative surgery and adjuvant radiation offer control rates up to 80–90%. External beam radiation doses are typically in the range of 50–54 Gy, and are limited by optic apparatus tolerance. Limited data exist for radiosurgery and intracystic radionuclide therapy. For select cases, radiosurgery may offer control rates of 85–90%. Intracystic radiation with yttrium-90 or phosphorus-32 to 200–250 Gy to the cyst wall may also be considered.

☙ CAUTION!

Expansion of the cystic component may occur during radiation treatment so patients should be imaged at least once during treatment to ensure that both the solid and cystic tumor components are encompassed within the radiation field. Expansion of the cystic component should be suspected and repeat imaging performed if symptoms worsen during treatment.

Side effects of treatment include pituitary dysfunction, often requiring growth hormone and thyroid hormone replacement, and sometimes sex hormone and glucocorticoid replacement. More rarely, diabetes insipidus or panhypopituitarism may ensue. Patients are also at risk of vision impairment.

Germ cell tumors

Germ cell tumors typically arise in the midline in the pineal or suprasellar region. These tumors fall into two categories: germinomas and nongerminomatous germ cell tumors (NGGCT). NGGCTs include yolk sac tumors, embryonal cancers, choriocarcinomas, teratomas, and mixed histology tumors. It is estimated that 5–15% of germinomas may be multifocal. NGGCTs exhibit elevated levels of alpha-fetoprotein (AFP) (yolk sac and embryonal cancers) and β human chorionic gonadotropin (β-hCG) (embryonal cancers and choriocarcinomas).

✋ CAUTION!

Germinomas lack AFP but may have mildly increased β-hCG of <100 IU/mL. Tumors with elevated AFP should be regarded as nongerminomatous germ cell tumors (NGGCTs).

Traditionally, germinomas were treated with craniospinal irradiation. However, studies have shown that, when combined with chemotherapy, more limited radiation fields may achieve similar control without the excess morbidity of neuraxis irradiation. Five-year overall survival is in the range of 80–90%. The radiation field encompasses the whole ventricle to 24–30 Gy with a boost to the primary to 45–50.4 Gy. Craniospinal irradiation is indicated for high risk patients with neuraxis involvement, multifocal presentation, or subependymal spread. The current protocol seeks to determine whether intensified chemotherapy with involved field radiation is sufficient in patients with a complete response.

NGGCTs are more aggressive, with 5-year survival of 20–40%. These tumors require multimodality therapy with maximal surgical resection followed by cisplatin-based chemotherapy and radiation. In the absence of spinal involvement, patients receive consolidative radiation to the primary tumor to 50.4–54 Gy. With spinal involvement, patients receive craniospinal irradiation to 30–36 Gy with involved field boost to 50.4–54 Gy.

Palliation

Brain metastases

Patients with brain metastases have several treatment options, depending on the number, location, and size of metastases, and prognosis and performance status of the patient. Options include surgery and adjuvant whole brain radiation or radiosurgery, whole brain radiation alone, radiosurgery alone, or whole brain radiation with radiosurgery boost. Surgery can have dual roles in decompression and obtaining tissue for diagnosis. Interestingly, in a study of patients undergoing surgery for suspected brain metastasis, 11% of patients were found to have no malignancy within the pathologic specimen.

EVIDENCE AT A GLANCE

1. The addition of whole brain treatment to surgery improves local control (90% vs. 54%) but not survival when compared with surgery alone. Because of the local control benefit of postoperative radiation, patients who undergo surgical resection of their brain metastasis should receive postoperative radiation. Studies suggest that adjuvant radiosurgery may be used to treat the tumor bed with a local control rate of 79%.

2. The addition of surgery to whole brain radiation provides both local control (80% vs. 48%) and survival (40 vs. 15 weeks) benefits compared with whole brain radiation alone. Similarly, in RTOG 9508, for patients with 1–4 brain metastases, the addition of radiosurgery boost to whole brain treatment improved

performance status (43% vs. 27%) and trended towards an improvement in overall survival (median 6.5 vs. 4.9 months, not statistically significant).

For select patients with small metastases, stereotactic radiosurgery may be considered. While direct comparisons of surgery and radiosurgery have not been performed, retrospective studies suggest comparable rates of local control. Radiosurgery offers a minimally invasive technique which may spare patients the neurocognitive decline associated with whole brain radiation.

EVIDENCE AT A GLANCE

The JROSG99-1 study showed comparable overall survival between patients with 1–4 brain metastases receiving radiosurgery alone compared with radiosurgery plus whole brain radiation (8 vs. 7.5 months) but slight decrement in new metastases (63.7% vs. 41.5%) and local control (72.5% vs. 88.7%).

For patients with 1–3 brain metastases, Chang *et al.* found improved survival (15.2 vs. 5.7 months) and neurocognitive function in radiosurgery patients compared with those who received radiosurgery and whole brain radiation, despite better local and whole brain control in the whole brain radiation arm. Retrospective data have further shown no decrement in survival in patients who underwent radiosurgery alone compared with those receiving whole brain and radiosurgery boost when allowing for salvage treatment. These data suggest that radiosurgery alone with close follow-up may be a reasonable option for some patients.

Typical whole brain radiation fractionations are 20 Gy in 5 fractions, 30 Gy in 10 fractions, 37.5 Gy in 15 fractions, and 40 Gy in 20 fractions. The fractionation schedule chosen depends on the patient's prognosis and performance status.

Acute side effects include extreme fatigue, alopecia, and brain edema which may require treatment with steroids. Late side effects include neurocognitive decline. The degree of neurotoxicity appears to be related to fraction size, with daily fractions >3 Gy causing more dementia. Radiosurgery may be performed with a Gamma Knife or with linear accelerators. Typical doses are in the range of 15–24 Gy in a single fraction.

Spine metastases

Metastases to the spine may cause compression fractures or compromise the spinal cord and nerve roots. As a consequence, they may cause significant pain and neurologic deficits. Spinal cord compression can cause motor or sensory deficits and loss of bowel or bladder function. The ability to restore function is inversely proportional to the amount of time the patient has been symptomatic and varies with the radiosensitivity of the tumor. Therefore, spinal cord compression is considered an oncologic emergency. Dexamethasone is given to reduce swelling and improve symptoms. Surgical decompression should be performed in patients with limited spine involvement, life expectancy >3 months, and good performance status.

EVIDENCE AT A GLANCE

A randomized trial comparing surgery with postoperative radiation therapy versus radiation alone showed improved rates of ambulation (84% vs. 57%) and durability of response (122 vs. 13 days), indicating that surgery is the preferred approach.

Spine metastases treated with external beam radiation alone can reduce pain in 70–90% of patients. Common fractionation regimens are 8 Gy in 1 fraction, 30 Gy in 10 fractions, and 37.5 Gy in 15 fractions. Comparisons of 8 Gy in 1 fraction, 20 Gy in 5 fractions, and 30 Gy in 10 fractions reveal similar rates of pain control and duration of control. However, patients treated in 1 fraction underwent repeat treatment more often.

Stereotactic radiosurgery is currently being investigated as a modality for treating spine metastases without cord compromise. Single institution studies report improved duration of pain control with stereotactic body radiosurgery without evidence of radiation myelitis. Doses range from 12.5–25 Gy in 1 fraction to 24 Gy in 3 fractions. The current RTOG 0631 trial compares 16 Gy in 1 fraction with stereotactic body radiosurgery with 8 Gy in 1 fraction with conventional external beam.

Selected bibliography

Bauman GS, Gaspar LE, Fisher BJ, Halperin EC, Macdonald DR, Cairncross JG. (1994) A prospective study of short-course radiotherapy in poor prognosis glioblastoma multiforme. *Int J Radiat Oncol Biol Phys* **29** (4), 835–9.

Broniscer A, Ke W, Fuller CE, Wu J, Gajjar A, Kun LE. (2004) Second neoplasms in pediatric patients with primary central nervous system tumors: the St. Jude Children's Research Hospital experience. *Cancer* **100** (10), 2246–52.

Chang EL, Wefel JS, Hess KR, Allen PK, Lang FF, Kornguth DG, *et al.* (2009) Neurocognition in patients with brain metastases treated with radiosurgery or radiosurgery plus whole-brain irradiation: a randomised controlled trial. *Lancet Oncol* **10** (11), 1037–44.

DeAngelis LM, Delattre JY, Posner JB. (1989) Radiation-induced dementia in patients cured of brain metastases. *Neurology* **39** (6), 789–96.

Duffner PK, Horowitz ME, Krischer JP, Friedman HS, Burger PC, Cohen ME, *et al.* (1993) Postoperative chemotherapy and delayed radiation in children less than three years of age with malignant brain tumors. *N Engl J Med* **328** (24), 1725–31.

Eleraky M, Papanastassiou I, Vrionis FD. (2010) Management of metastatic spine disease. *Curr Opin Support Palliat Care* **4** (3), 182–8.

Freeman CR, Farmer JP. (1998) Pediatric brain stem gliomas: a review. *Int J Radiat Oncol Biol Phys* **40** (2), 265–71.

Goldsmith BJ, Wara WM, Wilson CB, Larson DA. (1994) Postoperative irradiation for subtotally resected meningiomas: a retrospective analysis of 140 patients treated from 1967 to 1990. *J Neurosurg* **80** (2), 195–201.

Hartsell WF, Scott CB, Bruner DW, Scarantino CW, Ivker RA, Roach M 3rd, *et al.* (2005) Randomized trial of short- versus long-course radiotherapy for palliation of painful bone metastases. *J Natl Cancer Inst* **97** (11), 798–804.

Kiehna EN, Merchant TE. (2010) Radiation therapy for pediatric craniopharyngioma. *Neurosurg Focus* **28** (4), E10.

Merchant TE, Pollack IF, Loeffler JS. (2010) Brain tumors across the age spectrum: biology, therapy, and late effects. *Semin Radiat Oncol* **20** (1), 58–66.

Packer RJ, Ater J, Allen J, Phillips P, Geyer R, Nicholson HS, *et al.* (1997) Carboplatin and vincristine chemotherapy for children with newly diagnosed progressive low-grade gliomas. *J Neurosurg* **86** (5), 747–54.

Packer RJ, Vezina G. (2008) Management of and prognosis with medulloblastoma: therapy at a crossroads. *Arch Neurol* **65** (11), 1419–24.

Patchell RA, Tibbs PA, Walsh JW, Dempsey RJ, Maruyama Y, Kryscio RJ, *et al.* (1990) A randomized trial of surgery in the treatment of single metastases to the brain. *N Engl J Med* **322** (8), 494–500.

Patil CG, Pricola K, Garg SK, Bryant A, Black KL. (2010) Whole brain radiation therapy (WBRT) alone versus WBRT and radiosurgery for the treatment of brain metastases. *Cochrane Database Syst Rev* **6**, CD006121.

Phillips C, Guiney M, Smith J, Hughes P, Narayan K, Quong G. (2003) A randomized trial comparing 35 Gy in ten fractions with 60 Gy in 30 fractions of cerebral irradiation for glioblastoma multiforme and older patients with anaplastic astrocytoma. *Radiother Oncol* **68** (1), 23–6.

Regis J, Roche PH, Delsanti C, Thomassin JM, Ouaknine M, Gabert K, *et al.* (2007) Modern management of vestibular schwannomas. *Prog Neurol Surg* **20**, 129–41.

Snead FE, Amdur RJ, Morris CG, Mendenhall WM. (2008) Long-term outcomes of radiotherapy for pituitary adenomas. *Int J Radiat Oncol Biol Phys* **71** (4), 994–8.

Stupp R, Mason WP, van den Bent MJ, Weller M, Fisher B, Taphoorn MJ, *et al.* (2005) Radiother-

apy plus concomitant and adjuvant temozolomide for glioblastoma. *N Engl J Med* **352** (10),
987–96.

van den Bent MJ, Afra D, de Witte O, Ben
Hassel M, Schraub S, Hoang-Xuan K, *et al.*
(2005) Long-term efficacy of early versus
delayed radiotherapy for low-grade astrocytoma and oligodendroglioma in adults: the
EORTC 22845 randomised trial. *Lancet* **366**,
985–90.

5

General Aspects of Chemotherapy Including "Biologic Agents"

Jethro Hu[1] and Santosh Kesari[2]

[1]Johnnie L. Cochran Jr. Brain Tumor Center, Departments of Neurology and Neurosurgery, Cedars-Sinai Medical Center, Los Angeles, CA, USA
[2]Department of Neurosciences, Moores UCSD Cancer Center, University of California San Diego Health System, La Jolla, CA, USA

Introduction

The future of cancer therapy is chemotherapy. Surgery and radiation have been the mainstays of brain tumor treatment for decades, but it is chemotherapy that offers the potential for hitting a near-limitless number of molecular targets. As our knowledge of tumor biology grows, chemotherapy will be used in more patients, in more ways, for more tumor types.

This chapter provides a general overview of chemotherapy for brain tumors, touching upon the topics of drug delivery, drug development, "traditional" cytotoxic therapies, "newer" biologic agents, cancer stem cells, and even upon treatments that can be considered "chemotherapy" only in an abstract sense, namely immunotherapy and gene therapy. The information given here is by no means comprehensive, but should provide a framework for understanding the issues that are most relevant to using chemotherapy to treat patients with brain tumors.

Even as the promise and potential of chemotherapy is reviewed, it is important to be mindful of the frustrations of the past – for a long time, arguably up to and including today, chemother-apy has not worked very well for brain tumors. The reasons for this are numerous, but one of the biggest challenges is an obvious one: how do we get chemotherapy into the brain?

The challenge of drug delivery

The blood–brain barrier is a structural and physiologic marvel that regulates the composition of cerebrospinal fluid (CSF) and keeps potential neurotoxins at bay. Unfortunately, the defenses that evolved to keep toxic substances out also make it difficult for chemotherapeutic agents to get in. The endothelial cells that line cerebral capillaries are sealed together by tight junctions. Pericytes and astrocytic endfeet provide additional coverage. In addition to these structural barriers, drug-metabolizing enzymes and efflux pumps such as P-glycoprotein actively prevent unwelcome substrates (and many chemotherapeutic drugs) from entering the brain.

Traversing the blood–brain barrier is therefore a challenge few drugs are up to. All drugs greater than 180 kDa in size are excluded. (Vincristine, paclitaxel, and etoposide are over 400 kDa.) Plasma-protein bound drugs are excluded.

Neuro-oncology, First Edition. Edited by Roger J. Packer, David Schiff.

(Chlorambucil is 99% protein-bound.) Efflux pump substrates are excluded. For a compound to cross the blood–brain barrier, it must either be sufficiently liposoluble or have affinity for a carrier or receptor found on the cerebral endothelial cell. It has been estimated that only 2% of small molecular weight drugs (and no large molecular weight drugs) are able to penetrate an intact blood–brain barrier.

Though use of chemotherapeutic agents to treat brain tumor patients has grown, knowledge of whether these compounds are delivered to their targets remains limited. (Indeed, many of the drugs listed in the previous paragraph as being incapable of penetrating an intact blood–brain barrier are still used to treat brain tumors today.) For some drugs, pharmacokinetic studies have been performed to find the ratio between the concentration of drug in the CSF and its concentration in plasma – the CSF:plasma ratio. However, even this ratio is poorly reflective of how well a drug is distributed within a tumor following systemic delivery, as blood flow and interstitial pressure within a tumor can vary widely from region to region. Few studies evaluating intratumoral drug concentrations have been performed. Thus, any time a therapeutic clinical trial fails to produce the hoped-for results, asking whether a sufficient amount of drug reached its intended target is a legitimate question.

However, the blood–brain barrier may not always be an impediment to treatment. For example, monoclonal antibodies such as bevacizumab and rituximab are much too large to penetrate an intact blood–brain barrier, and yet they are routinely used to treat certain brain tumors. The utility of these drugs in spite of their large molecular weight is likely because of drug penetration at sites of blood–brain barrier breakdown, as well as drug effects that are independent of actual tumor penetration. Still, for many brain tumors (especially diffuse tumors like glioma), the blood–brain barrier is largely intact at the leading invasive edge of the tumor, which is, of course, the part of the tumor that is arguably most important to treat.

Several strategies are available for circumventing the blood–brain barrier. The most obvious is to choose a drug such as temozolomide with good CSF penetration. (Temozolomide has a CSF:plasma ratio of 0.2.) Alternatively, for drugs with poor CSF penetration, it may be possible to get chemotherapy into the brain simply by giving extremely high doses systemically, as is done with high dose intravenous methotrexate regimens. For drugs that are typically taken daily, pulse dosing is another potential method of getting more drug into the brain. Chemotherapy can also be delivered directly to the CNS intrathecally by lumbar puncture, or intraventricularly via Ommaya reservoir. Unfortunately, chemotherapy instilled directly into the CSF only penetrates a few millimeters into the parenchyma, which means that therapeutic drug concentrations are unlikely to be attained if bulky disease is present. Chemotherapy can also be placed in the resection cavity at the time of surgery. Intratumoral injection has been used in trials for gene therapy, immunotherapy, radioactive compounds, and conjugated toxins. Intracavitary BCNU-impregnated wafers (Gliadel®) are approved for the treatment of malignant glioma, though their use is not without drawbacks (see below.) A major concern with intratumoral injection is getting the therapeutic compound to every part of the residual tumor, especially as elevated and uneven pressure gradients within tumors prevent chemotherapy from diffusing freely. To overcome pressure gradients, some studies have utilized convection-enhanced delivery – the continuous delivery of a compound under positive pressure using catheters implanted into the tumor – but achieving uniform drug concentrations within a tumor is a challenge even with this strategy.

Another limitation of intratumoral therapies is the difficulty with giving repeated doses. Because giving chemotherapy systemically (PO or IV) is so much easier to do in clinical practice, a great deal of research has been performed to devise methods to improve delivery of systemic chemotherapy into brain tumors. An early method of doing this was to administer hyperosmolar therapy (e.g. intra-arterial mannitol) to increase blood–brain barrier permeability, providing a window for increased chemotherapy delivery. However, hyperosmolar therapy is technically demanding and not without risk. More recent efforts to permeabilize the blood–brain barrier transiently have focused on pharmacologic agents. The synthetic bradykinin antagonist RMP-7 was evaluated for this purpose. Results were modest, but next generation blood–brain barrier permeabilizers are in development. Alternatively, it may be possible to couple therapeutic compounds to ligands that take advantage of endogenous receptor-mediated endocytosis to cross the blood–brain barrier. For example, a taxane derivative conjugated to a peptide that binds lipoprotein receptor-related protein (LRP) receptor at the blood–brain barrier is currently in development. Solving the challenge of delivery will go a long ways toward solving the challenge of treating and curing brain tumors.

The drug development process: a long road

Before a compound can be evaluated in clinical trials, an Investigative New Drug (IND) application must be filed with the US Food and Drug Administration (FDA). Once approved, the compound is usually first studied in small phase I clinical trials that focus on establishing safety, assessing pharmacokinetics, and profiling toxicity. In contrast to non-oncology phase I trials that typically recruit healthy volunteers, drugs evaluated in oncology phase I trials are studied in patients with the relevant disease. Traditionally, the chief objective of phase I trials is to test progressively escalating doses of the new drug until a maximum tolerated dose (MTD) is established. (It has been argued that newer therapies that target a specific molecular function may have a "biologically effective dose" that is much lower than the MTD.) Drugs that are deemed safe in phase I studies may then proceed to phase II testing. Only at this point does evaluating drug efficacy become a primary goal. Many metrics for drug efficacy exist – overall survival is the gold standard, but radiographic response rates, biomarker assays, and time to tumor progression can all be used to evaluate efficacy. Drugs that show promise in phase II trials may then proceed to phase III testing. These trials are typically randomized, multi-institutional, and pit the investigative drug against an active control treatment (typically, standard therapy). If the phase III trials show positive results, the company can finally file

a New Drug Application with the FDA, which triggers FDA review.

This process takes time (typically, 12–15 years from drug discovery to marketing), is costly ($800 million to $2 billion per drug approved), and usually results in failure (only 5% of oncology IND applications progress beyond the investigational phase). Getting a drug approved to treat brain tumors is especially daunting. Unless specifically designed to treat brain tumors, most drugs are first tested in clinical trials that exclude patients with brain tumors.

Only 5% of adult cancer patients participate in clinical trials. A simple way to speed up drug development would be to enroll a higher percentage of patients in trials. However, eligibility restrictions often preclude patients from participating. Trials for glioblastoma, for example, are frequently restricted to patients with recurrent tumors, leaving fewer options for patients with tumors that have not yet recurred. Others trials place a cap on the number of recurrences, limiting options for patients with refractory disease. Patients with less common diagnoses also generally have fewer trial options to choose from.

Another way to make drug development more efficient is to develop better biomarkers or imaging correlates of treatment success or failure. Rather than wait the months to years necessary to calculate overall survival, biomarkers and imaging studies may provide information about drug efficacy in days to weeks, thereby not only accelerating the drug development process, but also giving patients who are unlikely to respond to the therapy a chance to try an alternative treatment. The development of robust, reproducible biomarkers and imaging correlates of response and failure is a major area of current research.

Cytotoxic chemotherapy

Cytotoxic vs. biologic therapy: potato, po-tah-to

As befits the name, cytotoxic drugs directly cause cell death. Biologic agents, in contrast, are designed to target specific proteins in order to modulate specific pathways. Cell death, if it occurs, is an indirect effect. Biologic therapies may stop tumor growth without causing cell death; for this reason, these therapies are sometimes referred to as "cytostatic."

Perhaps the simplest way to mentally differentiate cytotoxic drugs from biologic agents is to consider cytotoxic drugs as "old" and biologic agents as "new." This is a false dichotomy of course – new cytotoxic drugs are being developed all the time, and biologic agents have been around a while now. Whether anticancer biologic agents are technically "chemotherapy" is a minor semantic point. Defining chemotherapy more loosely as an anticancer therapy that involves administering patients some type of compound is more inclusive and ultimately more useful. After all, the goal – treating cancer – is the same, and reaching that goal frequently requires using both cytotoxic drugs and biologic agents.

Cytotoxic drugs interfere with cell division and DNA replication. The common element linking these drugs is that they are preferentially toxic to cells that divide rapidly, as cancer cells do. Furthermore, repair mechanisms that allow normal cells to survive cytotoxic insults are often lacking in cancer cells, rendering them more susceptible to injury. Common adverse effects of these drugs are a result of their effects on non-neoplastic rapidly dividing cells, such as those in the bone marrow (causing myelosuppression), the gastrointestinal tract (causing nausea, vomiting, mucositis, and diarrhea), and hair follicles (causing hair loss). Fatigue and malaise are also common, though usually not dose-limiting. Several cytotoxic drugs affect DNA; these drugs have the added risk of potentially being teratogenic and carcinogenic.

With a few important exceptions (e.g. temozolomide for gliomas, methotrexate for lymphoma), individual cytotoxic drugs are rarely used as first line therapy for brain tumors. However, several are still used as part of combination therapies or second line therapies. These drugs are also still used to treat rare tumors, in part because experience with newer drugs for these tumors is scant.

Adduct forming agents

Several chemotherapeutic drugs interfere with DNA replication and transcription by modifying the nitrogenous bases within DNA, resulting in mutations that lead to cell death via apoptosis.

The largest class of adduct forming drugs are the "alkylating agents" – so called because they attach alkyl groups to DNA. Cyclophosphamide and ifosfamide fall into this category. Both of these drugs are nitrogen mustards, and are occasionally used in multiagent regimens to treat neuroectodermal tumors such as medulloblastoma. To lower the potential risk of hemorrhagic cystitis with these drugs, aggressive IV hydration and 2-mercaptoethane sulfonate sodium (mesna) are typically given.

Nitrosoureas are another type of alkylating agent. Two drugs in this category – lomustine and carmustine – were previously used extensively in the treatment of brain tumors because their lipophilicity allows them to cross the blood–brain barrier more readily than most other cytotoxic drugs. Lomustine (also known as CCNU, or N-(2-chloroethyl)-N-cyclohexyl-N-nitrosourea), is an orally bioavailable nitrosourea that is still used as second line therapy for several brain tumors. It is typically given every 6 weeks, as the blood count nadir usually occurs 5–6 weeks following administration. Idiopathic pulmonary fibrosis and nephrotoxicity can also occur; the risk of these complications increases with cumulative dosing. Carmustine (also known as BCNU, or N,N-bis(2-chloroethyl)-N-nitroso-urea) can be given intravenously, but is unique in that it can also be implanted in the brain at the time of surgery in the form of a carmustine wafer (Gliadel). Carmustine wafers are an FDA-approved treatment for patients with newly diagnosed malignant glioma, but use has declined as other therapies have become more prevalent. Postoperative wound healing complications and a substantial local inflammatory response (which can be difficult to distinguish from tumor recurrence by imaging) can occur with carmustine wafers.

The most widely used chemotherapy drug for primary brain tumors is temozolomide (Temodar® in the United States, Temodal® in Europe), a derivative of the alkylating agent dacarbazine. Temozolomide is a prodrug that is converted to its active form MTIC (3-methyl-(triazen-1-yl)imidazole-4-carboxamide) at physiologic pH. Along with radiation, temozolomide is considered first line therapy for malignant glioma, largely replacing the earlier PCV regimen (procarbazine, CCNU, vincristine – procarbazine is also an alkylating agent). Advantages of temozolomide include good oral bioavailability, good CSF penetration, and general tolerability. Temozolomide is typically taken daily during fractionated radiation, followed by 4-week cycles in which it is given for 5 consecutive days followed by 23 days off. It is important to recognize that increased enhancement on magnetic resonance imaging (MRI) scans performed shortly after treatment with concurrent radiation and temozolomide does not necessarily signify tumor progression. Very often, this imaging finding actually represents a positive treatment effect known as "pseudoprogression." Distinguishing pseudoprogression from true tumor progression can be difficult, and is an area of active research.

Adverse effects with temozolomide such as nausea, fatigue, and constipation are typically mild. Myelosuppression, particularly thrombocytopenia, can occur, but is usually readily managed with dose delays or reductions. Occasionally, prolonged thrombocytopenia can be seen. Because of its activity and ease of use, temozolomide is also frequently used to treat brain tumors other than malignant glioma. In some cases, temozolomide is being used even prior to radiation therapy, in order to spare patients the adverse effects of radiation as long as possible.

The DNA damage caused by alkylating agents like temozolomide can be repaired by the enzyme MGMT (O-6-methylguanine-DNA methyltransferase). Malignant gliomas that silence MGMT expression through methylation of the MGMT gene promoter are less able to repair damage caused by temozolomide, and are thus more susceptible to its effects. The ability of the MGMT enzyme to repair DNA damage may be diminished by frequent drug administration; thus, some neuro-oncologists advocate giving temozolomide in lower per-day doses more frequently (e.g. daily; or 21 days on, 7 days off). Such so-called "metronomic" or "dose-dense" schedules may overcome the ability of MGMT within tumor cells to repair DNA damage. Pharmacologic inhibitors of MGMT have also been evaluated, though with limited success thus far.

Cisplatin and carboplatin damage DNA by attaching platinum adducts, as opposed to alkyl groups. Both drugs are administered intravenously. Use of cisplatin is limited by its high emetogenicity, nephrotoxicity, neurotoxicity (primarily neuropathy), and otoxicity. However, as a component of the "Packer" regimen (vincristine during radiation, followed by cycles of cisplatin, lomustine, and vincristine), it is still frequently used to treat pediatric medulloblastoma. Carboplatin causes less nephrotoxicity and is less emetogenic, but myelosuppression can be significant and dose-limiting. Like cisplatin, carboplatin is often given in combination with other drugs when used to treat brain tumors.

Antimetabolites

Purine antagonists (e.g. fludarabine), fluoropyrimidines (e.g. 5-fluorouracil [5-FU] and its prodrug capecitabine), deoxycytidine analogs (e.g. cytarabine, gemcitabine), and folate antagonists (e.g. methotrexate, pemetrexed) all fall into the class of chemotherapy drugs known as antimetabolites. These drugs potently inhibit enzymes involved in DNA synthesis.

Most antimetabolites are not used for the treatment of CNS tumors, in part because of poor blood–brain barrier penetration. Methotrexate is an exception. At conventional doses (50–500 mg/m^2), methotrexate does not cross the blood–brain barrier. However, when given intravenously at high doses (3 g/m^2, up to 8 g/m^2), enough methotrexate is able to get into brain tumors to have a therapeutic effect. Not surprisingly, such high doses can be exceedingly toxic if not given properly. Methotrexate can cause nausea, mucositis, myelosuppression, and significant nephrotoxicity. These effects can be abrogated by administering leucovorin to "rescue" normal cells following exposure to high dose methotrexate. Treatment with high dose methotrexate is typically given in a hospital setting, where aggressive fluid hydration can be given and patients can be closely monitored. While inconvenient for patients (especially when given every 2 weeks during hospital stays that are typically 4–5 days at a time), high dose methotrexate is a very effective treatment for CNS lymphoma. In fact, chemotherapy for CNS lymphoma has advanced to the point that radiation therapy can usually be deferred.

Furthermore, when given appropriately, high dose methotrexate is also generally very well tolerated.

Methotrexate can also be administered intraocularly for ocular lymphoma, as well as intrathecally for patients with leptomeningeal disease. However, the twice-a-week administration necessary to have a therapeutic effect with intrathecal methotrexate often precludes its practical use.

Methotrexate is also potentially neurotoxic. Acute complications (e.g. encephalopathy) or subacute complications (e.g. a reversible stroke-like syndrome) are rare; however, long-term neurocognitive effects are common. These neurocognitive effects are much more severe in patients who have previously been treated with radiation. In fact, giving methotrexate following radiation is rarely advisable, especially in elderly patients.

Pemetrexed (Alimta®) is a newer antifolate agent that can potentially be given in the outpatient setting. However, few studies evaluating its efficacy for CNS lymphoma have been performed to date.

Cytarabine (also known as cytosine arabinoside or Ara-C) is occasionally used to treat CNS lymphoma as well, often in combination with methotrexate. Cerebellar toxicity is a known potentially serious toxicity of cytarabine. Cytarabine can also be given intrathecally, usually in its liposomal formulation (DepoCyt®). Unlike intrathecal methotrexate, intrathecal liposomal cytarabine is usually given once every 2 weeks, making it the more convenient option for patients receiving intrathecal chemotherapy. Intrathecal cytarabine can cause a chemical arachnoiditis; to minimize this risk, steroids should be given before and after injection for a period of 5 days.

☆ TIPS AND TRICKS

INTRATHECAL CHEMOTHERAPY
Before giving intrathecal chemotherapy

- Image the entire neuraxis (brain and spine) in order to assess total burden of disease and identify possible blockages in cerebrospinal fluid (CSF) flow.

- If there are concerns that CSF flow may be disrupted, a CSF radionuclide cisternogram (CSF flow study) should be performed prior to giving intrathecal (IT) chemotherapy.
- Patients with leptomeningeal neoplastic disease may present with hydrocephalus. This should be managed with steroids when possible (e.g. 4 mg dexamethasone b.i.d. to start), and placing a shunt (the risk of peritoneal spread of malignancy is actually low). Shunts with on–off valves are available, and can be turned off for IT chemotherapy for short periods of time.

Indications

- Non-bulky leptomeningeal neoplastic disease (e.g. leptomeningeal disease documented by exam and CSF cytology, but without bulky deposits by imaging). IT chemotherapy only penetrates a 1–2 mm into tissue, and thus efficacy is poor for bulky, nodular disease.
- CNS chemoprophylaxis for aggressive hematologic malignancies.

Administration

- Placement of an Ommaya reservoir is generally preferred over serial lumbar punctures, especially if repeated instillations are planned. In addition to convenience, drug distribution throughout the leptomeninges is more uniform via an Ommaya reservoir.
- Maintain sterile precautions.
- Drape the surrounding area (to limit exposure should any chemotherapy spill).
- In general, the amount of CSF that is removed should equal the amount of volume that is instilled (chemotherapy volume plus flush).
- Inject slowly, keep bubbles up.
- Monitor response to therapy with CSF cytology.

Agents

- Cytarabine: 50 mg/dose 2–3 times per week. Use generally limited to hematologic malignancies.
- Liposomal cytarabine (DepoCyt): same dose as cytarabine, but given once every 2 weeks.
- Methotrexate: 10–12 mg twice per week.
- Thiotepa: 10 mg twice per week.

Very few studies have compared efficacy of these agents. Methotrexate may be more effective for leptomeningeal carcinomatosis from breast cancer, but choosing therapy is often guided more by convenience than anything else. Liposomal cytarabine, which only needs to be given once every 2 weeks, is therefore the most common choice.

Possible adverse events

- Risks of surgery to place Ommaya reservoir
- Risk of Ommaya-related complication (including 5–10% risk of infection)
- Chemotherapy-related adverse effects:
  - Cytarabine (both the liposomal and non-liposomal formulation) can cause a chemical arachnoiditis. Prevent by giving 4 mg dexamethasone b.i.d. for 5 days beginning 1–2 days before IT chemotherapy, or by administering IT hydrocortisone along with cytarabine.
  - Methotrexate can also cause arachnoiditis, as well as encephalopathy and myelopathy. It is metabolized systemically, and therefore can cause myelosuppression. To limit systemic toxicity, administer 10 mg leucovorin b.i.d. for 3 days concurrently. Methotrexate overdose can also be treated with glucarpidase.
  - Thiotepa can cause myelosuppression.

Topoisomerase inhibitors

The topoisomerase enzymes relieve torsional strain that develops during DNA replication and transcription. Disruption of these enzymes results in DNA strand breaks and eventual cell death. Topotecan and irinotecan belong to the class of drugs known as camptothecins. Both drugs inhibit topoisomerase I. Topotecan is not commonly used to treat brain tumors, although intrathecal topotecan has been used to treat leptomeningeal disease. Irinotecan was commonly given in conjunction with the antiangiogenic agent bevacizumab to treat patients with recurrent malignant glioma, as the original studies evaluating bevacizumab for use in brain tumor patients borrowed this drug combination from colorectal cancer treatment regimens. Subsequent studies demonstrated no significant improvement in efficacy with the combination, and ultimately bevacizumab received approval for recurrent glioblastoma as monotherapy. Newer camptothecins have been developed, but their efficacy for the treatment of brain tumors is uncertain.

Etoposide is a topoisomerase II inhibitor that is a component of several multidrug regimens used to treat a variety of tumors. It can be given either orally or intravenously. Adverse effects include nausea, myelosuppression, and diarrhea. Anthracyclines (e.g. doxorubicin) also disrupt topoisomerase II, but use of these drugs to treat brain tumors is rare.

Antimicrotubule agents

Taxanes and vinca alkaloids both cause cell death by disrupting microtubule assembly (a critical component of cell division), but they do so in contrasting ways. Taxanes (e.g. paclitaxel, docetaxel) promote uncontrolled polymerization of the tubulin dimers that form microtubules. Vinca alkaloids (e.g. vincristine), on the other hand, prevent polymerization. Both drug classes can cause a severe sensory predominant peripheral neuropathy. Vincristine is a component of several multiagent regimens for brain tumors (e.g. the "Packer regimen" for pediatric medulloblastoma), but use for glioma patients has declined as temozolomide has replaced PCV as standard therapy. The epothilones (e.g. patupilone) are a drug class with a mechanism of action similar to taxanes, but with a milder adverse effect profile. Patupilone is currently being evaluated in clinical trials for patients with brain metastases.

Signal transduction pathways, targeted therapy, and personalized medicine

The promise of chemotherapy lies in the belief that it is possible to take advantage of the mutations, epigenetic modifications, and signaling pathway dysregulation that differentiate cancer cells from normal cells for therapeutic gain. In 2002, Bernard Weinstein coined the term "oncogene addiction" to describe the idea that every cancer has its Achilles heel. Earlier convention held that the abnormalities in a malignancy were too numerous to be targeted individually. Thus, drug development focused on targeting cellular processes that are ubiquitous, such as DNA repair and cell division. By contrast, the "oncogene addiction" hypothesis holds that cancer cells can become dependent on a single oncogene for growth and survival, even when multiple other abnormalities are present.

The potential of this idea is best exemplified by the use of imatinib for the treatment of chronic myelogenous leukemia (CML). This disease is typified by a translocation between chromosomes 9 and 22 that results in the production of the Bcr-abl fusion protein, which functions as a constitutively active receptor tyrosine kinase. Imatinib was specifically designed to bind and inhibit the Bcr-abl kinase. Along with similarly designed drugs that were subsequently developed, imatinib has transformed CML from a fatal disease into a highly treatable one.

Such dramatic results have spurred on a new era of drug development, where the ultimate goal is to deliver "targeted therapy" and "personalized medicine." Rather than treat every patient with a given cancer the same way, the goal of personalized medicine is to use the tools of technology to analyze each patient's cancer and tailor therapy accordingly. Several FDA-approved oncologic drugs target specific proteins, and this number will keep growing. Many target oncogenic receptor tyrosine kinases such as Bcr-abl. Others target intracellular kinases, enzymes, or structural proteins. These targets and others are reviewed below.

Targeting receptor tyrosine kinases

Receptor tyrosine kinases are targets for many drugs used for cancer treatment (Plate 5.6, see plate section opposite p. 52). These receptors span the cell membrane and, in their normal wild-type form, are activated when ligand binds to the extracellular receptor domain. This binding triggers a conformational change in the receptor that leads to dimerization and activation of the intracellular kinase domain. The kinase domain phosphorylates tyrosine residues along the intracellular portion of the receptor, creating binding sites for proteins that activate downstream signal transduction pathways.

The human genome contains 90 receptor tyrosine kinase genes. Receptors with particular relevance to neuro-oncology include the epidermal growth factor receptor (EGFR), vascular endothelial growth factor receptor (VEGFR), platelet-derived growth factor receptor (PDGFR), and c-Met (which binds hepatocyte growth factor/scatter factor).

Aberrant activation of signal transduction pathways promotes the dysregulated growth and proliferation that drives cancer progression. Certain cancers, such as CML, are defined by overactivation of a specific receptor tyrosine kinase. Other cancers have subsets of patients with a specific overactive pathway. Sixty percent of gliomas, for example, show evidence of EGFR overactivation, either as the result of EGFR gene amplification or because of a mutation that results in a truncated protein with constitutive activity (known as EGFRvIII).

Targeting receptor tyrosine kinases and their downstream pathways – particularly when it is known which receptor pathway is overactivated – is therefore an appealing treatment strategy. To date, the two most common methods of inhibiting these receptors and their pathways are to use either small molecule inhibitors or monoclonal antibodies. Most small molecule inhibitors are designed to bind and occupy the active site of a receptor without causing further downstream signaling. Monoclonal antibodies are large molecules that can inhibit signaling either by binding up free ligand (e.g. bevacizumab) or by binding and inactivating the receptor directly (e.g. cetuximab). Rituximab, the first monoclonal antibody approved for use in the United States, binds the CD20 receptor found on the surface of B lymphocytes. It is used for the treatment of multiple hematologic malignancies, including CNS lymphoma.

Small molecule inhibitors have the theoretical advantage of being better able to penetrate the blood–brain barrier than large monoclonal antibodies, though data regarding CNS intratumoral penetration is scant even for small molecule inhibitors. (Whenever trials of these agents for brain tumor patients are unsuccessful, there is always the question of whether enough drug got into the tumors.) By virtue of their size, small molecule inhibitors are also capable of reaching intracellular targets, and thus are more versatile than monoclonal antibodies in this sense. Additionally, because the active sites of kinases are fairly well conserved, small molecule inhibitors usually bind to multiple targets with varying affinity. This lack of binding specificity can be advantageous – cancers with multiple overactive signaling pathways can potentially be treated with a single drug that targets all of them. However, the potential for adverse off-target effects also increases.

Monoclonal antibodies, on the other hand, bind their target with great specificity. In addition to their directly inhibitory effects, antibodies are also theoretically capable of activating an immune response against tumor – either antibody-dependent cellular cytotoxicity (ADCC) or complement-dependent cytotoxicity (CDC). However, the therapeutic relevance of this mode of action is uncertain, especially with regards to brain tumors.

In general, targeted therapies are well tolerated. Because they do not have a ubiquitous effect on rapidly dividing cells, targeted therapies tend to cause less myelosuppression. Nausea and fatigue are usually very manageable.

Vascular endothelial growth factor and antiangiogenic therapy

The VEGF family consists of five related glycoproteins that bind to VEGF receptor tyrosine kinases, of which there are three. VEGF signaling promotes angiogenesis, the process by which new blood vessels are formed from existing blood vessels. In healthy adults, angiogenesis has an important role in physiologic processes such as wound healing and the uterine cycle. In solid tumors, dysregulated VEGF signaling promotes tumor growth. VEGF increases migration and invasion of endothelial cells, augments homing of bone marrow-derived vascular precursor cells, and also increases blood vessel permeability. The cumulative effect of these functions is to increase tumor vascularity, even though actual blood flow within the tumor may be turbulent and inefficient. Despite the name, VEGF also has non-vascular effects that directly promote tumor cell survival, migration, and invasion. VEGF signaling can also indirectly promote tumor growth through local immune suppression.

The humanized monoclonal antibody bevacizumab is FDA-approved for the treatment of metastatic colorectal cancer, advanced non-small cell lung cancer, metastatic renal cell cancer, and recurrent glioblastoma. (The FDA recommended repealing its metastatic breast cancer indication in 2010.) Bevacizumab functions by binding circulating VEGF-A, thereby inhibiting VEGF signaling. Like other anti-VEGF drugs, bevacizumab is well tolerated, and does not cause the fatigue and myelosuppression that are commonly seen with cytotoxic agents. Potential adverse effects include hypertension (usually easily managed), proteinuria (generally reversible), impaired wound healing (which limits its use in the perioperative period; generally bevacizumab is not given within 4 weeks of surgery), and gastrointestinal perforation. Bleeding and thromboembolic complications are uncommon but potentially catastrophic. In fact, the fear of intracerebral hemorrhage or infarct was a major reason bevacizumab was not initially tested for use in CNS malignancies. Subsequent studies have demonstrated that this risk is small, even for patients on therapeutic anticoagulation.

Despite its inability to penetrate an intact blood–brain barrier, bevacizumab has transformed the treatment landscape for patients with malignant glioma. Prior to bevacizumab, patients with malignant glioma who failed initial therapy had to confront the reality that additional treatments were unlikely to provide significant benefit. With bevacizumab radiographic responses are not only possible, they are the norm. More importantly, patients feel better – adverse effects are typically minimal, and symptoms often improve. Because of its efficacy for malignant glioma, bevacizumab has become the de facto treatment for refractory CNS tumors of many types.

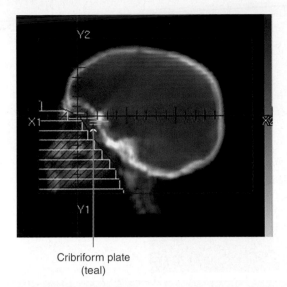

Cribriform plate
(teal)

Plate 4.1. Digital reconstruction of a whole brain radiation field. A lateral beam's eye view is shown. Multileaf collimators (white rectangles with stripes) shield the eyes and mouth. The cribriform plate is included in the radiation field.

Neuro-oncology, First Edition. Edited by Roger J. Packer, David Schiff.
© 2012 John Wiley & Sons, Ltd. Published 2012 by John Wiley & Sons, Ltd.

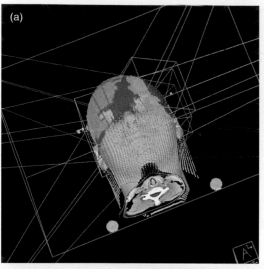

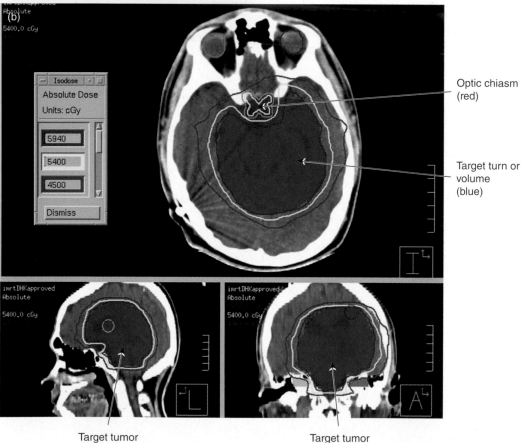

Optic chiasm
(red)

Target turn or
volume
(blue)

Target tumor
volume

Target tumor
volume

Plate 4.2. IMRT plan of 15-year-old boy with an anaplastic astrocytoma involving his left thalamus to a dose of 59.4 Gy. The patient was decompressed surgically and had a ventriculoperitoneal shunt placed. (a) Three-dimensional reconstruction showing seven-beam arrangement with each beam represented in a different color. (b) Axial (top), sagittal (bottom left), and coronal (bottom right) sections of treatment plan. The 59.4 and 54 Gy isodose lines conform to the tumor target volume. The optic chiasm is excluded from the high dose volume.

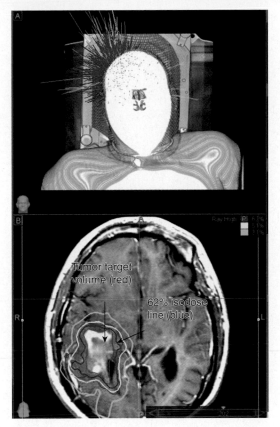

Plate 4.3. Stereotactic radiotherapy plan of a 19-year-old man with recurrent glioblastoma. The patient received 30 Gy in 5 fractions, treated to the 62% isodose line. Beams are shown as individual lines (upper panel) and result in conformal dose around the target (lower panel).

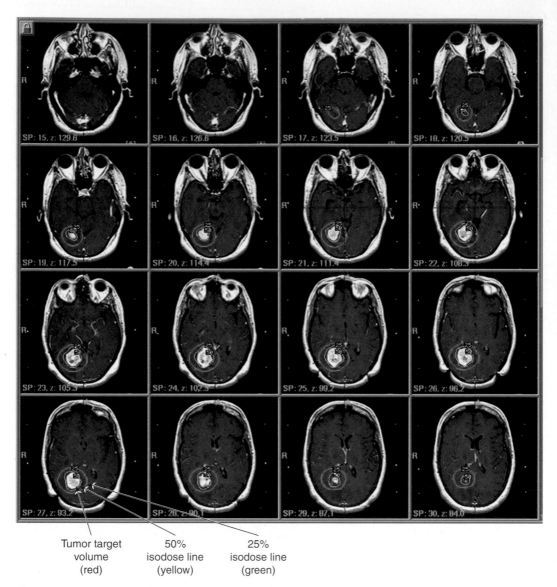

Tumor target	50%	25%
volume	isodose line	isodose line
(red)	(yellow)	(green)

Plate 4.4. Stereotactic radiosurgery plan for a patient with a lung cancer metastasis in the right occipital lobe presenting with left motor and sensory deficits. Axial magnetic resonance images with the radiation target and 50% and 25% isodose lines shown. The patient was treated to 15 Gy to the 50% isodose line in 1 fraction.

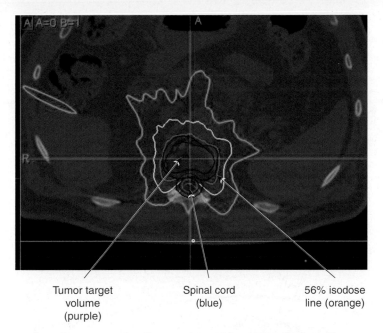

Tumor target volume (purple)   Spinal cord (blue)   56% isodose line (orange)

Plate 4.5. Stereotactic radiosurgery plan for a patient with metastatic thyroid cancer to the lumbar spine. Axial slice of radiation plan to the involved vertebral body for 16 Gy in 1 fraction. The 56% isodose line conforms to the target volume. The spinal cord is excluded from the high dose volume.

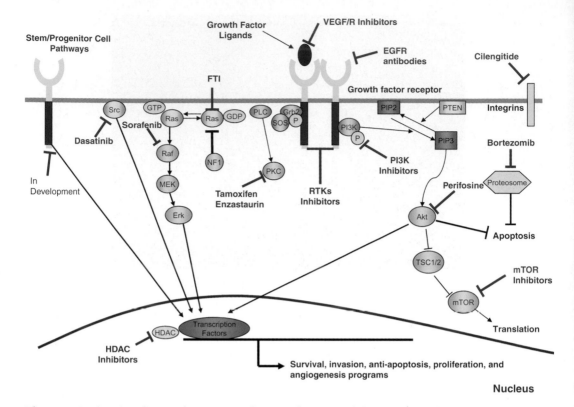

Plate 5.6. Major signaling pathways in malignant gliomas and the corresponding targeted agents in development for glioblastoma. RTK inhibitors that target epidermal growth factor receptor (EGFR) include gefitinib, erlotinib, lapatinib, BIBW2992, and vandetanib; those that target platelet-derived growth factor (PDGF) receptor include imatinib, dasatinib, and tandutinib; those that target vascular endothelial growth factor (VEGF) receptor include cediranib, pazopanib, sorafenib, sunitinib, vatalanib, vandetanib, and XL184. EGFR antibodies include cetuximab and panitumumab. Farnesyl transferase inhibitors (FTI) include lonafarnib and tipifarnib; HDAC inhibitors include depsipeptide, vorinostat, and LBH589; PI3K inhibitors include BEZ235 and XL765; mTOR inhibitors include sirolimus, temsirolimus, everolimus, and deforolimus; and VEGF receptor inhibitors include bevacizumab, aflibercept (VEGF-trap), and CT-322. Growth factor ligands include EGF, PDGF, IGF, TGF, HGF/SF, VEGF, and FGF. Stem-cell pathways include SHH, wingless family, and Notch. Akt denotes murine thymoma viral oncogene homologue (also known as protein kinase B). Erk, extracellular signal-regulated kinase; FGF, fibroblast growth factor; FTI, farnesyl transferase inhibitors; GDP, guanine diphosphate; Grb2, growth factor receptor-bound protein 2; GTP, guanine triphosphate; HDAC, histone deacetylase; HGF/SF, hepatocyte growth factor/scatter factor; IGF, insulin-like growth factor; MEK, mitogen-activated protein kinase kinase; mTOR, mammalian target of rapamycin; NF1, neurofibromin 1; P, phosphate; PIP2, phosphatidylinositol (4,5) biphosphate; PIP3, phosphatidylinositol 3,4,5-triphosphate; PI3K, phosphatidylinositol 3-kinase; PKC, protein kinase C; PLC, phospholipase C; PTEN, phosphatase and tensin homologue; Raf, v-raf 1 murine leukemia viral oncogene homologue 1; Ras, rat sarcoma viral oncogene homologue; RTK, receptor tyrosine kinase inhibitor; SHH, sonic hedgehog; SOS, son of sevenless; Src, sarcoma (Schmidt–Ruppin A-2) viral oncogene homologue; TGF, transforming growth factor family; TSC1 and 2, tuberous sclerosis gene 1 and 2. Blue text denotes inhibitors.

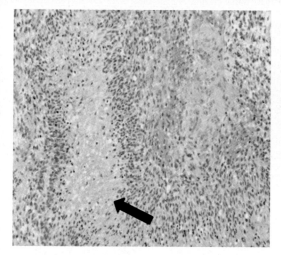

Plate 6.7. Histopathology of glioblastoma (GBM), demonstrating pseudopalisading necrosis (black arrow).

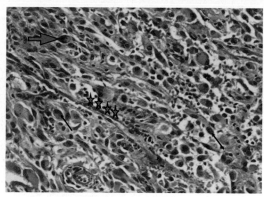

Plate 14.9. Anaplastic astrocytoma demonstrating dense cellular pattern with vascular proliferation (beneath the row of stars), nuclear atypia (thin arrow), and mitotic figures (block arrow). Courtesy of Dr Dimitris Agamanolis.

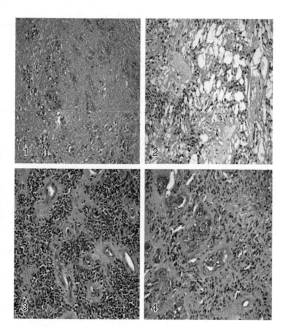

Plate 8.8. Tumor histology. 1, Subependymoma; 2, myxopapillary ependymoma; 3, ependymoma; 4, anaplastic ependymoma.

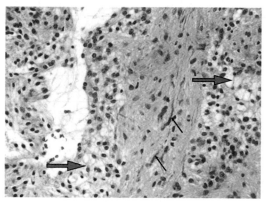

Plate 14.10. Pilocytic astrocytoma demonstrating pilocytic (threadlike) formations of the astrocytic component (bold arrows) and eosinophilic Rosenthal fibers (thin arrows). Courtesy of Dr Dimitris Agamanolis.

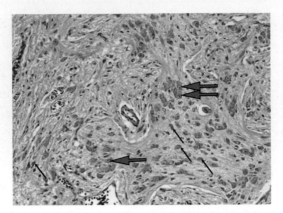

Plate 14.11. Ganglioglioma demonstrating clusters of mature appearing but disorganized ganglion cells (block arrows) found in the background of the more numerous and smaller neoplastic glial cells (thin arrows). Courtesy of Dr Dimitris Agamanolis.

Several other antiangiogenic drugs have been developed, though none are used as frequently for brain tumors as bevacizumab. FDA-approved small molecule multikinase inhibitors that bind to VEGF receptor include sorafenib and sunitinib; however, neither of these drugs has a particularly high affinity for the VEGF receptor. Several higher affinity small molecule VEGF receptor inhibitors are in development.

The antiangiogenic success story comes with qualifications. Anti-VEGF therapy does not cure brain tumors and, in fact, median survival benefit is modest in comparison to the dramatic improvements seen with traditional radiographic response metrics. (FDA approval of bevacizumab for recurrent glioblastoma was granted because of its effect on quality of life, not survival.) The impressive radiographic responses seen with anti-VEGF therapy may have more to do with effects on the vasculature (e.g. vasoconstriction, decreased vessel permeability) than actual anti-tumor effects – this phenomenon has been dubbed "pseudoresponse." Similarly, symptomatic improvement may be due more to antiedema than antitumor effects. It has been hypothesized that the benefit of anti-VEGF therapy may stem from its ability to "normalize" blood flow by pruning nascent inefficient vessels, a process that may improve chemotherapy delivery. Indeed, though approved as monotherapy, bevacizumab is frequently administered with other chemotherapeutic agents.

There is also evidence to suggest that anti-VEGF therapy can promote the development of diffuse invasive tumor, though this is still a point of controversy. Denied the ability to grow new blood vessels, tumors treated with anti-VEGF therapy may instead coopt existing native blood vessels. Tumors with this phenotype may be more resistant to other treatments. For this reason, anti-VEGF therapy is typically deferred until tumor recurrence, or given as part of a clinical trial if used as upfront therapy.

Epidermal growth factor receptor

The epidermal growth factor receptor (EGFR) is a tyrosine kinase that is capable of activating two major signal transduction pathways – the Ras pathway and the PI 3-kinase pathway – both of which are further discussed below. Aberrant EGFR activation, either via gene amplification or mutation, occurs in several malignancies. EGFR activation of the Ras pathway has been studied extensively in colorectal cancer and non-small cell lung cancer, while aberrant activation of the PI 3-kinase pathway appears to have a significant role in the pathogenesis of glioblastoma.

Commercially available EGFR inhibitors include the small molecule inhibitors erlotinib and gefitinib, as well as the monoclonal antibodies cetuximab, panitumumab, and nimotuzumab. None of these agents is currently FDA approved for the treatment of brain tumors, though several trials of these drugs, particularly erlotinib and gefinitib, have been performed or are underway. Additionally, a peptide vaccine against the constitutively active mutant receptor EGFRvIII is currently in development. A common adverse effect of treatment with EGFR inhibitors is rash, which occurs in approximately two-thirds of patients receiving such therapy. Usually the rash is easily managed, but occasionally dose reduction or discontinuation is necessary. Interestingly, patients who develop a rash typically have a good tumor response to therapy.

Not all tumors with overactive EGFR signaling are sensitive to treatment with EGFR inhibitors. If the signal transduction cascade triggered by EGFR is also aberrantly overactivated by some other mechanism, then overactivation by EGFR becomes redundant, and inhibiting EGFR does not sufficiently inhibit the downstream pathway enough to terminate tumor growth and proliferation. Colorectal cancer, for example, typically only responds to EGFR inhibition in tumors with normal wild-type KRAS (a member of the Ras family). Similarly, in glioblastoma, sensitivity to EGFR inhibition occurs only if the PI 3-kinase pathway is not otherwise overactivated (see below). These nuances highlight the importance and potential of molecular profiling. Drugs that appear to have little benefit when studied in an unselected population may actually have a profound effect if used in the specific subpopulation of patients that respond to them.

Platelet-derived growth factor receptor

The PDGF receptors (PDGF-Rα and PDGF-Rβ) have important roles in multiple signaling pathways that promote tumor growth and progression. PDGF signaling is complex – the four subunits of PDGF combine to form five ligands, and each has different signaling properties depending on which receptor it binds. Furthermore, PDGF binding to PDGFR releases more PDGF, creating autocrine (e.g. tumor cell to itself) and paracrine (e.g. endothelial cell to tumor cell) loops that further activate downstream signaling. PDGF-Rβ signaling promotes angiogenesis by stimulating VEGF expression in tumor endothelia and promoting vessel maturation via pericyte recruitment. PDGF-Rα signaling has a role in the development and maintenance of neural progenitor cells, and may function similarly to promote cancer stem cells. (See section on cancer stem cells below for more details.)

PDGFR gene amplification is present in 13% of glioblastoma. Small molecule inhibitors of PDGFR such as imatinib have been evaluated in brain tumor trials, primarily for the treatment of malignant gliomas and meningiomas. Results thus far have been modest, but it is not clear if this is due to a failure in principle or something else, such as lack of drug potency, inability of the drug to reach target tissue, or use of the drug in an unselected patient population. Newer small molecule inhibitors (e.g. nilotinib) are currently being evaluated. Monoclonal antibodies against PDGF are also being developed.

Targeting downstream signal transduction pathways

The downstream signal transduction pathways that are activated by aberrant receptor tyrosine kinase activity are too complex to be reviewed in detail here. However, reviewing some of the major players in these pathways helps provide a framework for understanding the rationale for using certain drugs and drug combinations.

The Ras/MAPK pathway

Activation of receptor tyrosine kinases such as EGFR and PDGFR leads to the activation of Ras, which then phosphorylates Raf, which then phosphorylates Mek, which then phosphorylates MAPK. Ras/MAPK pathway activation ultimately results in a host of changes that promote mitosis and proliferation. Effective Ras inhibitors have thus far been difficult to design. Because Ras activity is dependent on the addition of a farnesyl

moiety to the protein, drugs that inhibit the transfer of farnesyl groups – farnesyltransferase inhibitors such as tipifarnib and lonafarnib – have been evaluated in clinical trials for brain tumor patients. Results have been modest. The small molecule drug sorafenib inhibits Raf, VEGFR, and PDGFR, but use for CNS tumors has mostly been limited to small clinical trials.

The PI 3-kinase/Akt/mTOR pathway

Another commonly dysregulated signal transduction pathway in cancer is the PI 3-kinase pathway. This pathway governs a host of cellular processes that are important for growth and proliferation. In normal cells, the mediators of this pathway are held in check by regulatory enzymes and feedback inhibition. In cancer, the PI 3-kinase pathway can be overactivated either by aberrant receptor activation or by mutations and epigenetic modifications that directly affect the mediators of the pathway. PI 3-kinase phosphorylates the membrane phospholipid PIP2, forming PIP3. The enzyme Akt (also known as PKB) contains a domain that strongly binds to PIP3 and, in doing so, becomes activated along the cytosolic surface of the plasma membrane.

The PI 3-kinase pathway is negatively regulated by PTEN, a phosphatase with the reverse function of PI 3-kinase – it forms PIP2 by dephosphorylating PIP3. Because it counteracts PI 3-kinase, PTEN is a tumor suppressor, and loss of PTEN leads to aberrant activation of the PI 3-kinase pathway. In a sense, PTEN is the "brake" for the PI 3-kinase pathway, and loss of PTEN takes the brakes off. Several malignancies are characterized by the loss of PTEN expression, including glioma. In an elegant demonstration of the insights that can be gained by understanding signal transduction pathways, Mellinghoff *et al.* showed that glioblastoma patients with retained PTEN expression and aberrant EGFR pathway activation (resulting from the EGFRvIII mutation) were sensitive to the small molecule EGFR inhibitor erlotinib. Patients with tumors that had lost PTEN expression, on the other hand, were resistant to erlotinib treatment, presumably because the signaling pathway downstream from EGFR was already disinhibited by the loss of PTEN, rendering upstream inhibition of EGFR useless.

A major downstream mediator of PI 3-kinase/ Akt activation is the kinase mTOR. (Akt inhibits an inhibitor of mTOR.) mTOR integrates input from a number of upstream pathways, and in normal cells responds to factors such as nutrient levels and energy status, and determines the appropriate cellular response. mTOR inhibitors (such as sirolimus, temsirolimus, and everolimus) are used to treat cancer and to prevent transplant rejection. Several clinical trials investigating the use of these agents are ongoing, often in combination with other drugs. There are also drugs being developed that inhibit both PI 3-kinase and mTOR. As a class, mTOR inhibitors are particularly promising for the treatment for tuberous sclerosis. Tuberous sclerosis is characterized by mutations in either TSC1 or TSC2. As a complex, TSC1/TSC2 functions as a tumor suppressor that inhibits mTOR activity; the manifestations of tuberous sclerosis, therefore, are largely due to disinhibition of mTOR. In 2010, everolimus received FDA approval for the treatment of subependymal giant cell astrocytoma, a type of tumor found in patients with tuberous sclerosis.

mTOR is actually a key component of two multiprotein complexes: mTORC1 and mTORC2. The signaling pathway and drug inhibitors described above are in fact specific to mTORC1. mTORC2 has a positive feedback role on the PI 3-kinase/Akt pathway by activating Akt. Therefore, a complicating and potentially limiting feature of mTORC1-specific inhibitors is that they may accentuate mTORC2 activity, thereby activating the pathway the drug was designed to inhibit. Dual mTORC1/mTORC2 inhibitors are in development.

Other kinases, proteins, and targeted therapies

The list of potential oncologic drug targets continues to grow, only some of which are highlighted below.

HER-2/neu, a member of the EGFR family of receptors, is best known for its role in breast cancer, but a recent genomic screen revealed that 8% of glioblastomas possess mutations in *ERBB2*, the gene that codes for HER-2/neu. HER-2/neu-positive breast cancer patients treated with the anti-HER-2/neu monoclonal antibody trastuzumab have a greater risk of CNS metastasis, likely due in part to the inability of the monoclonal antibody to cross the blood–brain barrier. The EGFR/HER-2/neu inhibitor lapatinib has been evaluated for the treatment of brain metastases in patients with HER-2/neu-positive breast cancer, but the designated endpoint was not reached, even though some reductions in tumor size were noted.

The tyrosine kinase receptor c-Met has an important role in embryonal development, and has been implicated in cancer stem cell biology. Inhibitors of c-Met and its ligand HGF (hepatocyte growth factor) are in development.

The non-receptor tyrosine kinase Src activates multiple signaling pathways, many of which result in changes in the way cells interact with their extracellular environment. Src overactivation triggers integrin-dependent changes that lead to cell movement and proliferation, resulting in increased tumor invasiveness. The multikinase inhibitor dasatinib (which inhibits Src, PDGFR, c-Abl, c-Kit, and Eph kinases) is currently being studied in clinical trials for brain tumor patients. Another strategy to decrease invasiveness is to inhibit integrin signaling directly. Clinical trials of the $\alpha v\beta 3$ and $\alpha v\beta 5$ integrin inhibitor cilengitide are ongoing. Integrin signaling also has a role angiogenesis.

Protein kinase C β (PKC-β) has a role in both the VEGF and PI 3-kinase signaling pathways, and therefore represents an attractive therapeutic target. However, a phase III trial of the PKC-β inhibitor enzastaurin for patients with recurrent glioblastoma was disappointingly negative. The partial estrogen agonist tamoxifen is also a PKC inhibitor, but results of tamoxifen use in brain tumor patients have been modest.

DNA that is tightly bound to histones is not readily available for transcription. Binding affinity between histones and DNA is decreased by acetylation, and increased by the action of histone deacetylase enzymes. Inhibiting histone deacetylase with drugs such as vorinostat therefore opens up DNA so that it is accessible to other proteins. Making DNA more accessible may also make it more susceptible to the actions of chemotherapeutic agents that target DNA. It is worth noting that although histone deacetylase inhibitors target a specific enzyme, the downstream effects of this inhibition are nonspecific, and could include activation or deactivation of any number of genes.

Therapies on the horizon

As our knowledge of tumor biology expands, our therapeutic armamentarium has grown beyond the traditional confines of "chemotherapy," but it is still useful as a framework to discuss all of these treatments together.

Targeting cancer stem cells

In 2003, Singh *et al.* demonstrated that cancer cells with stem-like properties are present within brain tumors. Unlike the more differentiated cells that comprise the bulk of a tumor, cancer stem cells are capable of continual proliferation and self-renewal. Because these cells are relatively quiescent, they are resistant to radiation therapy and traditional cytotoxic chemotherapy. The importance of cancer stem cells is still a matter of debate – is the presence of these cells the reason why traditional therapies fail to prevent tumor recurrence? If so, future therapies must effectively target the cancer stem cell population, which means that traditional metrics of chemotherapy efficacy such as fractional cell kill may lose relevance. (Conversely, a therapy that has no effect on 99% of tumor cells but is able to kill cancer stem cells would be a huge breakthrough.) Complicating matters is the fact that cancer stem cells are not easily characterized. For gliomas, the transmembrane glycoprotein CD133 was initially used to define the stem cell subpopulation. Subsequent studies have identified cancer stem cell populations that are CD133-negative. In other words, even if it is clearly established that cancer stem cells are an important subpopulation of cells to target therapeutically, the exact identity of that target is not easily defined as of yet.

Normal stem cells are regulated by signaling pathways that have an important role in development. Prominent examples include the Sonic Hedgehog (SHH), Wnt, and Notch signaling pathways. Not surprisingly, dysregulation of these pathways can lead to the development of cancer stem cells. Interestingly, dysregulation in all three of these pathways has been implicated in the development of medulloblastoma, a tumor derived from stem cells or early progenitor cells in the external granule cell layer of the cerebellum. Inhibitors of SHH, Wnt, and Notch signaling pathways are in development.

Immunotherapy

With targeted personalized medicine as the goal, it should be noted that few if any pharmaceutical compounds are able to generate as robust, persistent, and "personalized" a response as the human immune system. In recognition of this, a great deal of research is being performed to elucidate methods to activate a patient's immune system against their own cancer. The therapeutic prostate cancer vaccine sipuleucel-T (Provenge®) received FDA approval in 2010; additional cancer immunotherapies are sure to follow.

Immunotherapy for brain tumors must overcome a special set of obstacles. The brain has traditionally been thought of as an immunologically privileged environment, because of the presence of the blood–brain barrier and the absence of draining lymphatics. Additionally, brain tumors, like other malignancies, suppress local immune response. And yet, histopathologic studies show that lymphocytes frequently infiltrate brain tumors, suggesting that this immunologic privilege can be surmounted.

Treatments specifically designed to promote a tumor-specific immune response include immune-priming adjuvant therapies (such as poly-ICLC, a toll-like receptor-3 ligand) and cancer cell vaccines. The simplest version of these vaccines consists of injections of lethally irradiated or formalin-fixed tumor cells with or without immune-stimulating adjuvants. A twist on this strategy is to combine killed tumor cells with cells that have been engineered to express immune-stimulating proteins (e.g. granulocyte–macrophage colony-stimulating factor [GM-CSF]).

It is now well-established that simply exposing tumor antigen to a patient is not sufficient to activate a robust antitumor response. The human immune system is best activated when antigen is presented by an antigen-presenting cell in lymphoid tissue. Dendritic cell vaccines attempt to recapitulate this pathway. These vaccines consist of a patient's dendritic cells, isolated via leukapheresis, that have been exposed either to a tumor-specific peptide (e.g. EGFRvIII), a pool of tumor antigens, or tumor lysate. Dendritic cells are potent antigen-presenting cells, and are able to track to lymph nodes following subcutaneous injection. Preliminary results of dendritic cell vaccines are promising; further studies are ongoing.

Gene therapy

Cancer gene therapy holds tremendous promise – as the means to insert and express basically any gene exists. Current antitumor strategies include introducing genes that promote apoptosis, or genes that code for an enzyme that converts a prodrug to its active form. The viral gene product thymidine kinase, for example, converts the prodrug ganciclovir into a molecule that causes DNA chain termination in replicating cells. Similarly, the gene for cytosine deaminase can be introduced to convert the prodrug 5-FC to the active drug 5-FU. Gene therapy can also be used to achieve some of the therapeutic goals mentioned above; for example, genes that stimulate an antitumor immune response or target cancer stem cells can be inserted. Yet significant obstacles remain, as evidenced by the fact that gene therapy is not yet available outside of a research setting. Gene therapy also is not without risk, as Jesse Gelsinger's death in 1999 (in a noncancer-related gene therapy trial) poignantly illustrates.

One of the major obstacles for gene therapy is delivery. In order for the therapeutic gene to get where it needs to go, intracavitary injection during surgery is typically required. Obviously, this severely limits the number of drug administrations that can be given to a brain tumor patient. Another aspect of gene therapy delivery that has yet to be optimized is choosing the right vector to carry the therapeutic gene. Nonreplicating viruses are less likely to produce an unwanted response in normal brain tissue. However, there is no way to infect every tumor cell during the injection process. Therapeutic efficacy for nonreplicating viral vectors is therefore dependent on the induction of a prominent "bystander effect," a term used to describe the spread of a therapeutic element (e.g. proapoptotic protein or active drug) to neighboring uninfected tumor cells. How actively this phenomenon occurs is not clear. Critics will note that the phase III trial of a nonreplicating adenovirus utilizing the viral thymidine kinase/ganciclovir strategy was disappointingly negative. Replicating viruses, on the other hand, are able to carry therapeutic genes to cells other than the ones they initially infected. These viruses are directly oncolytic in some cases. The challenge for replicating viruses is to engineer them so that they replicate efficiently, but only in tumor cells.

The future of chemotherapy

It is becoming clear that brain tumors, like most solid tumor malignancies, are extremely heterogeneous and therefore not likely to be amenable to universal cures with single agent therapy. Combination therapy is much more likely to be successful. But which combinations? How are they best tested? Clinical trials are "cleanest" when evaluating the effect of one drug at a time, but this may not be in the best interest of our patients. To test all the three-drug combinations that can be made from, say, a panel of five targeted drugs, it would be necessary to test 10 drug combinations. And this ignores all the possible permutations in dosing schedules that are available.

Ensuring widespread (ideally universal) access to chemotherapy is another daunting challenge. "Personalized" medicine is not cheap, and the billion dollar efforts of the pharmaceutical industry are generally not being spent with cost effectiveness in mind. Health care costs in the United States continue to escalate, but this is not a trend that is likely sustainable in the long run.

There is also a world on the periphery of chemotherapy with vast, largely unexplored potential – hundreds if not thousands of natural products and compounds may have antitumor activity, but their benefits are being sold (and likely oversold) to an eager patient population with little scrutiny or regulation. Determining which compounds are useful and which ones are not is yet another challenge that lies ahead.

☝ CAUTION!

SUPPLEMENTS
Natural compounds are a promising resource for cancer treatment. Drugs such as vincristine and paclitaxel are plant-derived. However:

- Studies suggest that only one-third of cancer patients tell physicians what supplements they are taking.
- Data regarding supplements are limited. Many patients believe that "natural" products are safe and do not have adverse effects.
- Many of the chemical compounds contained within supplements are unknown.
- All supplements may trigger allergic reactions.
- Product quality can vary widely. Supplements may be contaminated with microorganisms, pesticides, heavy metals, or other impurities.
- Supplements may be hepatotoxic, nephrotoxic, or cause gastrointestinal distress.
- Supplements may alter the metabolism of chemotherapeutic drugs. St John's wort, for example, induces CYP3A4, thus increasing metabolism and lowering the effective concentration of drugs such as irinotecan, imatinib, and docetaxel.
- Antioxidants may alter the effectiveness of radiation therapy and chemotherapeutic drugs that generate free radicals.
- Supplements such as feverfew, garlic, and gingko may have anticoagulant effects.

Selected bibliography

Batchelor T, Carson K, O'Neill A, Grossman SA, Alavi J, New P, *et al.* (2003) Treatment of primary CNS lymphoma with methotrexate and deferred radiotherapy: a report of NABTT 96-07. *J Clin Oncol* **21**, 1044–9.

Black KL, Yin D, Ong JM, Hu J, Konda BM, Wang X, *et al.* (2008) PDE5 inhibitors enhance tumor permeability and efficacy of chemotherapy in a rat brain tumor model. *Brain Res* **1230**, 290–302.

de Groot J, Milano V. (2009) Improving the prognosis for patients with glioblastoma: the rationale for targeting Src. *J Neurooncol* **95**, 151–63.

Dietrich J, Diamond EL, Kesari S. (2010) Glioma stem cell signaling: therapeutic opportunities and challenges. *Expert Rev Anticancer Ther* **10**, 709–22.

Hegi ME, Diserens AC, Gorlia T, Hamou MF, de Tribolet N, Weller M, *et al.* (2005) MGMT gene silencing and benefit from temozolomide in glioblastoma. *N Engl J Med* **352**, 997–1003.

Hegi ME, Liu L, Herman JG, Stupp R, Wick W, Weller M, *et al.* (2008) Correlation of O6-methylguanine methyltransferase (MGMT) promoter methylation with clinical outcomes in glioblastoma and clinical strategies to modulate MGMT activity. *J Clin Oncol* **26**, 4189–99.

Heimberger AB, Hlatky R, Suki D, Yang D, Weinberg J, Gilbert M, *et al.* (2005) Prognostic effect of epidermal growth factor receptor and EGFRvIII in glioblastoma multiforme patients. *Clin Cancer Res* **11**, 1462–6.

Jain RK. (2005) Normalization of tumor vasculature: an emerging concept in antiangiogenic therapy. *Science* **307**, 58–62.

Johnson LA, Sampson JH. (2010) Immunotherapy approaches for malignant glioma from 2007 to 2009. *Curr Neurol Neurosci Rep* **10**, 259–66.

Mellinghoff IK, Wang MY, Vivanco I, Haas-Kogan DA, Zhu S, Dia EQ, *et al.* (2005) Molecular determinants of the response of glioblastomas to EGFR kinase inhibitors. *N Engl J Med* **353**, 2012–24.

Norden AD, Young GS, Setayesh K, Muzikansky A, Klufas R, Ross GL, *et al.* (2008) Bevacizumab for recurrent malignant gliomas: efficacy, toxicity, and patterns of recurrence. *Neurology* **70**, 779–87.

Packer RJ, Sutton LN, Elterman R, Lange B, Goldwein J, Nicholson HS, *et al.* (1994) Outcome for children with medulloblastoma treated with radiation and cisplatin, CCNU, and vincristine chemotherapy. *J Neurosurg* **81**, 690–8.

Pardridge WM. (2003) Blood–brain barrier drug targeting: the future of brain drug development. *Mol Interv* **3**, 90–105, 51.

Prados MD, Schold SC Jr, Fine HA, Jaeckle K, Hochberg F, Mechtier L, *et al.* (2003) A randomized, double-blind, placebo-controlled, phase 2 study of RMP-7 in combination with carboplatin administered intravenously for the treatment of recurrent malignant glioma. *Neuro Oncol* **5**, 96–103.

Rainov NG. (2000) A phase III clinical evaluation of herpes simplex virus type 1 thymidine kinase and ganciclovir gene therapy as an adjuvant to surgical resection and radiation in adults with previously untreated glioblastoma multiforme. *Hum Gene Ther* **11**, 2389–401.

Singh SK, Clarke ID, Terasaki M, Bonn VE, Hawkins C, Squire J, *et al.* (2003) Identification of a cancer stem cell in human brain tumors. *Cancer Res* **63**, 5821–8.

Stewart DJ, Whitney SN, Kurzrock R. (2010) Equipoise lost: ethics, costs, and the regulation of cancer clinical research. *J Clin Oncol* **28**, 2925–35.

Thomas FC, Taskar K, Rudraraju V, Goda S, Thorsheim HR, Gaasch JA, *et al.* (2009) Uptake of ANG1005, a novel paclitaxel derivative, through the blood–brain barrier into brain and experimental brain metastases of breast cancer. *Pharm Res* **26**, 2486–94.

Vredenburgh JJ, Desjardins A, Herndon JE, Dowell JM, Reardon DA, Quinn JA, *et al.* (2007) Phase II trial of bevacizumab and irinotecan in recurrent malignant glioma. *Clin Cancer Res* **13**, 1253–9.

Weinstein IB. (2002) Cancer: addiction to oncogenes: the Achilles heal of cancer. *Science* **297**, 63–4.

Wick W, Puduvalli VK, Chamberlain MC, van den Bent MJ, Carpentier AF, Cher LM, *et al.* (2010) Phase III study of enzastaurin compared with lomustine in the treatment of recurrent intracranial glioblastoma. *J Clin Oncol* **28**, 1168–74.

Part II

Adult Nervous System Tumors

6

Malignant Gliomas in Adulthood

Michael Ivan, Matthew Tate and Jennifer L. Clarke

Department of Neurological Surgery, University of California, San Francisco, CA, USA

Introduction

In the United States, approximately 60,000 primary brain tumors are predicted to have been diagnosed in 2010, of which one-third are gliomas. Gliomas comprise 80% of malignant brain tumors, with approximately 14,000 new cases each year in the United States. The incidence of glioblastoma (GBM), the most common malignant glioma, increases with age, with the highest rates in the 75–84 year age group. GBMs are 1.6 times more common in males than females and more than twice as common among white than black people. The majority of malignant gliomas are comprised of GBM (60–70%, World Health Organization [WHO] grade IV), anaplastic astrocytoma (AA) (10–15%, WHO grade III), and anaplastic oligoastrocytoma (AOA) and anaplastic oligodendroglioma (AO) (10%, WHO grade III). Though gliomas can manifest in any area of the central nervous system, they are located supratentorially in 70% of affected adults. In children, however, 70% are infratentorial.

The standard of care for GBM includes maximal surgical resection followed by radiotherapy (RT) with concurrent and adjuvant temozolomide (TMZ) therapy. Even with aggressive therapy, prognosis for malignant glioma remains poor, with a median survival for GBM of 15 months in the phase III clinical trial that demonstrated the efficacy of TMZ. The relative survival estimates for GBM are quite low; less than 5% of patients diagnosed between 1995 and 2006 survived 5 years after diagnosis.

Recent advances in basic tumor biology have led to a number of promising targeted agents that are currently in clinical trials. Most notable is bevacizumab, a vascular endothelial growth factor (VEGF) inhibitor, which was recently given accelerated approval by the US Food and Drug Administration (FDA) for treatment of recurrent GBM based on encouraging phase II trials. In addition, improvements in surgical management, molecular characterization, and radiation oncology methods allow for more accurate clinical management and prognostication. This review begins with a discussion of the clinical features of malignant glioma, focusing on characteristic features, pathogenesis, and principles of management for both newly diagnosed and recurrent malignant glioma. Current protocols will then be examined for monitoring response to treatment, which is becoming particularly relevant with the emergence of biologic agents such as bevacizumab. Finally, recent advancements in the basic and clinical sciences are discussed and their potential translation to clinical neuro-oncology.

Neuro-oncology, First Edition. Edited by Roger J. Packer, David Schiff.

Clinical features

Clinical presentation of malignant glioma varies greatly. The most common symptom for any type of brain tumor is headaches, which are typically worse in the morning or when lying flat if caused by elevated intracranial pressure. Ultimately, the location of the tumor and its effect on the surrounding anatomy (via direct cortical neuronal dysfunction and/or altered transmission of adjacent white matter pathways) determines the neurologic deficit. For example, tumors located in the frontal cortex may have focal motor weakness, while dominant parietal and temporal tumors can cause various types of language dysfunction. Seizures are common as a result of cortical irritation. Other potential symptoms include memory loss, spasticity, muscle slowing, visual symptoms, cranial nerve deficits, cognitive decline, and personality changes.

Tumor pathology and grading

Astrocytes, glial cells which have many roles in the neuronal microenvironment, morphologically resemble the cell types in and may give rise to astrocytomas and GBMs. Oligodendrogliomas are a type of glioma with cells that morphologically resemble oligodendrocytes, whose primary function is to facilitate rapid transmission of electrical signals in the central nervous system via production of myelin. Whether gliomas develop from relatively undifferentiated "stem"/progenitor cells or from de-differentiation of more mature cells remains an area of active research. Morphologically, malignant gliomas are histologically heterogeneous, highly vascular tumors that often have extensive areas of necrosis and hypoxia. They also have a tendency to infiltrate extensively into surrounding brain tissue.

The WHO grades glial tumors based on histologic features (grades I–IV). Malignant gliomas are WHO grade III or IV tumors. These "high grade" tumors have worse survival than their "low grade" counterparts because of accelerated growth rates and invasiveness. Grade III astrocytomas are anaplastic astrocytomas (AAs), and grade IV astrocytomas are GBMs (Plate 6.7, see plate section opposite p. 52). There are variants of GBM, including gliosarcoma and giant cell glioblastoma, which also have a poor prognosis. Oligodendrogliomas are also characterized using the WHO grading scale, except only grades II and III are used (Table 6.1).

Extraneural metastasis has been reported, but is rare enough that systemic staging for distant metastases is not routinely done in cases of malignant glioma, in contrast to most other cancers.

Molecular pathology

In addition to gliomas initially diagnosed as grade III or IV, termed *de novo* or primary high grade glioma, some lower grade gliomas (typically grade II) may transform to a higher grade tumor over time. These tumors are referred to as secondary high grade gliomas. Primary GBMs typically present with a rapid progression of symptoms, while secondary GBMs can present more slowly and are more often seen in younger patients. Recently, it has been reported that up to 74% of low grade astrocytomas progress to high grade at some point. This process also occurs with oligodendrogliomas, but with less frequency. Ongoing research is investigating genetic differences between primary and secondary GBMs to evaluate if they are indeed different disease entities and thus may require distinct treatment strategies.

Targeting new therapies and predicting glioma progression and recurrence first requires an understanding of the molecular pathways and signals that are present in tumor cells. Several acquired (i.e. not inherited) genetic mutations have been found in malignant gliomas that deregulate growth and corrupt DNA repair, some of which can be found in low grade gliomas as well (Table 6.2).

The majority of anaplastic oligodendrogliomas (AOs) are characterized by combined loss of chromosomal arms 1p and 19q, as described below. In addition, with progression from low grade to high grade oligodendroglioma, defects have been demonstrated in PTEN, Rb, and p53.

Risk factors

The exact causes of malignant gliomas are not well understood. There have been numerous studies investigating possible environmental risk factors for brain tumors, but to date none

Table 6.1. World Health Organization (WHO) histologic features of glial tumors. Adapted from Louis DN (ed.) (2007) *WHO Classification of Tumours of the Central Nervous System*. IARC, Lyon.

Tumor grade	Nomenclature	Histologic features
Astrocytomas		
Grade II	Diffuse astrocytoma	Well-differentiated fibrillary or gemistocytic astrocytes; moderately increased cellularity; occasional nuclear atypia
Grade III	Anaplastic astrocytoma	Increased cellularity, nuclear atypia, and mitotic activity relative to grade II
Grade IV	Glioblastoma	In addition to grade III features, microvascular proliferation and/or pseudopalisading necrosis (see also Plate 6.7)
Oligodendrogliomas		
Grade II	Oligodendroglioma	Monomorphic cells with round nuclei and perinuclear halo (fried egg) appearance due to an artifact from tumor processing; "chicken-wire" vasculature; may have microcalcifications; may have occasional mitosis present
Grade III	Anaplastic oligodendroglioma	Cells retain some grade II features, but more poorly differentiated cell types, prominent mitotic activity; may have microvascular proliferation and/or necrosis
Grade III	Anaplastic Oligoastrocytoma	Mixed tumor type with both cell types involved; if necrosis present, more likely to be glioblastoma with oligodendroglial component

have demonstrated a direct link between environmental factors and malignant glioma, including cell phone usage. The one exception is exposure to ionizing radiation, which is a risk factor for many cancer types. Moreover, only 5% of cases of malignant glioma have a known heritable cause. Such hereditary syndromes include neurofibromatosis 1, adenomatous polyposis syndromes, and Li–Fraumeni familial cancer syndrome (inherited p53 mutations).

Prognostic factors

In considering overall patient prognosis, one must consider tumor growth rate, extent of operative excision, histologic features, Karnofsky performance status (KPS; Table 6.3) on presentation, patient age, tumor burden, and location. Other important prognostic factors include molecular markers; these have been a growing area of research because this knowledge will not only improve our ability to predict outcome, but also increase our ability to detect recurrence, predict response to chemotherapy, and follow disease progression (Table 6.4). One example is the co-deletion of chromosomal arms 1p and 19q in AOs, which predicts a favorable response to chemotherapy. Without this co-deletion the tumors are relatively more treatment-resistant with a worsened prognosis, especially when a p53 mutation is also noted.

> ★ **TIPS AND TRICKS**
>
> In any grade II or III tumor with an oligodendroglial component, even if it is only a small one, it is worth ordering fluorescence *in situ* hybridization (FISH) testing to look for loss of one copy of the 1p chromosomal arm and one copy of the 19q chromosomal arm, a condition commonly referred to as "1p/19q co-deletion" or "1p/19q loss of heterozygosity

(LOH)." However, if a tumor is purely astrocytic, it is probably not worth ordering the test. If 1p/19q LOH is present, this may indicate that the tumor is relatively more sensitive to treatment with either radiation or chemotherapy.

In addition, methylation of the promoter for O^6-methylguanine-DNA methyltransferase (MGMT) has been shown to be associated with improved survival in patients with GBM. The *MGMT* gene specifically encodes a protein that acts to repair DNA by removing the alkyl group from the O^6 position of guanine, where typical DNA alkylation occurs.

Diagnosis

Initial work-up for malignant gliomas includes imaging with magnetic resonance imaging (MRI).

On MRI, high grade gliomas typically enhance with gadolinium as a result of alteration of the blood–brain barrier in the main tumor mass (Figure 6.1). In addition, high grade tumors often have central necrosis and edema. Surrounding edema and/or non-enhancing, infiltrative tumor can be seen when looking at T2 or fluid attenuated inversion recovery (FLAIR) sequences. Magnetic resonance proton spectroscopy can also be useful to further characterize abnormalities seen on anatomic imaging. The combination of an elevated choline peak, because of increased membrane turnover, and a decreased *N*-acetyl-aspartate peak resulting from loss of neuronal cellularity, is not specific, but raises suspicion for tumor in the right clinical setting. Other MRI sequences can also help to narrow the diagnosis. For instance, increased vessel permeability can be noted on magnetic resonance perfusion imaging. In certain cases, when the tumor is infiltrating near motor or speech centers, MRI with

Table 6.2. Acquired genetic mutations in glioblastoma.

Genetic mutation	Normal function	Seen in primary glioblastoma	Seen in secondary glioblastoma
Tumor suppressor protein 53 (p53)	DNA repair , apoptosis regulation	Yes	Yes
Phosphatase and tensin homolog (PTEN)	Assists in cell destruction	Yes	Yes
Epidermal growth factor receptor (EGFR) overexpression	Cell proliferation	Yes	
Loss of heterozygosity on chromosome 10q (most frequent genetic alteration in GBM)	Location of several tumor suppressor genes	Yes	Yes
p16 deletion/mutation	Cyclin dependent kinase 4 inhibitor	Yes	Yes
Overexpression of platelet-derived growth factor receptor (PDGFR)	Glial cell development		Yes
Retinoblastoma (Rb)	Tumor suppressor		Yes
Isocitrate dehydrogenase (IDH) 1 and 2 (associated with a more favorable prognosis, also seen in low grade tumors)	Cellular intermediate metabolism		Yes

Table 6.3. Karnofsky Performance Status (KPS) Scale.

Karnofsky Performance Status	
100	Normal, no complaints, no evidence of disease
90	Able to carry on normal activity, minor signs or symptoms of disease
80	Normal activity with effort, some signs or symptoms of disease
70	Cares for self. Unable to carry on normal activity or do active work
60	Requires occasional assistance, but is able to care for most of own needs
50	Requires considerable assistance and frequent medical care
40	Disabled, requires special care and assistance
30	Severely disabled, hospitalization is indicated although death is not imminent
20	Hospitalization necessary, very sick, active supportive treatment necessary
10	Moribund, fatal processes progressing rapidly
0	Dead

Table 6.4. Positive prognostic factors in malignant glioma.

Clinical/ demographic factors	Younger age
	Good performance status (high KPS*)
	Extent of surgical resection of tumor
Tumor type/ molecular markers	Grade III (vs. grade IV) Oligodendroglial histology (vs. astrocytic) 1p/19q chromosomal loss of heterozygosity Methylation of the promoter for the *MGMT* gene Mutation of IDH1/2

KPS, Karnofsky Performance Status (see Table 6.3).

Ultimately, surgical biopsy or resection is needed to establish a definitive diagnosis. This can be done either stereotactically, via needle through a burr hole, or via an open craniotomy. Both cases require an operation and thus neurosurgical intervention. More conservative surgical approaches (i.e. biopsy) are sometimes prone to sampling error because of the heterogeneous nature of these tumors. Attention should be paid to the selection of biopsy site, and a pathologic diagnosis of lower grade glioma should be reviewed carefully if the clinical picture or imaging is more consistent with a higher grade tumor.

Treatment and outcomes

Treatment plans for malignant gliomas require a multidisciplinary approach combining several teams' treatment modalities. Options for malignant gliomas vary depending on tumor burden, location, grade, rate of growth, patient neurologic function and co-morbidities, and family and/or patient goals of care. The challenges of treatment in malignant glioma patients are eloquent tumor location, delivery of therapeutic drugs across the blood–brain barrier, and the intrinsic treatment resistance of these tumors.

Surgical treatment

Surgery is typically recommended, though a true curative resection cannot be achieved with

diffusion tensor imaging (DTI) or functional MRI (fMRI) may aid in demonstrating the location of the tumor relative to eloquent structures and/or pathways in the context of surgical planning.

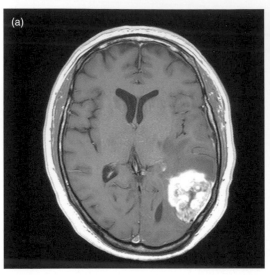
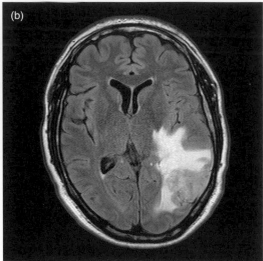

Figure 6.1. A 61-year-old man with a glioblastoma (GBM). (a) T1-weighted gadolinium-enhanced image. (b) T2-weighted FLAIR image.

malignant gliomas because of their invasive nature. The role of surgery is:

1 to obtain tissue for diagnosis;
2 to debulk the tumor to alleviate mass effect; and
3 to maximally resect the tumor to allow for the most effective adjuvant therapy.

Extensive resections become more challenging in situations when the tumor is in or adjacent to eloquent brain regions (motor, speech, white matter tracts, and brainstem) and compromise of neurologic function is in question. In these cases, intraoperative functional mapping of motor or language function may decrease morbidity. For tumors with extensive bilateral or multifocal involvement a more limited surgical biopsy may be preferable. Though overall surgical mortality is low (1–2% for tumor resection surgery), occasionally extensive surgery may be contraindicated because of a patient's co-morbidities and overall health condition.

During surgery, in addition to resection of tumor, a potential treatment option is the implantation of biodegradable impregnated polymer wafers containing carmustine (Gliadel® wafer) into the tumor bed. One clinical trial showed modest increase in survival from 11.6 to 13.9 months compared to radiotherapy alone.

Radiotherapy

After surgery, subsequent treatment with radiotherapy has been shown to prolong patient survival. Fractionated focal radiotherapy, in doses of approximately 60 Gy (30–33 fractions of 1.8–2 Gy given 5 days per week), showed increased survival from 17 to 26 weeks compared to surgery alone. In the elderly population (age over 70 years), radiotherapy was superior to supportive care. An abbreviated course of radiotherapy can be used in the older population or in patients with poor performance status, as they often tolerate standard radiotherapy less well than other patients.

> ### SCIENCE REVISITED
>
> Radiation damages cellular DNA, leading to cell death when DNA replication is attempted during cell division. The total dose of radiation is divided into daily fractions, with 30–33 total fractions generally used to treat malignant gliomas; usually one fraction is approximately 1.8–2 Gy (or 180–200 cGy). Fractionating the radiation like this is thought to allow healthy cells with presumably intact

repair mechanisms to recover, while cancer cells (which have presumably lost many of their error control processes) cannot recover and instead go on to die.

Chemotherapy for glioblastoma

TMZ, a DNA methylating agent, has been found to improve median survival in GBM patients when combined with initial radiation. Specifically, radiation therapy plus concurrent low dose daily TMZ, followed by 6 months of adjuvant TMZ, demonstrated a significant increase in median survival by almost 3 months relative to patients treated with radiation therapy alone. This study only enrolled patients up to 70 years of age, so no data are available for patients aged over 70.

EVIDENCE AT A GLANCE

The seminal clinical trial showing the benefit of combining temozolomide (TMZ) with radiation for initial treatment of glioblastoma (GBM) was published by Stupp *et al.* in the *New England Journal of Medicine* in 2005. Patients up to 70 years old were randomized to either radiation alone or radiation with TMZ (75 mg/m^2/day concurrent with radiation, followed by a larger dose given 5 days in a row every 4 weeks for six cycles). In the arm with TMZ and radiation, median overall survival increased from 12 to 14.6 months, and the percentage of patients still alive at 2 years increased from 10% to 26%. On the basis of this trial, TMZ and radiation became the standard of care for initial treatment of GBM.

Prior to TMZ, individual trials of adjuvant nitrosourea treatment did not show clear benefit, though subsequent meta-analysis has demonstrated modest efficacy for this family of drugs also.

A subset of GBM patients have *MGMT* promoter methylation, a positive prognostic factor. These patients, when treated with TMZ, had a survival of 21.7 months, whereas patients whose tumors did not have promoter methylation had a mean survival of 12.7 months. That said, patients with tumors lacking *MGMT* promoter methylation may still benefit from treatment with TMZ and combined treatment remains the standard of care for all patients with GBM.

Chemotherapy for anaplastic gliomas

As with GBMs, standard therapy initially begins with maximal surgical resection and radiotherapy to 60 Gy after surgery, but the value of concomitant and/or adjuvant chemotherapy with TMZ has not yet been tested prospectively in anaplastic gliomas. Randomized clinical trials failed to demonstrate prolonged survival with a combination of radiation and procarbazine/lomustine/vincristine (PCV) chemotherapy in newly diagnosed AOA and AO, although progression-free survival was prolonged. Time to second treatment failure (i.e. failure of both chemotherapy and radiation) was similar whether patients were initially treated with chemotherapy (followed by RT at first progression) or treated initially with RT (followed by chemotherapy at progression) in another randomized trial. Interestingly, a subset of oligoastrocytomas and oligodendrogliomas with 1p/19q co-deletion have a much higher response rate to PCV (up to 100%) compared with response rates of 23–31% without, leading some to consider chemotherapy alone for initial treatment of co-deleted anaplastic tumors.

Supportive care

Corticosteroids, typically dexamethasone, are often initiated for treatment of tumor-associated edema when tumor diagnosis is made and the patient is symptomatic. Improvement in clinical symptoms can occur quickly and can be sustained for several weeks, allowing surgical intervention and initiation of definitive treatment. Once surgical intervention is completed, the corticosteroids can usually be tapered off. During the use of corticosteroids, blood glucose should be carefully monitored, especially in the patients with pre-existing diabetes. Long-term steroids have multiple other potential side effects, including gastrointestinal upset and (rarely) perforation, redistribution of body fat, proximal myopathy, osteoporosis and compression fractures, and opportunistic infections, including *Pneumocystis jirovecii* pneumonia. Calcium supplementation and prophylaxis against *Pneumocystis* should be considered, as should acid blockers if stomach upset is present.

When seizures occur as the presenting symptom or during treatment of malignant gliomas, antiepileptic medication should be prescribed. In asymptomatic patients, prophylactic anticonvulsants are not clearly indicated. First generation anticonvulsants (phenytoin, carbamazepine, phenobarbital) are strong inducers of the hepatic cytochrome P450 enzyme system, and increase metabolism of many chemotherapy agents (though, fortunately, not TMZ). Therefore, later generation, non-enzyme-inducing drugs such as levetiracetam are preferred.

In addition, it should be remembered that patients with malignant gliomas, as with many other types of cancer, have an increased risk for venous thromboembolism due to hypercoagulability. Patients should be monitored carefully for signs of thrombosis, with a low threshold for undertaking evaluation if a patient develops limb swelling or respiratory distress. If a patient is diagnosed with deep venous thrombosis, either in an extremity or a pulmonary embolus, anticoagulation should be considered. There is a risk of hemorrhage into a patient's malignant glioma, as these are highly vascular tumors. The relative risks and benefits of anticoagulation must be weighed in each individual case, but it is often still appropriate to treat these patients with anticoagulation. Low molecular weight heparinoids are often preferred over warfarin for treatment of cancer-associated thromboembolism.

Recurrent disease

Tumor recurrence is nearly universal, and treatment at recurrence depends both on the prior treatment received and on the patient's physical condition and goals. The median time to progression for GBM after treatment with radiotherapy and TMZ in the phase III study was 6.9 months. If chemotherapy was not given as part of initial treatment, some benefit has been seen with cytotoxic therapy, particularly with TMZ.

The antiangiogenic agent bevacizumab was granted accelerated approval by the FDA in May 2009 for use in recurrent GBM. Whether combined with irinotecan or given alone, bevacizumab improved 6-month progression-free survival in recurrent GBM, compared with patients treated with TMZ. Further clinical trials are ongoing, and this agent is becoming a mainstay treatment for GBM recurrence in the United States. Repeat surgery and implantation of carmustine-impregnated wafers is another approved treatment that may prolong survival in selected patients.

Monitoring response to therapy

The most widely used tool for assessment of response to treatment in malignant glioma is known as the Macdonald criteria, although most recently a new set of criteria has been proposed by the Response Assessment in Neuro-Oncology (RANO) Working Group. Using this scheme, which incorporates imaging (contrast-enhanced MRI/CT) and patient parameters (corticosteroid dose, clinical course), the response is categorized (Table 6.5). While the Macdonald criteria serve as a reasonable and objective method of monitoring response which allows for comparison between studies, they have a number of limitations. Measurement of irregularly shaped tumors, multifocal tumors, or tumors at the wall of cysts and/or surgical cavities is often difficult. In addition, under the Macdonald scheme, an increase in enhancement automatically qualifies as progression. However, contrast enhancement is not specific to tumor regrowth and can be seen with any process that alters blood–brain barrier permeability, such as postoperative changes (e.g. ischemia), inflammation, and reactions to radiation (see below). Conversely, a reduction in enhancement that does not necessarily mean tumor response can be observed with antiangiogenic therapy or corticosteroids. Moreover, lack of enhancement does not guarantee a lack of tumor progression. In the following sections, important aspects of monitoring response in malignant glioma patients are addressed that are not adequately addressed in the traditional Macdonald criteria: (a) non-tumoral enhancement (pseudoprogression, radiation necrosis); and (b) non-enhancing tumor (pseudoresponse, non-enhancing tumor progression).

Table 6.5. Macdonald and Response Assessment in Neuro-Oncology (RANO) criteria.

Response	Imaging findings	Steroids	Clinical status
Macdonald criteria			
Complete	MRI with no new lesions and resolution of all original lesions for at least 4 weeks	No corticosteroids	Stable/improved clinically
Partial	≥50% decrease in size of all lesions for at least 4 weeks, no new lesions	Stable/decreased corticosteroid dose	Stable/improved clinically
Stable	Any situation not fitting other categories	N/A	Stable/improved clinically
Progression	≥25% increase in size of lesions, any new lesion	N/A	Stable (if imaging worse) or clinical deterioration (regardless of imaging findings)
RANO criteria			
Complete	MRI with no new lesions and resolution of all original lesions for at least 4 weeks, and stable/improved T2/FLAIR lesions	No corticosteroids	Stable/improved clinically
Partial	≥50% decrease in size of sum of products of all lesions for at least 4 weeks, no new lesions, and stable/improved T2/FLAIR lesions	Stable/decreased corticosteroid dose	Stable/improved clinically
Stable	Any situation not fitting other categories	N/A	Stable/improved clinically
Progression <12 weeks after finishing XRT/TMZ	Must show new enhancement outside the high dose radiation field (e.g. outside the 80% isodose line), due to concern about pseudoprogression	N/A	Clinical worsening alone is not enough to call progression
Progression ≥12 weeks after finishing XRT/TMZ	New enhancement outside radiation field, *or* An increase by ≥25% in size in sum of products of all lesions, *or* Clear progression of nonmeasurable disease, *or* For patients on antiangiogenic therapy, significant increase in T2/FLAIR nonenhancing lesion(s) without other explanation for the increase (e.g. effect of radiation, seizures)	Increase in steroid dose alone is not enough to call progression unless in the absence of clinical worsening	Clinical worsening alone is enough to call progression but not to allow enrollment into a new study

FLAIR, fluid attenuated inversion recovery; MRI, magnetic resonance imaging; TMZ, temozolomide; XRT, radiotherapy.

Pseudoprogression

The standard of care for newly diagnosed GBM patients includes maximal surgical resection followed by radiation with concurrent and adjuvant TMZ. Given this stable regimen and careful surveillance MRI scans, we now know that 20–30% of patients will develop contrast enhancement shortly after treatment that stabilizes or improves over weeks. However, there is another fraction of patients who have new or increased enhancement that continues to get worse because of actual progression of tumor. The phenomenon of enhancement without tumor growth is termed pseudoprogression and is likely a result of tumor vasculature alteration by radiation that is potentiated by TMZ. While patients with pseudoprogession are typically asymptomatic, when extensive it can be associated with clinical deterioration, making it difficult to differentiate from tumor progression. Pseudoprogression complicates assessment of tumor progression in the immediate post-treatment window and may bias the results of clinical trials for recurrent disease because of incorrect enrollment of stable patients into these trials. Thus, in the initial months following standard therapy completion, contrast enhancement must be interpreted with caution.

In the new set of criteria by RANO, different definitions for progression have been proposed depending on the timing after completion of chemoradiotherapy (Table 6.5): <12 weeks (new enhancement outside of radiation field or unequivocal histopathologic diagnosis by tissue sampling) vs. ≥12 weeks (new enhancement outside of radiation field, increase by ≥25% tumor size, clinical deterioration, or increased T2 and/ or FLAIR signal for patients receiving antiangiogenic therapy and stable and/or increasing steroid dose). Of note, clinical worsening and/ or increased enhancement within the radiation field are not sufficient for the diagnosis of recurrence in patients <12 weeks post-chemoradiation under this scheme. The assumption is that time will resolve the nontumoral enhancement. In addition to temporal factors, molecular signatures of tumors may aid in distinguishing true progression from pseudoprogression. For example, malignant glioma patients with *MGMT* promoter methylation appear to have a higher rate of pseudoprogession than those with tumors lacking *MGMT* promoter methylation.

Radiation necrosis

Radiation necrosis (RN) is defined as permanent destruction of neural tissue following focal radiation. Along with pseudoprogression, it is a major cause of post-treatment enhancement in the absence of tumor recurrence and thus complicates monitoring of tumor progression. Fortunately, RN is only seen in 5% of patients undergoing standard radiotherapy for malignant glioma and is thus much less common than pseudoprogression. Also, the time course of RN (months to years after chemoradiotherapy) is distinct from pseudoprogression (limited to the first few months following therapy). However, as with pseudoprogression, the difficulty lies in distinguishing RN from recurrent tumor. Positron emission tomography, magnetic resonance spectroscopy, and perfusion imaging modalities have shown promise in delineating RN from true tumor recurrence, but all lack the adequate sensitivity and specificity profile to warrant routine clinical use at this time. Definitive diagnosis requires direct surgical biopsy.

Pseudoresponse

With the implementation of antiangiogenic agents such as bevacizumab into clinical practice, oncologists are observing a decrease in tumor enhancement as early as 1–2 days after administration in 25–50% of patients. While this finding may indeed represent a substantial cytotoxic response within the tumor, the rapidity of the change and the lack of a significant survival benefit argue that it may be a "pseudoresponse" that reflects an alteration of the local tumor vascular bed permeability rather than true tumor killing. Thus, a conservative interpretation of decreased enhancement is warranted unless stable for >4 weeks, as is suggested in both the Macdonald and the RANO criteria.

Non-enhancing tumor progression

Non-enhancing tumor progression can be difficult to appreciate, leading to a delay in diagnosis and treatment. This phenomenon is particularly prevalent in grade III malignant gliomas such as AAs, where a significant portion of the tumor may be non-enhancing. In addition, progression without enhancement can also occur as a mode of failure of antiangiogenic drugs. While increased T2/FLAIR intensity may be used to identify non-enhancing tumor, this characteristic is difficult to interpret following radiation and/or antiangiogenic therapies, which can independently alter T2/FLAIR intensity. However, certain characteristics of T2/FLAIR changes, such as increasing area over time, mass effect, and presence outside of field of radiation, favor tumor progression over treatment effects.

Experimental therapies

Traditional chemotherapeutics

In part as a result of recent data that *MGMT* methylation positively correlates with response to TMZ (suggesting an inability of tumors with methylated *MGMT* to repair TMZ-induced DNA repair), there are currently multiple trials investigating manipulation of DNA repair pathways to increase efficacy of TMZ. Specific strategies include enzyme depletion (TMZ dose-intensive schemes), treatment with MGMT inhibitors, and treatment with inhibitors of poly(ADP-ribose) polymerase (PARP), another DNA repair enzyme.

Molecularly targeted therapy

Given the recent elucidation of a number of molecular substrates involved in glioma growth, a number of targeted pharmacologic agents are under development. The major categories of molecular targets in glioma include cell surface growth factor receptors, intracellular signaling molecules, and angiogenesis mediators.

Among the growth factor receptor family of molecules, epidermal growth factor receptor (EGFR) and platelet-derived growth factor receptor (PDGFR) are among the most studied in the context of glioma progression. EGFR is known to be amplified in almost half of primary GBMs and many GBMs have a specific mutation imparting constitutive activation of the receptor EGFRvIII. The molecular alterations result in increased proliferation and invasiveness while inhibiting apoptosis. Likewise, PDGFR expression is elevated in many gliomas and promotes unchecked proliferation. Both EGFR and PDGFR inhibitors have shown activity in preclinical glioma models but have thus far failed to demonstrate a significant impact in clinical trials.

The most studied intracellular targets for malignant glioma are mediators of the PI3K/Akt/mTOR pathway. Increased receptor activity (EGFR, PDGFR) leading to overstimulation of the pathway and loss of PTEN (a tumor suppressor) are two common alterations seen in glioma. Another intracellular pathway that has been investigated is the Ras/MAPK pathway.

Epigenetic machinery presents another set of intracellular targets for glioma therapy. Recent data demonstrated a mild improvement in progression-free survival in recurrent GBM patients treated with a histone deacetylase inhibitor.

Immunotherapy

It is now appreciated that brain tumors do indeed stimulate a systemic immune response, and several strategies are being investigated to augment the native antitumor response. One such strategy involves widespread stimulation of the immune response by administration of double-stranded RNA (typically seen in viruses) such as poly-ICLC, which causes a generic pro-tumoricidal release of cytokines and interferon-γ. Another strategy involves administration of EGFRvIII, a tumor-specific antigen, as part of a classic vaccine protocol in EGFRvIII-expressing GBM. Other vaccine strategies under investigation include adoptive immune transfer (priming a patient's effector T cells *ex vivo* with tumor antigen followed by transfer back to the patient), local delivery of antigen by injection, and dendritic cell-based vaccines.

Surgery

The goals of surgical resection in malignant glioma are: (a) tissue diagnosis, (b) relief of mass effect, (c) seizure reduction, and (d) cytoreduction while minimizing morbidity (particularly preserving motor and language function). Recent evidence suggests that extent of resection correlates with improved survival, and a number of advances have allowed for more aggressive surgical resection. Image-guided surgery allowing precise three-dimensional navigation is now a routine part of tumor surgery. In addition, incorporation of fMRI and DTI data with traditional

MRI sequences allows for improved preoperative planning and avoidance of eloquent structures during resection. A recent phase III trial has also demonstrated that intraoperative administration of 5-aminolevulinic acid, which delineates tumor tissue by fluorescence of the metabolite protoporphyrin IX, improves the gross total resection rate relative to conventional surgical methods (65% in treatment arm vs. 35% in conventional arm).

Radiation therapy

Radiation therapy has a long-standing role in the treatment of malignant brain tumors. Typical protocols involve radiation to a target area encompassing the entire FLAIR signal abnormality and a 2-cm margin initially (2 Gy/day for 23 days), followed by a boost to the enhancing area and a 2-cm surrounding margin (2 Gy/day for 7 days). Given the improved accuracy of imaging studies used for planning as well as intraprocedural algorithms that correct for patient positioning, it is likely that the margin surrounding target volumes can be reduced, thereby reducing radiation dose to surrounding structures without compromising local control. In addition to technical advances in radiotherapy, given the known benefit of radiation therapy in high grade glioma and the proposed radiosensitizing mechanism of TMZ-induced tumor reduction, recent efforts have aimed at identifying additional agents that may increase sensitivity to radiation.

Conclusions

High grade gliomas represent the majority of malignant brain tumors in adults and are associated with poor outcomes. However, advances in surgical and medical therapies over the past few decades have resulted in a modest improvement in overall survival. Further, new insights into the biologic basis of glioma growth have identified a number of exciting targeted therapeutic interventions which are reflected in the number and variety of clinical trials in progress for high grade glioma.

Selected bibliography

Batchelor TT, Sorensen AG, di Tomaso E, Zhang WT, Duda DG, Cohen KS, *et al.* (2007) AZD2171, a pan-VEGF receptor tyrosine kinase inhibitor, normalizes tumor vasculature and alleviates edema in glioblastoma patients. *Cancer Cell* **11** (1), 83–95.

Berger MS, Hadjipanayis CG. (2007) Surgery of intrinsic cerebral tumors. *Neurosurgery* **61** (1 Suppl), 279–304; discussion 304–5.

Brandes AA, Franceschi E, Tosoni A, Blatt V, Pession A, Tallini G, *et al.* (2008) MGMT promoter methylation status can predict the incidence and outcome of pseudoprogression after concomitant radiochemotherapy in newly diagnosed glioblastoma patients. *J Clin Oncol* **26** (13), 2192–7.

Burdett S, Stewart L. (2003) Chemotherapy for high-grade glioma. *Neuroepidemiology* **22** (6), 366.

CBTRUS (2010) CBTRUS Statistical Report: Primary brain and central nervous system tumors diagnosed in the United States in 2004–2006. Central Brain Tumor Registry of the United States, Hinsdale, IL. Available at: www.cbtrus.org

Clarke J, Butowski N, Chang S. (2010) Recent advances in therapy for glioblastoma. *Arch Neurol* **67** (3), 279–83.

Dubey RB, Hanmandlu M, Gupta SK. (2010) Risk of brain tumors from wireless phone use. *J Comput Assist Tomogr* **34** (6), 799–807.

Galanis E, Jaaeckle KA, Maurer MJ, Reid JM, Ames MM, Hardwick JS, *et al.* (2009) Phase II trial of vorinostat in recurrent glioblastoma multiforme: a north central cancer treatment group study. *J Clin Oncol* **27** (12), 2052–8.

Glantz MJ, Cole BF, Forsyth PA, Recht LD, Wen PY, Chamberlain MC, *et al.* (2000) Practice parameter: anticonvulsant prophylaxis in patients with newly diagnosed brain tumors. Report of the Quality Standards Subcommittee of the American Academy of Neurology. *Neurology* **54** (10), 1886–93.

Hegi ME, Diserens AC, Gorlia T, Hamou MF, de Tribolet N, Weller M, *et al.* (2005) MGMT gene silencing and benefit from temozolomide in glioblastoma. *N Engl J Med* **352** (10), 997–1003.

Iwamoto FM, Fine HA. (2010) Bevacizumab for malignant gliomas. *Arch Neurol* **67** (3), 285–8.

Jaeckle KA, Decker PA, Ballman KV, Flynn PJ, Giannini C, Scheithauer BW, *et al.* (2010) Transformation of low grade glioma and correlation with outcome: an NCCTG database analysis. *J Neurooncol* **104** (1), 253–9.

Khasraw M, Lassman AB. (2010) Advances in the treatment of malignant gliomas. *Curr Oncol Rep* **12** (1), 26–33.

Louis DN (ed.) (2007) *WHO Classification of Tumours of the Central Nervous System*. IARC, Lyon.

Macdonald DR, Cascino TL, Schold SC Jr, Cairncross JG. (1990) Response criteria for phase II studies of supratentorial malignant glioma. *J Clin Oncol* **8** (7), 1277–80.

National Cancer Institute (2010) *Adult brain tumor treatment (PQR): Glioblastoma*. National Cancer Institute, July 8, 2010. Available from: http://www.cancer.gov/.

Quon H, Abdulkarim B. (2008) Adjuvant treatment of anaplastic oligodendrogliomas and oligoastrocytomas. *Cochrane Database Syst Rev* **2**, CD007104.

Stummer W, Pichlmeier U, Meinel T, Wiestler OD, Zanella F, Reulen HJ; ALA-Glioma Study Group. (2006) Fluorescence-guided surgery with 5-aminolevulinic acid for resection of malignant glioma: a randomised controlled multicentre phase III trial. *Lancet Oncol* **7** (5), 392–401.

Stupp R, Tonn JC, Brada M, Pentheroudakis G; ESMO Guidelines Working Group (2010) High-grade malignant glioma: ESMO Clinical Practice Guidelines for diagnosis, treatment and follow-up. *Ann Oncol* **21** (Suppl 5), 190–3.

Stupp R, Mason WP, van den Bent MJ, Weller M, Fisher B, Taphoorn MJ, *et al.* (2005) Radiotherapy plus concomitant and adjuvant temozolomide for glioblastoma. *N Engl J Med* **352** (10), 987–96.

Van Meir EG, Hadjipanayis CG, Norden AD, Shu HK, Wen PY, Olson JJ. Exciting new advances in neuro-oncology: the avenue to a cure for malignant glioma. *CA Cancer J Clin* **60** (3), 166–93.

Wen PY, Kesari S. (2008) Malignant gliomas in adults. *N Engl J Med* **359** (5), 492–507.

Wen PY, Macdonald DR, Reardon DA, Cloughesy TF, Sorensen AG, Galanis E, *et al.* (2010) Updated response assessment criteria for high-grade gliomas: response assessment in neuro-oncology working group. *J Clin Oncol* **28** (11), 1963–72.

Wen PY, Norden AD, Drappatz J, Quant E. (2010) Response assessment challenges in clinical trials of gliomas. *Curr Oncol Rep* **12** (1), 68–75.

Yan H, Parsons DW, Jin G, McLendon R, Rasheed BA, Yuan W, *et al.* (2009) IDH1 and IDH2 mutations in gliomas. *N Engl J Med* **360** (8), 765–73.

7

Low Grade Gliomas and Oligodendrogliomas in Adulthood

Derek R. Johnson[1] and Kurt A. Jaeckle[2]

[1]Department of Neurology, Mayo Clinic, Rochester, MN, USA
[2]Department of Neurology, Mayo Clinic, Jacksonville, FL, USA

Introduction

Low grade gliomas (LGG) are slow-growing primary brain tumors which typically affect young adults. Approximately 2000 adults in the United States are diagnosed with LGG annually. Although the term "malignant glioma" is typically reserved for World Health Organization (WHO) grade III and IV tumors, LGG are not clinically benign. Because of their infiltrating growth pattern, LGG are not curable via surgery, and most patients eventually succumb to tumor-related complications. LGG can manifest in a number of different ways, with new onset seizures often heralding the diagnosis. Although imaging can be suggestive of LGG, pathologic confirmation of tumor remains the diagnostic "gold standard."

Treatment of LGG is controversial, and varying strategies for initial management are employed, including observation, resection, radiation, and/ or chemotherapy. Median survival after diagnosis depends on LGG subtype. Patients with favorable subtypes may live many years. Given the potential for prolonged survival, quality of life and preservation of cognition are important considerations when planning LGG treatment, as the relatively long survival increases the likelihood of encountering late treatment-related toxicity.

Definition

In its broadest construction, the term low grade glioma (LGG) can be used to refer to all WHO grade I and II gliomas. While this terminology is useful in separating these tumors from more aggressive WHO grade III and IV "high grade" gliomas, it obscures the significant differences between WHO grade I and WHO grade II tumors. Notably, WHO grade I gliomas are typically well-circumscribed tumors that present in childhood and are quite rare in adults, while WHO grade II gliomas are infiltrating primary neuroectodermal brain tumors of adulthood. As such, when referring to adult patients, the term LGG is typically used in reference to WHO grade II tumors such as astrocytomas, oligodendrogliomas, and oligoastrocytomas. This more limited definition of LGG will be used in this chapter.

Epidemiology

The majority of gliomas are high grade (WHO grades III and IV) at time of diagnosis; only about 15% are low grade (WHO grade II). Approximately 2000 adults are diagnosed with LGG each year in the United States. The age-adjusted incidence rate of LGG is approximately 1 per 100,000 person-years. LGGs in adults are most frequently

Neuro-oncology, First Edition. Edited by Roger J. Packer, David Schiff.

diagnosed in the fourth or fifth decades of life, younger than the typical age of diagnosis for malignant gliomas. LGG, like all infiltrating gliomas, are more common among men, with a male to female ratio of 1.18:1 for WHO grade II astrocytoma.

Risk factors

There are no clearly identified environmental or historical risk factors for glioma other than exposure to a high level of ionizing radiation, such as in therapeutic irradiation. Low levels of irradiation, such as from dental X-rays, have not been shown to increase the risk of glioma. A variety of other environmental and occupational risk factors have been proposed based on case–control and cohort studies, but these remain to be validated. Recently, there has been interest in a possible role for cellular telephone use as a glioma risk factor. Currently, no proof of this association has been published. Cohort studies have provided evidence that greater adult height and greater body mass index (BMI) in adolescence are associated with increased glioma risk. These studies primarily included patients with high grade glioma, and it is not clear to what extent the results apply to LGG.

Familial cancer syndromes such as neurofibromatosis are responsible for only a small proportion of all gliomas. Recently, several germline single nucleotide polymorphisms (SNPs) have been associated with risk of LGG. For example, polymorphisms in the region of 8q24.21 (rs4295627, CCDC26) are significantly more common in patients with WHO grade II oligodendroglioma and oligoastrocytoma than in control subjects.

Clinical presentation

LGGs are slowly growing tumors, and may be present for years prior to diagnosis. Clinical manifestations depend on the tumor location, but seizures are the most common presenting symptom. While a new onset of generalized seizure almost invariably leads to rapid medical evaluation, patients sometimes experience focal seizures or seizure auras for long periods before presenting for care.

Focal neurologic deficits, which may be subtle, are the most common initial nonseizure manifestation of LGG. The nature of the deficits will vary significantly as a function of tumor location. LGG located in the nondominant frontal lobe may grow quite large prior to the development of symptoms. Presentation with symptoms of elevated intracranial pressure, such as headache, is relatively uncommon in LGG. It is not unusual for LGG to be discovered incidentally on head imaging obtained for (unrelated) headache or vertigo.

Natural history and treatment outcome

WHO grade II gliomas are sometimes referred to as "benign" gliomas, but LGG is not clinically benign, frequently causing significant symptoms and mortality via progressive growth. The time to progression (TTP) is defined as the time from diagnosis to tumor growth for patients initially observed, or the time from first treatment until tumor growth in patients initially treated. Given enough time, tumor progression is almost inevitable. In the clinical trial RTOG 9802, patients younger than age 40 who had undergone gross total resection of their tumor – the group of patients thought to have the best prognosis – were observed until progression. In this group, 18% had progressed by 2 years, and by 5 years 50% of patients had progressed. LGG can progress in two ways: by growing as a WHO grade II tumor and via "transformation" into higher grade (WHO grade III or IV) glioma. The typical nature of tumor progression differs as a function of tumor histology, with oligodendroglial tumors remaining WHO grade II at recurrence more frequently than astrocytomas or mixed oligoastrocytomas.

Most patients diagnosed with LGG will eventually succumb to the tumor, although long-term survivorship is much more common in LGG than in higher grade tumors. The 2011 Statistical Report of the Central Brain Tumor Registry of the United States reports that 2-year, 5-year, and 10-year relative survival rates for low grade astrocytoma are 60%, 48%, and 39%, respectively. The 2-year, 5-year, and 10-year relative survival rates for low grade oligodendroglioma are 90%, 79%, and 64%, respectively. Table 7.1 displays 2-year and 5-year overall survival rates by tumor morphology and patient age group.

Several patient level and tumor level factors are predictive of outcome. Two prognostic factor

Table 7.1. Two-year and five-year survival rates for low grade gliomas, by age group at time of diagnosis and histologic type. Source: Surveillance, Epidemiology, and End Results (SEER) Program (www.seer.cancer.gov).

Morphology	Survival (years)	Patient age at diagnosis		
		20–39 years	40–59 years	60+ years
Astrocytoma	2	84.4%	53.5%	16.9%
	5	60.3%	37.3%	5.5%
Mixed glioma	2	87.6%	72.2%	32.8%
	5	68.9%	51.3%	16.5%
Oligodendroglioma	2	94.2%	85.0%	56.4%
	5	83.2%	70.0%	35.9%

scoring schemes have become widely used. A European Organization for Research and Treatment of Cancer (EORTC) analysis of several large trials showed that age ≥40 years, astrocytoma histology, tumor ≥6 cm in maximum dimension, tumor crossing midline, and the presence of a neurologic deficit before surgery were unfavorable prognostic factors. Patients with two or fewer of these factors had a median survival of 7.72 years, whereas patient with three or more of these factors had a median survival of 3.2 years. An alternative University of California at San Francisco Low-Grade Glioma Prognostic Scoring System employs a 0–4 grading scale, with points given for less favorable variables, including Karnofsky performance status (KPS) ≤80, patient age >50 years, tumor diameter >4 cm, and tumor involving a presumed eloquent location. Patients with a score of 1 have a 5-year survival probability of 0.98, while patients with a score of 4 have only a 0.46 5-year survival probability.

The role of tumor morphology and molecular pathology in predicting tumor behavior is becoming clearer with time. Oligodendrogliomas tend to be more indolent than astrocytomas, and are associated with longer survival. One of the first genetic alterations noted to be predictive of outcome was co-deletion of chromosome regions on 1p and 19q. Tumors carrying 1p/19q co-deletion, almost always oligodendrogliomas or mixed oligoastrocytomas, have a better prognosis than tumors not carrying this co-deletion. Recently, mutations in the enzyme isocitrate dehydrogenase (IDH) have been found to be an early alteration in the genesis of LGG. IDH mutation is found in most LGG, regardless of mor-

phology. Tumors containing IDH mutations have a better prognosis than tumors without these mutations, and patients whose tumors contain both IDH mutation and 1p/19q co-deletion seem to do better than those with IDH mutation alone. Methylation of the gene for the DNA repair enzyme O^6-methylguanine-DNA methyltransferase (MGMT) is a marker of interest in high grade glioma. Methylation of MGMT results in reduced DNA repair capacity and theoretically a greater susceptibility to chemotherapy. A retrospective review of patients with LGG demonstrated that MGMT methylation is associated with improved tumor response and progression-free survival following chemotherapy; however, other studies have not confirmed this. The importance of these biologic markers in predicting outcome and response to therapy must await further clarification within the context of future randomized clinical trials.

Diagnosis

Imaging

✋ CAUTION!

HINTS ON AVOIDING PROBLEMS
Lack of contrast enhancement on magnetic resonance imaging (MRI) does not reliably distinguish low grade gliomas from other glial tumors. Grade II gliomas occasionally enhance, and high grade gliomas may not show enhancement.

Currently, magnetic resonance imaging (MRI) is the primary diagnostic tool used to identify sus-

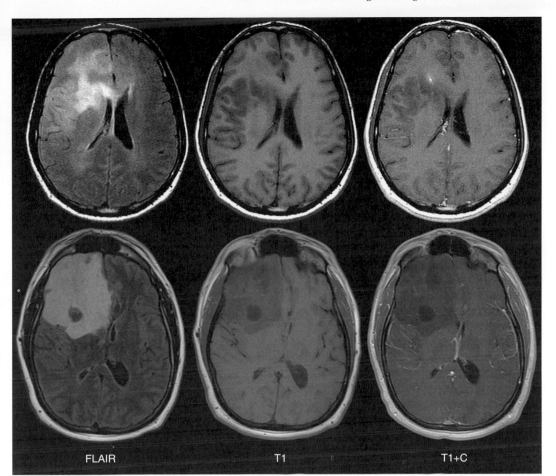

FLAIR   T1   T1+C

Figure 7.1. Characteristic magnetic resonance imaging (MRI) findings of low grade astrocytoma and oligodendroglioma. Specific details of the characteristics are described fully in the text.

pected LGG because these tumors are typically isointense on computed tomography (CT) scan but visible on MRI as hyperintense abnormalities on T2-weighted images that are hypointense on T1-weighted images. Figure 7.1 demonstrates characteristic MRI findings of low grade astrocytoma and oligodendroglioma. WHO grade II LGG classically do not enhance on post-gadolinium MRI, but lack of enhancement is not synonymous with LGG; some WHO grade II gliomas display faint enhancement. Significant enhancement may suggest either a WHO grade I tumor, such as pilocytic astrocytoma, or a malignant (WHO grade III or IV) glioma, depending on the pattern and other tumor characteristics. Rare WHO grade II glioma variants such as pleomorphic xanthastrocytoma, which typically present in childhood, may display marked enhancement

and still have a favorable clinical course. CT scan remains useful for the detection of tumor calcification, which is more frequent in oligodendroglial tumors than in pure astrocytic tumors. Although calcification generally suggests an indolent tumor biology, it should be remembered that calcification can remain in an LGG that has transformed to WHO grade III–IV.

While MRI is a sensitive test for LGG, the characteristic changes associated with LGG lack specificity. The imaging differential diagnosis of LGG may include chronic ischemic changes, central nervous system (CNS) viral infections, autoimmune encephalitic processes, and congenital abnormalities. These diagnoses can often be distinguished on the basis of clinical history and laboratory evaluation, or by evolution of findings on serial imaging.

Laboratory testing

No blood or cerebrospinal fluid (CSF) testing is clinically available to confirm the diagnosis of LGG. Laboratory testing is only indicated in situations where the patient presentation is thought to potentially represent an alternative diagnosis such as infection or inflammation, and should be aimed at confirming or excluding the alternative diagnosis.

Pathology and molecular pathology

Ultimately, the diagnosis of LGG can only be made via pathology. Whenever possible, primary brain tumors should be examined by an experienced neuropathologist, as there may be a significant rate of nonconcordance between neuropathologists and general pathologists.

The WHO guidelines are used to classify primary brain tumors according to grade and morphology. WHO grade II infiltrating gliomas are classified by morphology into three primary categories: astrocytoma, oligodendroglioma, and oligoastrocytoma (mixed tumors). The distinction between a "pure" oligodendroglioma or astrocytoma and a "mixed" oligodendroglioma is not well defined in the literature. For example, a glioma with a dominant oligodendroglial component and a minor astrocytic component may be called an oligodendroglioma by some neuropathologists and oligoastrocytoma by others.

Criteria to classify an infiltrating glioma as grade II are defined by the WHO. A WHO grade II astrocytoma is characterized by well-differentiated astrocytes with increased cellularity relative to normal brain, often with nuclear atypia, but without necrosis or microvascular proliferation. Mitotic activity is usually not seen, but the presence of a single mitosis in a relatively large tumor sample (i.e. not simply a stereotactic biopsy) is compatible with the diagnosis of grade II astrocytoma. WHO grade II oligodendrogliomas display a characteristic "fried egg" or "honeycomb" appearance in formalin-fixed paraffin-embedded sections. This finding is an artifact of tissue fixation, and is not seen in smear preparations or frozen section. Nuclear atypia may be prominent, and mitotic activity is absent or low. As in astrocytoma, high mitotic activity, necrosis, and microvascular proliferation are signs of progression to a higher grade tumor.

Glioma often contain areas that appear to represent differing grades of tumor, and the portion with the highest grade defines the grade of the entire neoplasm, even if it composes a minority of the tumor mass. Thus, it is possible for a biopsy to under-grade a tumor by sampling a low grade portion of a tumor that is truly high grade.

Symptom management

Seizure control

In patients presenting with seizure, long-term antiepileptic therapy is warranted. Duration of therapy is controversial; some physicians advocate lifelong therapy, but others routinely attempt to discontinue anticonvulsant drug therapy after tumor resection and an appropriate seizure-free period. The issue of prophylactic anticonvulsant therapy in patients with glioma and no history of seizure has been assessed in several clinical trials. No benefit of prophylactic anticonvulsant therapy was seen in any individual trial, or in meta-analysis. Of note, all of the randomized trials used older anticonvulsant agents, such as phenytoin and valproic acid, rather than the anticonvulsants currently in wide use in patients with brain tumors, such as levetiracetam. The American Academy of Neurology has issued a practice guideline stating that prophylactic anticonvulsants should not be used routinely in patients with newly diagnosed brain tumors, because of lack of efficacy in preventing first seizures and the potential for anticonvulsant-related side effects. Further, in patients who have not had a seizure, tapering and discontinuing anticonvulsants after the first week following brain surgery is appropriate, particularly in stable patients and those who are experiencing anticonvulsant-related side effects.

Edema and mass effect

Low grade glioma is significantly less likely than high grade glioma to produce a substantial amount of peritumoral edema. Whereas the T2/FLAIR abnormality surrounding the enhancing core of a glioblastoma is typically vasogenic edema that can be partially ameliorated with corticosteroid therapy, the T2/FLAIR abnormality of LGG often represents tumor infiltration that does not respond significantly to steroid therapy. Occasionally, tumors in the midbrain region may cause obstructive hydrocephalus requiring a CSF diversion procedure. Either ventriculoperitoneal shunting or third ventriculostomy can be considered, depending on the tumor location and the preference of the surgeon.

Tumor-directed therapy

Surgery

There are three primary rationales for surgery in patients with LGG: to establish a diagnosis, to debulk tumors causing significant mass effect, and potentially to improve outcome if extensive resection can be performed. Currently, there is no noninvasive way to definitively diagnose LGG, so surgery is usually necessary for diagnostic purposes. Only rarely is biopsy deferred in favor of treatment without tissue diagnosis. In patients with asymptomatic or minimally symptomatic brain lesions strongly suspected to represent LGG, an initial strategy of observation rather than surgery is occasionally employed. In one report, patients with suspected LGG who were observed until symptomatic or radiographic progression were compared with patients who received early surgery and radiation. No differences were seen in survival or quality of life between these two groups. When the strategy of initial observation is chosen, close clinical and radiographic follow-up is required. Observation remains a controversial approach, given the high likelihood of tumor progression and concern that the ability to achieve an extensive tumor resection may be compromised by tumor growth. In the absence of a strong contraindication to surgery, most neuro-oncologists and neurosurgeons recommend early treatment.

Diagnostic surgery can take the form of stereotactic needle biopsy or open resection, and there are risks and benefits to both approaches. Needle biopsy has the advantage of low morbidity and short recovery time. The in-hospital morbidity following brain biopsy is often quoted as less than 1%, but analysis of healthcare databases suggests this may be an underestimate. A potential disadvantage of needle biopsy is the possibility of obtaining nondiagnostic or nonrepresentative tissue. In addition, tumors often display significant heterogeneity, and a biopsy that shows WHO grade II glioma does not exclude the possibility that other regions of the tumor meet criteria for high grade glioma. A variety of presurgical functional imaging tests to predict and target suspected areas of high grade glioma within a background of LGG are currently being evaluated, but their value remains unclear. Biopsy also has the disadvantage of not allowing debulking, which is necessary if a tumor has significant mass effect.

Surgery is the initial therapeutic intervention in patient with tumors accessible to gross total or near-total resection. For LGG, gross total resection is defined as removal of all areas of tumor-related T2/FLAIR abnormality. Gross total resection does not lead to cure of LGG, as microscopically identifiable neoplasm usually extends beyond the area of imaging abnormality. Considerable retrospective data suggest that extensive tumor resection (i.e. 80–90% resection or greater) is associated with longer survival than biopsy or subtotal resection. For example, one study reported that patients with LGG and at least 90% extent of resection (EOR) had a 91% 8-year overall survival rate, whereas patients with less than a 90% EOR had a 60% 8-year overall survival rate. Volumetric measurement of residual LGG after surgery may be a better measure of extent of resection than proportion of tumor removed, but the limited availability of the technique and technical issues with obtaining this measure have prevented it from entering wide use at this time. When gross total resection of all tumor visible on MRI is achieved, some clinicians will advocate a strategy of observation, and defer further treatment until the time of tumor recurrence.

A variety of operative and imaging techniques may help surgeons safely achieve extensive tumor resection. Preoperative imaging with techniques such as functional MRI and diffusion tensor tractography can help in the localization of brain areas critical for language and movement, allowing them to be spared. Surgeons' subjective intraoperative impressions of extent of resection may be inaccurate, and intraoperative MRI facilitates visualization of residual tumor while there is still an opportunity for further resection. For tumors in eloquent areas of the brain, awake craniotomy with cortical mapping is a valuable tool to minimize the risk of surgery-induced neurologic deficits.

Radiation

Radiation therapy is often used as the initial post-operative treatment of LGG. This is especially true in patients with residual tumor after surgery, as they are at high risk of early progression, and it is clear that tumor progression is associated with cognitive and functional decline as well as mortality. Randomized trials have established that low dose radiation (50–54 Gy) is as effective as higher doses.

Radiation therapy has both short-term and long-term potential complications. Short-term complications tend to be self-limited, and include radiation-related alopecia, skin irritation, and fatigue, which can be significant. The potential long-term complication of radiation that is of most concern to patients is cognitive decline. A longitudinal study of patients with LGG suggests that in the first several years after diagnosis, the primary predictor of cognitive decline is the presence or absence of tumor progression rather than radiation history. In the longer term, patients without tumor progression who received radiation are more likely to show a progressive cognitive decline than patients without tumor progression who did not receive radiation. At a mean follow-up time of 12 years after initial diagnosis, patients treated with radiation displayed deficits in attentional functioning, executive functioning, and information processing speed. Ongoing randomized trials to examine cognitive function from time of diagnosis to death as well as duration of survival will provide a more nuanced understanding of the relative pros and cons of different treatment strategies.

Patients with glioma of any grade typically receive only a single course of radiation therapy, because of the issue of cumulative toxicity. However, there is some literature supporting salvage hypofractionated re-irradiation in patients with recurrent primary glioblastoma. In principle, this strategy may also be useful in LGG, particularly following transformation from LGG into a secondary high grade glioma, and when recurrent tumor extends beyond the original treatment field. Re-irradiation is also considered in patients with recurrent disease who either refuse chemotherapy or cannot receive additional treatment because of hematologic or other toxicity.

Generally, when LGG recurs after radiation, chemotherapy is often proposed prior to re-irradiation. It is important to point out that no chemotherapy agent or regimen to date has been approved by the US Food and Drug Administration (FDA) for the indication of recurrent adult LGG.

Chemotherapy

The optimal role for chemotherapy in the treatment of LGG has yet to be defined. Previously, chemotherapy was typically reserved for treatment of progression after radiation therapy, but more recently up-front chemotherapy strategies are becoming more widely investigated.

Much of the older published data involved nitrosourea-based regimens, either procarbazine, lomustine, and vincristine (PCV) given in combination, or lomustine monotherapy. Nitrosourea regimens have activity against LGG as demonstrated by a significant rate of radiographic response. The RTOG 9802 study explored the role of chemotherapy as an addition to radiation in the initial therapy of LGG. In this trial, high risk patients, defined as those aged 40 years or older or those with residual tumor after resection, were randomized to radiation alone or radiation followed by six cycles of PCV. Patients receiving combined chemoradiotherapy had a statistically significant increased progression-free survival, and a trend towards improved overall survival. In subset analysis of patients alive at 2 years following initial treatment, those treated with combined chemoradiotherapy were more likely to become 5-year survivors than patients treated with radiation alone. The duration of nitrosourea therapy is limited by cumulative toxicity, but ongoing decreases in tumor size can be seen for years following discontinuation of chemotherapy.

Temozolomide (TMZ) chemotherapy is part of the standard-of-care regimen for treatment of glioblastoma, and, although not FDA approved for LGG, in practice it has displaced nitrosourea-based regimens in the treatment of LGG. While there has not been a head-to-head trial of TMZ versus PCV in LGG, many clinicians favor TMZ because of perceived similar efficacy and superior tolerability. There are several ongoing international phase III trials that promise to provide further information about the role of TMZ in LGG treatment.

Molecularly targeted therapies are also being investigated, primarily as treatment for progressive LGG. Relative to the literature on targeted therapies for high grade glioma, little has been published on this topic. A phase II trial of imatinib, a tyrosine kinase inhibitor with activity against *bcr-abl*, c-*kit*, and platelet-derived growth factor receptor (PDGFR) in combination with hydroxyurea showed therapy was well tolerated and associated with encouraging activity. This finding has yet to be confirmed in larger trials, and neither agent is FDA approved for this indication.

Observation

An initial strategy of postoperative observation, "watchful waiting," following diagnosis has been proposed by some clinicians. The rationale for watchful waiting is that while radiation therapy has been shown to improve overall survival in subtotally resected tumors, the optimum timing of radiation is an ongoing controversy in neuro-oncology. The EORTC 22845 randomized trial compared initial observation after surgery with immediate radiation in patients aged 16–65 years with Karnofsky Performance Status of at least 60. This trial found that initial observation was associated with shorter progression-free survival (i.e. less time from initial diagnosis until tumor growth), but no difference in length of overall survival. Given the similar overall survival times associated with early and delayed radiation strategies, quality of life concerns are important in guiding therapy choices. Although in young children there are data supporting the delay of radiation therapy to prevent decline in cognitive and quality of life function, current data in adult LGG patients are insufficient to draw definitive conclusions regarding early vs. delayed radiation. Ongoing studies will address this issue formally.

In clinical practice, observation after initial surgery is typically reserved for patients thought to have a high likelihood of prolonged progression-free survival even in absence of radiation therapy. This group includes younger patients lacking substantive symptoms or signs who have undergone a gross total resection of their tumor.

Ongoing clinical trials

A number of factors have limited the conduct of clinical therapeutic trials in adult LGG. First, the relative rarity of these tumors makes accrual to large trials difficult. Secondly, the many proposed patient-level and tumor-level prognostic factors make defining treatment groups controversial. Finally, if the primary endpoint of overall survival is used, the long survival of these individuals requires trials that extend over many years before analysis, during which time the treatment approaches may become obsolete. The Response Assessment in Neuro-Oncology (RANO) Group recently published recommendations regarding appropriate assessments and endpoints for future LGG clinical trials. These include both imaging (e.g. standard MRI, functional MRI, PET) and clinical (e.g. quality of life, cognition, symptom burden) outcomes in addition to survival. If these recommendations are widely followed, future trials might identify surrogate endpoints that capture clinically relevant differences between treatments, and the uniform use of response criteria will facilitate comparison of results across studies.

Two current large phase III clinical trials will shed further light on the role of chemotherapy in LGG. The ECOG E3F05 study, which is currently enrolling patients, randomizes adult patients with LGG to radiation alone versus radiation with concurrent and adjuvant TMZ chemotherapy, and utilizes 5-year survival as the primary endpoint. EORTC/NCIC 22033-26033, which recently completed accrual, involved a randomization of patients to standard radiation versus daily low dose TMZ for 1 year. Both of these studies include detailed cognitive and quality of life assessments. Smaller phase II studies of targeted therapies, such as the mTOR inhibitor everolimus, and the VEGF receptor tyrosine kinase inhibitor vandetanib, are also ongoing.

Post-treatment follow-up

Following treatment of LGG, life-long follow-up is necessary. There is no standard approach to follow-up in terms of frequency of imaging. Some clinicians routinely image patients every 3 months for 1–2 years, then every 6 months for several years, then annually thereafter, but there is relatively wide variation in the frequency of follow-up in clinical practice.

MRI is the imaging modality most frequently used to follow LGG patients over time. While MRI is more sensitive than any other imaging tool for this purpose, proper interpretation of MRI imaging may not be straightforward. Formal LGG response criteria for clinical use have not yet been established, and the Macdonald criteria, which were developed to assess the response of glioblastoma in clinical trials, are difficult to apply to LGG, as the criteria do not formally address noncontrast enhancing disease. Further, subtle changes in tumor size may be difficult to appreciate on imaging, as they may be obscured by differences in imaging technique or head position. Even when clear change is seen, it may not represent tumor growth; increased T2/FLAIR signal can occur as an effect of radiation, and treated tumor can develop enhancement, falsely suggesting transformation into a higher grade lesion. Often, these changes should simply be followed closely, and if they do not stop growing or regress after an appropriate interval further treatment or surgical intervention for tissue diagnosis can be considered. Novel functional imaging and cognitive measures that monitor for progression, such as those being considered by RANO, will require validation within the context of prospective clinical trials.

Reproductive issues

LGG often occur in young patients still in their reproductive years. The effects of chemotherapeutic agents on long-term fertility are unclear, and patients of childbearing potential should be advised of this potential adverse effect prior to initiation of therapy. A number of fertility preservation techniques are available, including cryopreservation of embryos, oocytes, or sperm. Referral to a reproductive specialist to discuss fertility preservation strategies is advised if future fertility is a patient concern.

Conclusions

LGG in adults are a difficult clinical problem and carry a poorer prognosis than is generally recognized. They are rarely curable with surgery, radiation, or chemotherapy, and most patients with LGG ultimately succumb to the disease. Currently, outside of radiotherapy, there is no universally accepted standard of care for LGG, and strategies are divergent, ranging from initial simple observation to relatively aggressive management with surgery followed by chemotherapy and radiation. The identification of molecular markers that are prognostic or predictive of response to specific therapies may facilitate the selection of subsets of patients most likely to benefit from these treatments. The long-term survival of many of these patients has increased the focus on the preservation of quality of life and cognitive status in clinical therapeutic studies.

Selected bibliography

Benson VS, Pirie K, Green J, Casabonne D, Beral V; Million Women Study Collaborators (2008) Lifestyle factors and primary glioma and meningioma tumours in the Million Women Study cohort. *Br J Cancer* **99** (1), 185–90.

Central Brain Tumor Registry of the United States. Available from: http://www.cbtrus.org/2011-NPCR-SEER/WEB-0407-Report-3-3-2011.pdf (Last accessed March 1, 2011)

Chang EF, Clark A, Jensen RL, Bernstein M, Guha A, Carrabba G, *et al.* (2009) Multiinstitutional validation of the University of California at San Francisco Low-Grade Glioma Prognostic Scoring System. Clinical article. *J Neurosurg* **111** (2), 203–10.

Douw L, Klein M, Fagel SS, van den Heuvel J, Taphoorn MJ, Aaronson NK, *et al.* (2009) Cognitive and radiological effects of radiotherapy in patients with low-grade glioma: long-term follow-up. *Lancet Neurol* **8** (9), 810–8.

Glantz MJ, Cole BF, Forsyth PA, Recht LD, Wen PY, Chamberlain MC, *et al.* (2000) Practice parameter: anticonvulsant prophylaxis in patients with newly diagnosed brain tumors. Report of the Quality Standards Subcommittee of the American Academy of Neurology. *Neurology* **54** (10), 1886–93.

Houillier C, Wang X, Kaloshi G, Mokhtari K, Guillevin R, Laffaire J, *et al.* (2010) IDH1 or IDH2 mutations predict longer survival and response to temozolomide in low-grade gliomas. *Neurology* **75** (17), 1560–6.

Jaeckle KA, Decker PA, Ballman KV, Flynn PJ, Giannini C, Scheithauer BW, et al. (2011) Transformation of low grade glioma and correlation with outcome: an NCCTG database analysis. *J Neurooncol* **104**, 253–9.

Jenkins RB, Wrensch MR, Johnson DR, Fridley BL, Decker PA, Xiao Y, et al. (2011) Distinct germ line polymorphisms underlie glioma morphologic heterogeneity. *Cancer Genet* **204** (1), 13–8.

Louis DN, Ohgaki H, Wiestler OD, et al. (eds) (2007) *WHO Classification of Tumours of the Central Nervous System*, 4th edn. IARC Press, Lyon.

Pignatti F, van den Bent M, Curran D, Debruyne C, Sylvester R, Therasse P, et al. (2002) Prognostic factors for survival in adult patients with cerebral low-grade glioma. *J Clin Oncol* **20** (8), 2076–84.

Shaw EG, Berkey B, Coons SW, Brachman D, Buckner JC, Stelzer KJ, et al. (2006) Initial report of Radiation Therapy Oncology Group (RTOG) 9802: Prospective studies in adult low-grade glioma (LGG). *J Clin Oncol* **24** (June 20 suppl; abstr 1500).

Shaw EG, Wang M, Coons SW, et al. (2008) Final report of Radiation Therapy Oncology Group (RTOG) protocol 9802: Radiation therapy (RT) versus RT + procarbazine, CCNU, and vincristine (PCV) chemotherapy for adult low-grade glioma (LGG). *J Clin Oncol* **26** (May 20 suppl; abstr 2006).

Smith JS, Chang EF, Lamborn KR, Chang SM, Prados MD, Cha S, et al. (2008) Role of extent of resection in the long-term outcome of low-grade hemispheric gliomas. *J Clin Oncol* **26** (8), 1338–45.

van den Bent MJ, Afra D, de Witte O, Ben Hassel M, Schraub S, Hoang-Xuan K, et al. (2005) Long-term efficacy of early versus delayed radiotherapy for low-grade astrocytoma and oligodendroglioma in adults: the EORTC 22845 randomised trial. *Lancet* **366** (9490), 985–90.

van den Bent MJ, Wefel JS, Schiff D, Taphoorn MJ, Jaeckle K, Junck L, et al. (2011) Response assessment in neuro-oncology (a report of the RANO group): assessment of outcome in trials of diffuse low-grade gliomas. *Lancet Oncol* **12**(6), 583–93.

8

Ependymomas

Kanwal P. S. Raghav[1] **and Mark R. Gilbert**[2]

[1]Department of Medical Oncology, The University of Texas MD Anderson Cancer Center, Houston, TX, USA
[2]Department of Neuro-Oncology, The University of Texas MD Anderson Cancer Center, Houston, TX, USA

Introduction

Ependymomas are rare neuroepithelial tumors. Bailey published the first descriptive case series of "ependymal gliomas" in January 1924, relating 11 cases of tumors presumably arising from ependymal cells. As the name implies, ependymomas are thought to arise from ependymal cells within the central nervous system (CNS). They can occur along or adjacent to the entire neuraxis (cerebral ventricles and central canal). Intracranial ependymomas, mostly seen in children, present as intraventricular or parenchymal lesions. Spinal ependymomas, usually seen in adults, present as either intramedullary masses or exophytic masses at conus medullaris or cauda equina. Approximately 90% of all ependymomas in the pediatric setting are intracranial while 75% of ependymomas seen in adults are spinal in location. Ependymomas are distinct from ependymoblastomas, which are considered to be primitive neuroectodermal tumors (PNET); however, there are ependymoma variants such as myxopapillary ependymomas considered to be related, although with distinctive clinical characteristics.

Ependymomas are rare malignancies. Despite this rarity, patients with these malignancies clearly benefit from early diagnosis and intervention, making it imperative for neurologists and oncologists to have a comprehensive understanding of the biology, diagnosis, and management of these rare neoplasms. This chapter describes the profile, pathology, presentation, and management of these tumors.

Epidemiology

A total of 1,529,560 new cancer cases will be diagnosed in the United States in 2010. Approximately 22,020 (1.4%) among these are primary nervous system tumors. Ependymomas are exceptionally rare and represent only 2.1% of all primary (CNS) malignancies in all age groups. They are more commonly seen in pediatric population (8–10% of primary CNS cancers) and are infrequent in adults (less than 4% of adult primary CNS cancers). Ependymomas are the third most common type of pediatric brain tumors after pilocytic astrocytomas and medulloblastomas. Ependymomas are also the most common primary tumor of the spinal cord, accounting for 25% of all cases.

Ependymomas are classified as glial tumors that are thought to arise from ependymal cells that line the ventricular system. Ependymal cells are embryologically derived from primitive neuroectoderm. The mechanism and genetics behind oncogenic transformation of these ependymal cells is not known. Taylor *et al.* identi-

Neuro-oncology, First Edition. Edited by Roger J. Packer, David Schiff.

fied a population of radial glia cells as candidate stem cells for ependymomas.

Notably greater than 70% of all supratentorial ependymomas are parenchymal in location and do not arise in the ventricular system. Hahn *et al.* in their case series of 1316 intracranial tumors showed a 3.4% (46 cases) incidence of ependymomas. Nearly 43% (20) were supratentorial and, among these, 17 cases (85%) were extraventricular. These ependymomas are thought to arise from embryonic ependymal cortical rests.

Ependymal tumors occur along the neural axis. The sites include the intracranial periventricular region (infratentorial and supratentorial), spinal cord (intramedullary), and conus medullaris and cauda equina regions. The anatomic location varies with age. Most pediatric ependymomas arise intracranially. Among intracranial tumors, infratentorial location is more common. The posterior fossa is the most common site in infants and children. Within the posterior fossa, the most frequent location is the fourth ventricle. Adult ependymomas arise mostly in the spinal cord. About half of all spinal cord lesions are found in lumbosacral region and "cauda" region, although many of these tumors are the myxopapillary variant. Among typical ependymomas and anaplastic ependymomas of the spinal cord, the cervical region is the most common site of origin. A large case series of 101 patients described by Mork and Loken illustrates this anatomic distribution (Figure 8.1). The series confirmed that ependymomas constituted 1.2% (48 of 4054) of primary intracranial tumors and 32% (53 of 164) of intraspinal tumors.

Extraneural ectopic sites as presentation of primary ependymomas such as ovaries, peritoneum, and mediastinum have been reported in literature. Extraneural metastasis (ENM) is rare. A review of 81 ependymomas at Memorial Sloan–Kettering Cancer Center, New York, showed only five (6.2%) cases had ENM. ENM may involve lung, thoracic lymph nodes, pleura, bone, peritoneum, and liver.

All ependymomas can give rise to cerebrospinal fluid (CSF) dissemination. Vanuytsel and Brada reported a 6.9% incidence of spinal seeding in ependymomas. The likelihood of dissemination increased with higher grade, infratentorial location, and poor control of primary lesions. Spinal cord ependymomas have a relatively low risk of dissemination. Because of this risk of dissemination, staging of the CNS is recommended especially for posterior fossa ependymomas and anaplastic grade. Following the established paradigm for medulloblastomas, analysis of CSF should be performed no earlier than 2 weeks after surgery. The frequency of surveillance of the spine for evidence of dissemination in patients with ependymomas remains uncertain.

Age is a major determinant of site of presentation. Intracranial tumors are most commonly seen in children. Spinal ependymomas are common in adults and rarely occur in children younger than 15 years. The age-specific incidence shows a bimodal distribution, with the

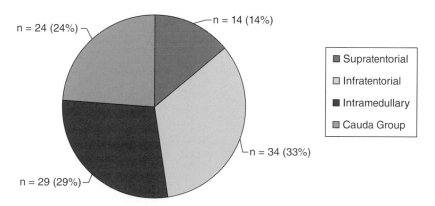

Figure 8.1. Distribution of ependymomas by site. (Reproduced from Mork SJ, Loken AC. Ependymoma: a follow-up study of 101 cases. Cancer. 1977 Aug; 40 (2): 907–15. PMID: 890671 with permission of John Wiley & Sons.)

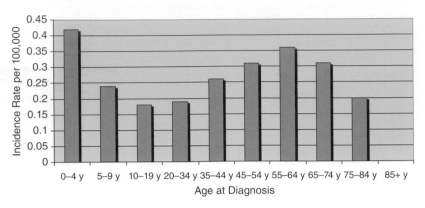

Figure 8.2. Age-specific incidence rate for ependymomas.

first peak occurring at early age (0–4 years) and a second peak in the third or fourth decade of life (Figure 8.2).

In multiple case series, the mean age of presentation was 16.4–23.4 years for intracranial and 40–41 years for spinal ependymomas. In pediatric populations, the mean age of presentation was 4–5 years. For intracranial tumors, the mean age of diagnosis is lower for infratentorial (14.5–15.4 years) than supratentorial (18.8–22 years) lesions. White people are somewhat more commonly affected than black individuals. The age-adjusted incidence rate per 100,000 person-years is 0.27 in white people and 0.16 in African-Americans. Overall, there is no sex predilection of these tumors. The age-adjusted incidence rate per 100,000 person-years is 0.26 in males and 0.25 in females. In adults, the male and female distribution is equal. In children with intracranial ependymomas, a slight male preponderance (1.3:1) is seen. Supratentorial intracranial lesions occur more commonly in females (2:1) and infratentorial lesions occur more commonly in males (1.3:1).

Most ependymomas are sporadic malignancies. Rarely, they may be seen in relation with neurofibromatosis type 2 (NF-2). Ependymomas are found in 3–6% of patients diagnosed with NF-2.

Classification

Ependymal tumors have been classified by the World Health Organization (WHO) in 2007 into four major subtypes (Table 8.1). Grade II ependy-momas are further divided into cellular papillary, clear cell, and tanycytic varieties.

Grade I tumors are biologically distinct from grade II and III tumors. Grade I (myxopapillary ependymomas and subependymomas) tumors are noninvasive. These do not infiltrate surrounding brain or spinal cord and rarely undergo malignant transformation into a higher grade tumor. They have high cure rates following complete surgical excision. Grade II ependymomas frequently undergo malignant transformation to grade III tumors and have a lower rate of cure, even with extensive resection. Anaplastic ependymomas are extensively infiltrative and are seldom cured with surgical resection.

Despite published grading criteria, particularly for pediatric ependymomas, controversy remains regarding the prognostic implications of the grading system.

Pathology

Ependymal tumors are composed of tan to gray soft tissue. They are often well demarcated from the surrounding parenchyma (except anaplastic ependymomas, which show evidence of frank intraparenchymal invasion). They may have associated hemorrhage, necrosis, and calcification.

Ependymomas exhibit diverse cytomorphologic characteristics (Table 8.2). Elongated fibrillary glial-type cells and epithelioid cells may be seen. Low grade lesions show tumor cells with monomorphic round to oval nuclei containing finely dispersed chromatin. High grade neo-

Table 8.1. World Health Organization (WHO) classification of ependymomas. (Reproduced from Mork SJ, Loken AC. Ependymoma: a follow-up study of 101 cases. Cancer. 1977 Aug; 40 (2): 907–15. PMID: 890671 with permission of John Wiley & Sons.)

Grade	Tumor type	Age	Location	Biology	Malignant transformation	Cure rate
I	Myxopapillary ependymoma	Young adults	Spinal cord (conus/cauda)	Non-infiltrative	Rare	High
I	Subependymoma	Elderly	Ventricles (IV>Lateral>III)	Non-infiltrative Indolent	Rare	Often an incidental finding at autopsy
II	Ependymoma	Children Adults	Spinal cord	Infiltrative	Frequent	Low
III	Anaplastic ependymoma	Children	Supratentorial	Infiltrative	–	Rare

Table 8.2. Histologic characteristics of ependymomas.

Grade	Tumor type	Histologic characteristics
I	Myxopapillary ependymomas	Pseudopapillary structures (cuboidal ependymal cells radially arranged surrounding a myxoid stroma with mucin and central blood vessel) Tumor cells surrounded by mucoid material Mucin-rich microcysts Collagen balls or balloons (unique to this ependymoma variant; small fibrillary rounded eosinophilic structures with reticulin)
I	Subependymoma	Nodular appearance at low power Poorly formed or absent perivascular pseudorosettes Hypocellular Background highly fibrillary with cystic changes
II	Ependymoma	Cellular (monotonous highly cellular appearance) Papillary (central vascular core surrounded by cylindrical cells) Clear cell (regularly arranged cells with clear cytoplasm and inconspicuous perivascular rosettes) Tanycytic (elongated spindle-shaped cells with eosinophilic fibrillary processes arranged in fascicles and prominent pseudorosettes)
III	Anaplastic ependymoma	Hypercellularity Hyperchromatic and pleomorphic nuclei Abundant mitosis Pseudopalisading necrosis Microvascular proliferation Ependymal rosettes absent

plasms show polymorphic, irregular, and hyperchromatic nuclei. The so-called "combined" tumors (with multiple grades seen) should be graded according to the highest grade component present.

Hallmark histology consists of perivascular pseudorosettes (Plate 8.8, see plate section opposite p. 52). These are anuclear perivascular zones with radially arranged ependymal cell processes directed towards central blood vessels. The second characteristic attribute is presence of ependymal rosettes. Unlike pseudorosettes, ependymal rosettes are composed of epithelioid cuboidal to columnar cells arranged around a central lumen. Perivascular pseudorosettes are more commonly observed on histopathology than ependymal rosettes. However, the latter are more specific for ependymomas. Perivascular pseudorosettes are stained positively with antibodies targeting vimentin and glial fibrillary acidic protein (GFAP).

Subependymomas are slow-growing lesions (grade I). As a result they are primarily discovered as autopsy findings. When presenting clinically, the symptoms are brought about by ventricular obstruction or hemorrhages. Many pathologists believe that subependymomas should not be grouped with ependymomas, although occasional tumors are comprised of a mixture of these two histologies.

Myxopapillary ependymomas are also slow-growing tumors. Clinically, they manifest as chronic back pain. These tumors are typically in the lower aspect of the spinal cord or cauda equina. They may be encapsulated, thereby allowing complete tumor removal.

Grade II ependymomas are further divided into four types: cellular ependymomas, clear cell ependymomas, papillary ependymomas, and tanycytic ependymomas. As their name suggests, cellular ependymomas are highly cellular lesions and papillary ependymomas are characterized by a papillary architecture. Clear cell ependymomas are seen predominantly in the supratentorial compartment in young adults. Histologically, they resemble oligodendrogliomas. Tanycytic ependymomas are rare.

Anaplastic ependymomas are designated as grade III gliomas by the World Health Organization classification schema. High rates of mitosis and widespread cellular pleomorphism with prominent angiogenesis, often with loss of the pseudorosettes seen with grade II ependymomas, are the hallmarks of anaplastic ependymomas. These tumors are associated with rapid growth and decreased survival.

Immunohistochemistry

Ependymal tumors have universally positive staining for S100, GFAP, vimentin, and neural cell adhesion molecule (NCAM) or CD56. Absence of GFAP staining should prompt search for another diagnosis. Epithelial membrane antigen (EMA) staining often shows a characteristic punctuate dot-type pattern. EMA staining is not seen in the myxopapillary variant.

Molecular biology

The understanding of molecular pathology of ependymomas has been limited by the relative rarity of the disease and lack of appropriate laboratory models, although recent publications suggest that this is an area that is garnering increasing interest. Ependymomas represent a genetically and clinically heterogeneous group of neoplasms. This heterogeneity amplifies with differences in both tumor location and patient age. The most frequent chromosomal abnormalities observed include losses on chromosomes 6q, 17p, and 22q, and gains on 1q and 9q. Chromosome 9q33-34 is gained in 30% of ependymomas. Recent data also suggest occurrence of an ependymoma tumor suppressor gene on chromosome 22. Specific genetic mutations are uncommon with the exception of NF2, often in the setting of loss of heterozygosity (LOH) of chromosome arm 22q and mutations of MEN1 along with 11q LOH.

Presentation

The symptoms observed result from disruption of physiologic neural pathways and subsequently functions. This produces both local and distant effects. The specific symptoms depend on location of tumor. Broadly, they can be described as either cranial or spinal symptoms.

Tumors can cause symptoms from ventricular involvement resulting in increased intracranial pressure (ICP) and hydrocephalus. Patients often complain of headaches, nausea/vomiting, diplopia, vision loss, lethargy, vertigo, and dizziness. Focal neurologic symptoms such as hemiparesis may also be reported. Uncommonly, patients may present with seizures.

Spinal symptoms

The most frequent manifestation is pain. This is typically nocturnal, unremitting, and gnawing in character. The location of pain may be indicative of the anatomic site of the tumor. Back pain and/or neck pain is the presenting symptom in about 63% of patients with a spinal cord tumor.

Distal symptoms arise as a result of disruption of spinal cord pathways. Sensory dysesthesias, motor weakness, and sphincter dysfunction may occur, consistent with the intraparenchymal (intramedullary) location of the tumor. These symptoms may begin unilaterally and then can evolve into bilateral symptoms. Patients may frequently complain of gait disturbance.

Physical examination

In spinal cord tumors, weakness (63%), sensory alterations (63%), hyperreflexia (42%), and spasticity (31%) are the most common findings. Papilledema is the most frequent physical examination findings in patients with intracranial tumors.

Diagnosis

Imaging has a pivotal role in diagnosis, assessing response to treatment and surveillance of patients with ependymomas. Computed tomography (CT) scanning is often the initial imaging modality to evaluate for a suspected intracranial space-occupying lesion because of the rapid acquisition of imaging and favorable cost. However, CT is limited with respect to ependymomas because of its inability to define precise anatomic details. Therefore, magnetic resonance imaging (MRI) is preferred (Figure 8.3).

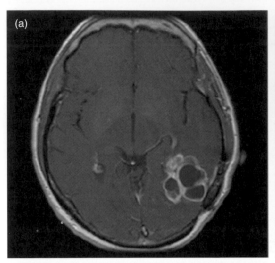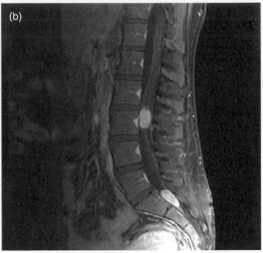

Figure 8.3. Magnetic resonance imaging of ependymoma. (a) T1 post contrast image demonstrating a left parietal anaplastic ependymoma. (b) T1 post contrast sagittal image demonstrating two regions of spinal cord ependymoma. The inferior lesion is likely a drop metastasis.

Management

A consensus regarding management of ependymomas is lacking. The present approach to treatment has been largely consolidated from experience with more common pediatric ependymomas. Two large retrospective reviews in adults show that the basic principles of management hold true in both adult and pediatric patients. The benefit of maximum surgical resection is irrefutable. Therefore, treatment is gross total resection. In spinal ependymomas, removal of tumor while conserving the integrity of tumor capsule is vital to prevent any dissemination. Tumors not amenable to surgery are treated with stereotactic radiosurgery or fractionated external beam radiation therapy (EBRT). Adjuvant radiation should be given in patients with post surgical residual disease irrespective of tumor grade. Adjuvant radiation should also be given for anaplastic ependymomas irrespective of extent of surgical resection. Craniospinal radiotherapy is not indicated for nondisseminated ependymomas. In children, totally resected posterior fossa ependymomas are treated with conformed radiotherapy; there is no consensus whether pediatric totally resected supratentorial ependymomas require radiotherapy. A review of 152 patients from the French Neurosurgical Centers study supports the above principles. Multivariate analysis revealed that overall survival rates and risk of recurrence were associated with histologic grade ($P < 0.001$), extent of surgery ($P = 0.006$), patient's age ($P = 0.004$), and patient's Karnofsky performance status ($P = 0.03$). Radiotherapy resulted in beneficial effect for incompletely resected low grade ependymomas and to a lesser extent for completely removed high grade tumors.

Role of chemotherapy

There is no evidence to suggest the addition of chemotherapy to radiotherapy improves survival. Chemotherapy does not have any proven effect on outcomes of spinal cord ependymomas. Chemotherapy may be beneficial in deferring radiotherapy in children younger than 5 years. This approach may be preferable because radiotherapy has the potential to cause developmental neurologic damage resulting in cognitive impairment, endocrinopathy, and risk of second malignancy. At present, chemotherapy is thus principally to be given in the clinical trial setting and is essentially investigational. A variety of chemotherapeutic agents – etoposide and temozolomide – have shown activity in this disease; however, data are insufficient. Targeted agents have not been investigated extensively in ependymomas.

Treatment of refractory disease

Recurrent disease may be managed by re-resection followed by re-irradiation with either conventional EBRT or a more focused radiation therapy. The risk of radiation toxicity (myelopathy) increases with repeated treatment.

Prognosis

Prognosis is good, with >80% 5-year disease-free survival. Location of tumor is the most significant prognostic factor for ependymomas. Less significant factors are grade and age. Histologically, number of mitosis, necrosis, and age >16 years are significant prognostic factors for supratentorial ependymomas. For supratentorial lesions, subependymoma is associated with longer survival. The 5-year and 10-year overall survival rates for intracranial adult ependymomas are 84.8 and 76.5% for all grades. In spinal ependymomas, surgery results in a 5 and 10-year progression-free survival of 89% and 84%, respectively. Preoperative neurologic status is an independent predictor of functional outcome in these patients.

Future directions

The rarity of the disease has to date limited our ability to conduct large-scale clinical trials or single-institution investigations in ependymomas. However, collaborative approach is likely to yield better results in future. The Collaborative Ependymoma Research Network (CERN) (www.cern-foundation.org) has been established to conduct collaborative projects to gather information on the treatment strategies and develop new treatment strategies based on clinical trials to improve survival and outcome. Ongoing trials with chemotherapy will most likely outline the role of chemotherapy in ependymomas in the near future. Studies are needed to characterize the molecular alterations and to assess their impact on pathogenesis and prognosis. This may result in delineating molecular profile of ependymomas and, it is hoped, in development of novel therapeutic targets and both standardized and personalized treatment strategies.

Selected bibliography

Boström A, von Lehe M, Hartmann W, Pietsch T, Feuss M, Boström JP, Schramm J, et al. (2011) Surgery for spinal cord ependymomas: outcome and prognostic factors. *Neurosurgery* **68** (2), 302–8.

Chamberlain MC, Johnston SK. (2009) Temozolomide for recurrent intracranial supratentorial platinum-refractory ependymoma. *Cancer* **115** (20), 4775–82.

Gilbert MR, Ruda R, Soffietti R. (2010) Ependymomas in adults. *Curr Neurol Neurosci Rep* **10** (3), 240–7. (Review)

Godfraind C. (2009) Classification and controversies in pathology of ependymomas. *Childs Nerv Syst* **25** (10), 1185–93. (Review)

Grill J, Le Deley MC, Gambarelli D, Raquin MA, Couanet D, Pierre-Kahn A, et al.; French Society of Pediatric Oncology. (2001) Postoperative chemotherapy without irradiation for ependymoma in children under 5 years of age: a multicenter trial of the French Society of Pediatric Oncology. *J Clin Oncol* **19** (5), 1288–96.

Grundy RG, Wilne SA, Weston CL, Robinson K, Lashford LS, Ironside J, et al.; Children's Cancer and Leukaemia Group (formerly UKCCSG) Brain Tumour Committee (2007) Primary postoperative chemotherapy without radiotherapy for intracranial ependymoma in children: the UKCCSG/SIOP prospective study. *Lancet Oncol* **8** (8), 696–705.

Hahn F, Schapiro R, Okawara SF. (1975) Supratentorial ependymomas. *Neuroradiology* **10**, 5–13.

Healey EA, Barnes PD, Kupsky WJ, Scott RM, Sallan SE, Black PM, et al. (1991) The prognostic significance of postoperative residual tumor in ependymoma. *Neurosurgery* **28** (5), 666–71; discussion 671–2.

Jaing TH, Wang HS, Tsay PK, Tseng CK, Jung SM, Lin KL, et al. (2004) Multivariate analysis of clinical prognostic factors in children with intracranial ependymomas. *J Neurooncol* **68** (3), 255–61.

Johnson RA, Wright KD, Poppleton H, Mohankumar KM, Finkelstein D, Pounds SB, et al. (2010) Cross-species genomics matches driver mutations and cell compartments to model ependymoma. *Nature* **466**, 632–6.

Mack SC, Taylor MD. (2009) The genetic and epigenetic basis of ependymoma. *Childs Nerv Syst* **25** (10), 1195–201. (Review)

Merchant TE, Li C, Xiong X, Kun LE, Boop FA, Sanford RA. (2009) Conformal radiotherapy after surgery for paediatric ependymoma: a prospective study. *Lancet Oncol* **10** (3), 258–66.

Metellus P, Barrie M, Figarella-Branger D, Chinot O, Giorgi R, Gouvernet J, *et al.* (2007) Multicentric French study on adult intracranial ependymomas: prognostic factors analysis and therapeutic considerations from a cohort of 152 patients. *Brain* **13** (Pt 5), 1338–49.

Mork SJ, Loken AC. (1977) Ependymoma: a follow-up study of 101 cases. *Cancer* **40** (2), 907–15.

Puget S, Grill J, Valent A, Bieche I, Dantas-Barbosa C, Kauffmann A, *et al.* (2009) Candidate genes on chromosome 9q33-34 involved in the progression of childhood ependymomas. *J Clin Oncol* **27** (11), 1884–92.

Robertson PL, Zeltzer PM, Boyett JM, Rorke LB, Allen JC, Geyer JR, *et al.* (1998) Survival and prognostic factors following radiation therapy and chemotherapy for ependymomas in children: a report of the Children's Cancer Group. *J Neurosurg* **88** (4), 695–703.

Rogers L, Pueschel J, Spetzler R, Shapiro W, Coons S, Thomas T, *et al.* (2005) Is gross-total resection sufficient treatment for posterior fossa ependymomas? *J Neurosurg* **102** (4), 629–36.

Shaw EG, Evans RG, Scheithauer BW, Ilstrup DM, Earle JD. (1986) Radiotherapeutic management of adult intraspinal ependymomas. *Int J Radiat Oncol Biol Phys* **12** (3), 323–7.

Sun B, Wang C, Wang J, Liu A. (2003) MRI features of intramedullary spinal cord ependymomas. *J Neuroimaging* **13** (4), 346–51.

Surveillance Epidemiology and End Results (SEER) database. Incidence projections are based on rates from the North American Association of Central Cancer Registries (NAACCR) from 1995–2006. Available at: http://seer.cancer.gov (Last accessed November 12, 2010.)

Taylor MD, Poppleton H, Fuller C, Su X, Liu Y, Jensen P, *et al.* (2005) Radial glia cells are candidate stem cells of ependymoma. *Cancer Cell* **8** (4), 323–35.

Vanuytsel L, Brada M. (1991) The role of prophylactic spinal irradiation in localized intracranial ependymoma. *Int J Radiat Oncol Biol Phys* **21** (3), 825–30.

9

Germ Cell Tumors and Other Pineal Region Tumors

Geneviève Legault and Jeffrey C. Allen

Departments of Pediatrics and Neurology, NYU Langone Medical Center, New York, NY, USA

Introduction

Pineal region tumors comprise 3–5% of pediatric central nervous system (CNS) tumors and 0.4% of adult CNS tumors. Pineal region tumors consist of a diverse group of tumors with regard to age of onset, pathology, treatment, and prognosis. The origin of these tumors relates to the anatomic diversity of this region and the poorly understood role this region has in the ontogeny of the CNS. Several types of tumors arise in this region. Germ cell tumors (GCT) range histologically from mature variants (teratoma, dermoid cysts) to more aggressive variants (germinoma, mixed malignant germ cell tumors [MMGCT], immature teratomas). Pineal parenchymal tumors (PPT) of varying aggressivity arise in the pineal gland, a derivative of neuroectodermal tissue. Adjacent glial tissue may give rise to astrocytomas and ependymomas. GCT are the most common histology in children and young adults, followed by PPT and gliomas, although the frequencies vary with age as shown by Al-Hussaini *et al.* and illustrated in Table 9.1.

Germ cell tumors

Epidemiology and incidence

The incidence of GCT varies by geography and ethnicity, with an incidence of 3% of all intracranial childhood tumors in the Western hemisphere and as high as 15% in Japan. Aggressive GCT are divided into two histologic subgroups that are highly prognostic: germinomas and MMGCT or nongerminomatous germ cell tumors (NGGCTs). The latter group usually consists of a combination of several different histologies such as germinoma, embryonal carcinoma, choriocarcinoma, endodermal sinus tumor, and occasionally mature or immature teratoma. The World Health Organization classifies CNS GCT into choriocarcinomas, embryonal carcinoma, germinomas, mixed germ cell tumors, teratomas (immature, mature, teratoma with malignant transformation) and yolk sac tumors. All GCTs are biologically malignant except for mature teratomas. Germinomas are the most common histology in most series, representing 76% of the total number of cases, leaving 7% teratoma, 2% embryonal carcinoma, 0.5% choriocarcinoma, 1% yolk sac tumor, and a remainder of 13.5% mixed tumors. For secreting MMGCT, a contemporary approach is to use fluid tumor markers alone and forgo histologic confirmation for assigning treatment alternatives. This appears to be the practice in Canada in a recent national review. In 66% of the patients with a secreting MMGCT, the diagnosis was made with markers alone without a biopsy.

Neuro-oncology, First Edition. Edited by Roger J. Packer, David Schiff.

Table 9.1. Distribution of pineal region tumor histologies by age. (Adapted with kind permission from Springer Science + Business Media: Al-Hussaini M, Sultan I, Abuirmileh N, Jaradat I, Qaddoumi I. (2009) Pineal gland tumors: experience from the SEER database. J Neurooncol 94 (3), 351–8.)

	GCT	Glioma	PPT	Others
Children (n = 355)	237 (66.8)	9 (2.5)	96 (27.0)	13 (3.7)
Adults (n = 278)	136 (48.9)	23 (8.3)	91 (32.7)	28 (10.1)

Values are n (%). GCT, germ cell tumor; PPT, pineal parenchymal tumor.

GCT more commonly arise in the first and second decades of life, with a median age at diagnosis of 11.6 years of age. Approximately 90% of the patients present before 20 years of age but less than 3% of the cases occur in children under 5 years of age. GCT in very young children tend to arise in atypical locations and are usually comprised of mixed histologies including mature and immature teratomas. In older children and young adults, the histologic subtypes vary by site of origin. For example, an equal mix of pure germinomas and MMGCT arise in the suprasellar region but pure germinomas are more common in the pineal region. The sex distribution also varies by site. The male to female ratio in the pineal region is approximately 10:1 and in the suprasellar region is 1:1. There may be a genetic predisposition to CNS GCT as they arise more frequently in *ras* pathway disorders such as neurofibromatosis type 1 and Noonan syndrome, Klinefelter syndrome (47XXY karyotype), Down syndrome (trisomy 21) and certain Asian populations.

GCT probably arise from developmental rests of primordial germ cells, which may reside in gonads, CNS, or elsewhere in the body such as in the mediastinum. In the CNS, the tumors predominate in midline locations. The pineal region is the most common site in 53.7% of patients, followed by the suprasellar region in 30.6%, the basal ganglia in 5%, and other locations in 2.5%. In 8.3% of cases, the tumor appears to arise synchronously in both the pineal and suprasellar regions, constituting the bifocal or multifocal presentation. The majority of patients with bifocal GCT have pure germinoma histology.

Clinical presentation

The clinical manifestations of CNS GCT relate to their histologic type and location. Germinomas tend to present with a more protracted course, often over years. Diabetes insipidus (DI) is often the first symptom in suprasellar primaries and eventually other endocrine deficiencies and impairments in visual acuity may occur. The diagnosis is often delayed in patients with protracted prodromes, especially when diagnostic imaging is inconclusive. Basal ganglia and thalamic germinoma can present with hemiparesis, movement disorder, precocious puberty, and cognitive or mental status change. Patients with isolated pineal GCT have a shorter prodrome relating primarily to symptoms of raised intracranial pressure, prompting neuroimaging. Signs and symptoms of Parinaud syndrome (convergence-retraction nystagmus, altered vertical gaze, and impaired pupillary response to light) may be present related to dorsal midbrain and aqueductal compression.

Diagnosis

The neuroimaging characteristics of CNS GCT are largely nonspecific and diagnosis is suspected more by the location and clinical presentation. Pineal masses can be found incidentally in 1.4–10% of cases. Computed tomography (CT) scan is often the initial screening radiologic investigation. A symptomatic pineal region tumor often presents with hydrocephalus. There may be intratumoral calcifications or hemorrhage and the mass is usually circumscribed, hyperdense, and enhances with contrast. Contrast enhanced magnetic resonance imaging (MRI) of the brain and spine is a more sensitive tool for assessing the size, degree of infiltration or edema of the adjacent brain parenchyma, presence of an occult suprasellar mass, and evidence of intraventricular and/or spinal metastases. The pineal tumor is usually isointense to hyperintense to normal brain on a T1-weighted sequence and

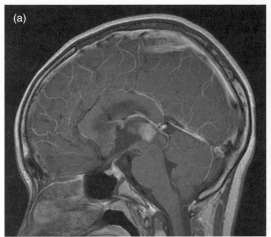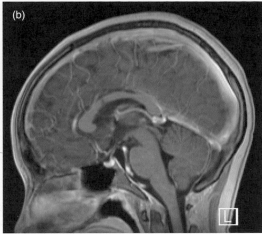

Figure 9.1. Neuroimaging of a germ cell tumor. An 11-year-old male with a biopsy-proven pineal pure germinoma. (a) Sagittal view in a T1-weighted image showing the enhancing pineal tumor with mild secondary hydrocephalus. (b) Similar sagittal plane in a T1-weighted image with contrast after four cycles of chemotherapy with carboplatin and etoposide showing complete resolution of the pineal germinoma prior to radiotherapy.

intratumoral cysts or calcification may be present. Following gadolinium administration, the tumor enhances as shown in Figure 9.1. Subependymal spread may be identified along the walls of the third or lateral ventricles. Restricted diffusion may be observed. More heterogeneous patterns of enhancement are typical of mixed malignant GCT. Infiltrative GCT of the basal ganglia may cause ipsilateral atrophy, edema, and a patchy enhancement. Findings on magnetic resonance spectroscopy (MRS) include an increase in the choline peak and decrease in the N-acetyl-aspartate (NAA) peak. Because of the tumor propensity to disseminate through the CSF, it is imperative to include neuroimaging of the entire neuraxis, which identifies leptomeningeal metastases in 10–30% of cases.

☝ CAUTION!

Diabetes insipidus can antecede magnetic resonance imaging (MRI) evidence of enlargement of the infundibulum by several months to years. Patients with acquired diabetes insipidus should be followed prospectively with serial MRI and endocrine evaluations. Langerhans cell histiocytosis remains in the differential diagnosis but is less common.

Serum and CSF tumor markers

The investigation of the patient suspected of harboring a CNS GCT includes the search for associated tumor markers (the β subunit of human chorionic gonadotropin [β-hCG] and alpha-fetoprotein [AFP]) in the serum and CSF. Quantitative assessments of these fluid proteins may aid in determining the diagnosis, response to therapy, and the duration of remission. In most cases, the initial serum assays are noninformative, especially in germinoma. Serial ventricular CSF assays are not practical and not available at diagnosis in all patients so most of the published guidelines on the use of these markers in CSF relate to lumbar CSF values. Thus, as part of the initial staging evaluation following the surgical control of raised intracranial pressure by an external ventricular drainage (EVD) or ventriculo-peritoneal (VP) shunt, a lumbar puncture can usually be safely performed for CSF cytology and tumor markers. A concomitant serum level of the same hormones should be obtained. If it can be done safely, a preoperative analysis is preferred. Alternatively, specimens should be collected 2–3 weeks after surgery to avoid cytology false positives. The distinction between a pure germinoma and a mixed secreting GCT is clinically meaningful as the prognosis and treatment plan will vary. Specifically, pure germinomas are more radio- and chemosensitive, whereas mixed secreting GCT require more intensive therapy. A marked elevation of AFP level alone in either serum or lumbar CSF is usually the signature of yolk sac or endodermal tumor component. Elevations of AFP and β-hCG are usually associated with embryonal carcinoma components and high values of β-hCG alone occur in choriocarcinoma. The diagnosis of a pure germinoma can only be entertained with a normal AFP value in serum and CSF and relatively low levels of β-hCG (<50–100 mIU/mL).

Most contemporary European and North American clinical trials have arbitrarily set an upper limit of CSF or serum β-hCG level of 50 mIU/mL above which any tumor, even in the setting of a biopsy-proven pure germinoma, has been regarded as containing MMGCT elements and treated as such. A Japanese Pediatric Brain Tumor Study Group, however, found no statistically significant difference in 5-year survival and recurrence rates between low secreting pure germinoma and high secreting β-hCG, either in the serum or CSF with levels ≤200 mIU/mL in children with pathologically confirmed pure germinoma treated with combinations of chemotherapy and radiation therapy.

If biopsied, a major challenge to making an accurate histologic diagnosis is the very small tissue samples delivered by an endoscopic biopsy. Pure germinomas have a classic biphasic cell pattern consisting of a population of large, uniform, undifferentiated cells, resembling primordial germinal elements and a variable perivascular infiltrate of small lymphocytes. Supportive immunohistochemistry confirms membrane immunoreactivity for c-*kit* (CD 117) and nuclear positivity for OCT4. Cytoplasmic identification of placental alkaline phosphatase (PLAP) is less constant and β-hCG is variable. Embryonal carcinoma resembles a highly neoplastic primitive embryo with large pleomorphic totipotential cells forming nests and sheets. It may share immunoreactivity for PLAP, OCT 4, AFP, and β-hCG but lacks c-*kit* expression. Choriocarcinoma contains syncytiotrophoblastic giant cells and cytotrophoblastic components. Giant syncytiotrophoblastic cells are normally immunoreactive for β-hCG. Yolk sac tumor (endodermal

sinus tumor) consists of primitive-appearing epithelial cells proliferating in sheets or more commonly in a reticular pattern. Strongly eosinophilic periodic acid–Schiff (PAS) positive (glycogen-rich) globules are diagnostic. The epithelial elements demonstrate characteristic strong immunohistochemistry positivity for AFP and negativity for c-*kit* and OCT4. Teratomas retain the differentiation pattern of all three primitive embryonic cell layers. Mature teratomas are characterized by the presence of fully differentiated components. Immature teratoma is defined by its variable portions of incompletely differentiated elements of diverse organ lineages. Immunohistochemistry patterns reflect the differentiated somatic counterparts. Genetic imbalances have been identified in GCT, including gains in 12p, 8q, 1q regions, and X chromosome and losses in 11q, 18q, and 13. Some tumors harbor mutations of c-*kit*.

Management

For patients with isolated pineal region tumors, histologic documentation of a specific GCT variant with supportive serum and CSF tumor markers followed by a third ventriculostomy, MRI, and CSF cytologic staging prepares the patient for definitive therapy. Given the sensitivity of pure germinoma to radiotherapy and chemotherapy, resection is not necessary or recommended. If an MMGCT is suspected based on fluid tumor markers, then a resection of the tumor either at diagnosis or after several courses of chemotherapy may contribute to curative treatment.

An endocrinologic survey should be routinely performed in all patients suspected of having a pineal or suprasellar region tumor prior to initiating therapy to assess the need for hormone replacement. This survey would include thyroid stimulating hormone (TSH), free thyroxine (T4) level, adrenocorticotropic hormone (ACTH), AM cortisol, follicle stimulating hormone (FSH), luteinizing hormone (LH), free testosterone, prolactin, insulin-like growth factor 1 (IGF-1), electrolytes, and urine specific gravity. Baseline visual field examinations in patients with suprasellar disease and neuropsychologic evaluations are also recommended.

Treatment assignments should be based on histology and/or tumor markers. Patients with high values of β-hCG (>200 mIU/mL) in serum and/or CSF or elevations of AFP should be treated as having MMGCT, regardless of histology. Patients with normal AFP in the CSF and β-hCG <50 mIU/mL in serum and CSF with histologic verification of a germinoma can be treated as having a pure germinoma. Pure germinomas are highly curable with high doses and extended volumes of radiation therapy (RT) alone, depending on the extent of disease at diagnosis. Over 80% of patients will experience a 5-year progression-free survival. Standard RT volumes for unifocal suprasellar or pineal region germinoma include whole ventricular (WVI) dose to 30 Gy with a boost to the primary tumor to 45 Gy. Patients with disseminated disease should receive 30 Gy to the craniospinal axis (CSI) and a boost to 45 Gy to measurable disease. Given the high cure rates, improving quality of life by decreasing long-term complications of therapy is a major objective.

Combining chemotherapy (CHT) with lower doses and volumes of RT appears to offer similar favorable outcomes. Germinomas are highly chemosensitve as well as confirmed by a high complete response to platinum-based CHT administered prior to RT. Several protocols have reduced the RT volume (involved field rather than whole ventricular) as well as the dose (5–30 Gy) to the tumor in patients with localized disease at diagnosis, sparing the patient some RT-related morbidity. However, a European germinoma study using this approach has found an increased incidence of ventricular relapse. Using chemotherapy alone without any RT has a high relapse rate. However, the majority of germinoma patients who relapse can be salvaged with additional chemotherapy and RT.

Current clinical trials in Europe and North America are attempting to establish a new standard of care for unifocal suprasellar or pineal disease using post surgery CHT for 2–4 courses with carboplatin and etoposide followed by reduced dose WV RT (18 Gy) with a boost to 30 Gy to the primary tumor. Bifocal GCT (pineal and suprasellar) pose a different challenge. Because the predominant histology in this syndrome is pure germinoma in several series, some institutions will forgo a biopsy and treat as a localized pure germinoma with WV RT alone or CHT followed by WV RT. Certain subsets of germinomas, including tumors located in the basal ganglia, have been considered at increased risk for recurrence and have traditionally been treated with larger RT volumes using either craniospinal or whole brain fields. Germinomas that contain syncytiotrophoblastic cells or show an elevated level of β-hCG have been associated with a slightly worse prognosis and higher rate of recurrence than pure germinoma lacking these characteristics when treated with irradiation alone. Therefore, recent treatment plans favor addressing these tumors as MMGCT and include adjuvant chemotherapy. Controversy remains about the upper limit of β-hCG level in serum or lumbar CSF associated with a pure germinoma.

MMGCT have a less favorable outcome following RT alone with a 5-year survival of 20–45% but the recent addition of chemotherapy and radical surgical resection has considerable improved 5-year survival rates which now approach 70–80% in several larger series. Treatment usually begins with multiple courses of CHT with drugs such as carboplatin, ifosfamide, and etoposide followed by CSI to maximum tolerable dose (36 Gy) with boosts to measurable disease (54 Gy). Following therapy, some patients with residual disease and normal tumor markers may harbor a "growing teratoma" and radical resection is often curative. Investigational studies for MMGCT are exploring lower RT volumes such as WV RT in patients with localized disease at diagnosis with successful pre-RT chemotherapy and normalization of tumor markers.

Post-treatment care

Patients are imaged at regular intervals for at least 5 years following treatment because GCT can recur late. Brain MRI alone should be alternated with brain and spine MRI. If the CSF tumor markers were abnormal at diagnosis, a lumbar puncture should be repeated for several years to confirm normal values. Serum assays are less reliable. Late effects involving endocrine and cognitive function require continual monitoring.

Pineal parenchyma tumors

PPT represent 14–27% of all pineal region neoplasms. PPT include pineocytoma, parenchymal tumor of indeterminate differentiation, and pineoblastoma.

Pineocytomas

Pineocytomas are slow-growing WHO grade I tumors accounting for 9% of all the PPT. They can affect patients of any age, but are more frequently seen in adults, with a mean age of 38 years. Unlike GCT, pineocytomas are found in males and females in equal proportions.

Clinical presentation

Pineocytomas can compress adjacent structures including the cerebral aqueduct, brainstem, and cerebellum and present with signs and symptoms similar to GCT, that is, intracranial hypertension, Parinaud syndrome, mental status changes, and brainstem deficits. Rarely, pineocytomas can present in an apoplectic manner from intratumoral hemorrhage.

Diagnosis

Their neuroimaging pattern is characterized by a well-demarcated hypodense globular mass on CT scan which homogeneously enhances with contrast. They can harbor calcifications and intratumoral cysts. On MRI, they usually appear hypointense to isointense on T1-weighted sequences, and hyperintense on T2, again with homogeneous enhancement. Hydrocephalus is frequently identified. Histologically, pineocytomas are well-differentiated, moderately cellular tumors containing uniform small pineocytes and occasional microcalcifications. These cells are often assembled in large pineocytomatous rosettes. Nuclei are usually round, and mitotic figures are rare. The typical immunohistochemistry pattern includes reactivity to neuron-specific enolase (NSE), synaptophysin, and neurofilament protein (NFP).

Management

Gross total resection has been set as the standard of care for these tumors, whenever possible. If this cannot be accomplished, adjuvant RT is frequently administered. Pineocytomas typically follow a benign course with a 5-year survival of 86–100%.

Pineal parenchymal tumors of intermediate differentiation

These tumors are of intermediate differentiation between a low grade pineocytoma and malignant pineoblastomas. They represent a relatively new entity, created to accommodate approximately 10% of all PPT with a WHO grade II or III. They occur throughout life, with a peak incidence in early adulthood. Unlike pineocytomas, they are slightly more frequently encountered in females.

Histology consists of moderately cellular tumors with mild to moderate nuclear atypia and a low to moderate mitotic activity (MIB-1 index of 3–10%). PPT of intermediate differentiation show positive immunohistochemistry for NSE and synaptophysin.

Management

Because this is a recently described entity, prognosis is difficult to assess and optimal treatment has yet to be fully clarified. Management alternatives include radical surgical resection and close MRI surveillance or involved field RT for incompletely resected disease. The benefits of adjuvant CHT are uncertain. Five-year survival rates range from 39 to 74%. Although local recurrence may occur, metastases are uncommon.

Pineoblastomas

Pineoblastomas constitute 81% of all PPT and represent the most aggressive form. These highly malignant primitive neuroectodermal tumors (PNET) are WHO grade IV. Although they can present at any age, pineoblastomas are much more frequent in children, arising primarily in the first two decades of life with a mean age of 12.6 years. There is a 2:1 male predominance.

Clinical presentation

Although the clinical presentation of pineoblastoma is similar to other pineal tumors, the symptomatic interval before diagnosis tends to be shorter and almost all patients seeking medical attention have signs of raised intracranial pressure.

Diagnosis

Pineoblastoma appears on brain CT scan as a poorly demarcated, homogenous, and enhancing mass. Calcifications are rarely seen. On MRI, they show a hypointense to isointense appearance with heterogeneous enhancement. CSF seeding may be identified in up to 15% at diagnosis when spine imaging is included in the evaluation.

The histology consists of highly cellular tumors with irregular hyperchromatic nuclei and limited amount of cytoplasm. They are morphologically identical to PNET in other locations such as medulloblastoma. Immunohistochemistry reactivity usually reflects the neuronal lineage of the tumor (i.e. synaptophysin, NFP, and NSE). Mitoses are frequent and the MIB-1 is high.

Management

Pineoblastoma may rarely be associated with congenital familial bilateral retinoblastoma and is then referred to as the trilateral retinoblastoma syndrome. Pineoblastomas have also been identified in patients with familial adenomatous polyposis. Given its rarity, most experimental protocols include pineoblastoma in the high risk PNET category. Infants may be treated with high dose CHT alone and older children receive craniospinal RT followed by adjuvant CHT. Prognosis varies according to known risk factors such as the degree of surgical resection, and the presence of leptomeningeal or intraventricular metastases. Treated aggressively, pineoblastoma patients have been reported to have a 5-year survival of approximately 50–58%. However, series of patients diagnosed in infancy report a poorer prognosis.

Other diagnostic entities that can be encountered in the pineal region include gliomas of any grade, including ependymoma, benign pineal cysts, and vascular lesions (arteriovenous or vein of Galen malformations, dural arteriovenous fistulas). Pineal cysts are common and are seen in 1.4–10% of MRIs. They are more frequent in women, with a male to female ratio of 1:3. In the vast majority they are asymptomatic, and usually identified incidentally. They appear as well-circumscribed fluid density lesions with a calcified rim and peripheral contrast enhancement, ranging in diameter from 10 to 15 mm. In over 75% of cases, the size of a pineal cyst remains stable over time. About 6% demonstrate interval growth on follow-up imaging.

Conclusions

Pineal region tumors encompass a range of diagnoses and treatment assignment requires a definitive diagnosis, based on a combination of histology and CSF tumor marker determination. For GCT, MMGCT can be diagnosed on the basis of elevations of tumor markers alone and radical surgical resection improves prognosis when followed by CHT and CSI. The definitive diagnosis of a pure germinoma requires histologic confirmation via endoscopy or open craniotomy. Complete CNS staging with brain and spine MRI and lumbar CSF analysis is critical for optimum treatment planning, regardless of diagnosis. Management considerations are evolving to not only improve prognosis, but also diminish late effects of therapy. The management of other tumors of the pineal region such as pineal parenchymal tumors is based on the grade and, like tumors of similar histology elsewhere in the CNS, their prognosis is relatively favorable.

Selected bibliography

Alapetite C, Brisse H, Patte C, Raquin MA, Gaboriaud G, Carrie C, *et al.* (2010) Pattern of relapse and outcome of non-metastatic germinoma patients treated with chemotherapy and limited field radiation: the SFOP experience. *Neuro Oncol* **12** (12), 1318–25.

Al-Hussaini M, Sultan I, Abuirmileh N, Jaradat I, Qaddoumi I. (2009) Pineal gland tumors: experience from the SEER database. *J Neurooncol* **94** (3), 351–8.

Allen JC, DaRosso RC, Donahue B, Nirenberg A. (1994) A phase II trial of preirradiation carboplatin in newly diagnosed germinoma of the central nervous system. *Cancer* **74** (3), 940–4.

Allen JC, Nisselbaum J, Epstein F, Rosen G, Schwartz MK. (1979) Alphafetoprotein and human chorionic gonadotropin determination in cerebrospinal fluid: an aid to the diagnosis and management of intracranial germ-cell tumors. *J Neurosurg* **51** (3), 368–74.

Balmaceda C, Heller G, Rosenblum M, Diez B, Villablanca JG, Kellie S, *et al.* (1996)

Chemotherapy without irradiation – a novel approach for newly diagnosed CNS germ cell tumors: results of an international cooperative trial. The First International Central Nervous System Germ Cell Tumor Study. *J Clin Oncol* **14** (11), 2908–15.

Cuccia V, Rodriguez F, Palma F, Zuccaro G. (2006) Pinealoblastomas in children. *Childs Nerv Syst* **22** (6), 577–85.

Dahiya S, Perry A. (2010) Pineal tumors. *Adv Anat Pathol* **17** (6), 419–27.

Dhall G, Khatua S, Finlay JL. (2010) Pineal region tumors in children. *Curr Opin Neurol* **23** (6), 576–82.

Echevarria ME, Fangusaro J, Goldman S. (2008) Pediatric central nervous system germ cell tumors: a review. *Oncologist* **13** (6), 690–9.

Gaillard F, Jones J. (2010) Masses of the pineal region: clinical presentation and radiographic features. *Postgrad Med J* **86** (1020), 597–607.

Hadziahmetovic M, Clarke JW, Cavaliere R, Mayr NA, Montebello JF, Grecula JC, *et al.* (2008) CNS germinomas: what is the best treatment strategy? *Expert Rev Neurother* **8** (10), 1527–36.

Keene D, Johnston D, Strother D, Fryer C, Carret AS, Crooks B, *et al.* (2007) Epidemiological survey of central nervous system germ cell tumors in Canadian children. *J Neurooncol* **82** (3), 289–95.

Kellie SJ, Boyce H, Dunkel IJ, Diez B, Rosenblum M, Brualdi L, *et al.* (2004) Primary chemotherapy for intracranial nongerminomatous germ cell tumors: results of the second international CNS germ cell study group protocol. *J Clin Oncol* **22** (5), 846–53.

Khatua S, Dhall G, O'Neil S, Jubran R, Villablanca JG, Marachelian A, *et al.* (2010) Treatment of primary CNS germinomatous germ cell tumors with chemotherapy prior to reduced dose whole ventricular and local boost irradiation. *Pediatr Blood Cancer* **55** (1), 42–6.

Khatua S, Phillips A, Fangusaro J, Bovan S, Dhall G, Finlay JL. (2011) Recurrent pure CNS germinoma with markedly elevated serum and cerebrospinal fluid human chorionic gonadotropin-beta (HCGbeta). *Pediatr Blood Cancer* **56** (5), 863–4.

Kochi M, Itoyama Y, Shiraishi S, Kitamura I, Marubayashi T, Ushio Y. (2003) Successful treatment of intracranial nongerminomatous malignant germ cell tumors by administering neoadjuvant chemotherapy and radiotherapy before excision of residual tumors. *J Neurosurg* **99** (1), 106–14.

Louis DN (ed.) (2007) *WHO Classification of Tumours of the Central Nervous System*, 4th edn. International Agency for Research on Cancer, Lyon.

Ogino H, Shibamoto Y, Takanaka T, Suzuki K, Ishihara S, Yamada T, *et al.* (2005) CNS germinoma with elevated serum human chorionic gonadotropin level: clinical characteristics and treatment outcome. *Int J Radiat Oncol Biol Phys* **62** (3), 803–8.

Pusztaszeri M, Pica A, Janzer R. (2006) Pineal parenchymal tumors of intermediate differentiation in adults: case report and literature review. *Neuropathology* **26** (2), 153–7.

Reddy AT, Wellons JC 3rd, Allen JC, Fiveash JB, Abdullatif H, Braune KW, *et al.* (2004) Refining the staging evaluation of pineal region germinoma using neuroendoscopy and the presence of preoperative diabetes insipidus. *Neuro Oncol* **6** (2), 127–33.

Schneider DT, Zahn S, Sievers S, Alemazkour K, Reifenberger G, Wiestler OD, *et al.* (2006) Molecular genetic analysis of central nervous system germ cell tumors with comparative genomic hybridization. *Mod Pathol* **19** (6), 864–73.

Sonoda Y, Kumabe T, Sugiyama S, Kanamori M, Yamashita Y, Saito R, *et al.* (2008) Germ cell tumors in the basal ganglia: problems of early diagnosis and treatment. *J Neurosurg Pediatr* **2** (2), 118–24.

Souweidane MM, Krieger MD, Weiner HL, Finlay JL. (2010) Surgical management of primary central nervous system germ cell tumors. Proceedings from the Second International Symposium on Central Nervous System Germ Cell Tumors. *J Neurosurg Pediatr* **6** (2), 125–30.

Srinivasan N, Pakala A, Mukkamalla C, Oswal A. (2010) Pineal germinoma. *South Med J* **103** (10), 1031–7.

Villano JL, Propp JM, Porter KR, Stewart AK, Valyi-Nagy T, Li X, *et al.* (2008) Malignant pineal germ-cell tumors: an analysis of cases from three tumor registries. *Neuro Oncol* **10** (2), 121–30.

10

Sellar Tumors: Pituitary Adenomas and Craniopharyngiomas

Robert G. Louis, Robert Dallapiazza and John A. Jane Jr

Department of Neurological Surgery, University of Virginia Health System, Charlottesville, VA, USA

Introduction

Pituitary tumors account for 10–15% of all intracranial neoplasms. These are relatively common tumors with an overall prevalence of 16.7% in autopsy and radiographic studies. This corresponds to an annual incidence of 0.5–8.2 per 100,000 persons. Interestingly, both autopsy studies and magnetic resonance imaging (MRI) series reveal an overall prevalence of approximately 10%. The prevalence and clinical presentation for each type of pituitary adenoma is summarized in Table 10.1. Tumors less than 1.0 cm in diameter are classified as microadenomas while those measuring 1 cm or larger are designated as macroadenomas. Pituitary tumors generally present either from a hypersecretory syndrome or due to mass effect. Nonfunctioning tumors generally cause compression of surrounding structures (e.g. optic apparatus or the normal pituitary gland) before they come to clinical attention. On the other hand, tumors that secrete biologically active hormones are more likely to cause symptoms and thus be diagnosed at a smaller size.

Imaging of sellar lesions

The differential diagnosis of sellar lesions is relatively broad and so a comprehensive approach must be employed. MRI is the diagnostic modality of choice for all types of pituitary tumors. The difficulty in diagnosing pituitary microadenomas is a result of several factors. MRI with contrast offers the best opportunity to visualize smaller tumors, which usually appear isointense to normal pituitary gland on both T1 and T2 weighted images. However, variability does exist and hemorrhage or necrosis may appear hyperintense. With gadolinium, pituitary adenomas are relatively hypointense, as they enhance more slowly than the richly vascular normal pituitary gland. A microadenoma will appear as a hypoenhancing, round, demarcated intrapituitary lesion, surrounded by a prominently enhancing, crescentic compressed rim of anterior pituitary. Up to 30% of microadenomas may only be seen with dynamic contrast enhanced MRI, with coronal thin section T1 weighted images obtained during contrast infusion. Other imaging modalities, including computed tomography (CT), are generally not helpful in the diagnosis of smaller tumors. In cases of suspected Cushing disease, where hypercortisolemic patients have a negative MRI but are suspected of harboring an adrenocorticotropic hormone (ACTH) secreting microadenoma, inferior petrosal sinus sampling may be particularly useful.

Neuro-oncology, First Edition. Edited by Roger J. Packer, David Schiff.

Table 10.1. Prevalence and clinical features of pituitary adenomas.

Tumor type	Prevalence	Clinical features
Non-functioning adenoma	25–35%	Mass effect results in visual disturbances, headaches, hypopituitarism, ophthalmoplegia
Prolactinoma	30–45%	Women: amenorrhea, galactorrhea Men: decreased libido, fatigue, impotence
Somatotroph adenoma	15%	*Adults* Acromegaly: frontal bossing, prognathism, nerve entrapments, macroglossia, increased hand and foot size *Children* Gigantism
Corticotroph adenoma	10%	Cushing disease: hypertension, hyperglycemia, obesity, hyperpigmentation, striae
Thyrotroph adenoma	1%	Hyperthyroidism: anxiety, palpitations, heat intolerance, weight loss, tremor

In contrast to microadenomas, where the normal gland is usually clearly visible, macroadenomas appear somewhat different. By definition, a macroadenoma is more than 1 cm in diameter, whereas a "giant" adenoma is more than 4 cm. Depending on their size, pituitary macroadenomas may appear as a combined intrasellar–suprasellar lesion without a separate identifiable pituitary gland. On CT, macroadenomas are of variable attenuation, but most commonly appear isodense to surrounding gray matter. Cyst formation and necrosis are relatively common and hemorrhage is seen in up to 10% of lesions. Calcification is uncommon, occurring in only 1–2% of macroadenomas. In contrast to microadenomas, CT can prove useful in macroadenomas where bony invasion and destruction alters the normal anatomy and may displace the carotid arteries. In these cases, a CT angiogram may be useful to delineate the bony and vascular anatomy. Most commonly, macroadenomas appear isointense on both T1 and T2 weighted images. Occasionally, cyst formation and hemorrhage may alter these characteristics and confer internal heterogeneity. With gadolinium, almost all moderately enhance, while few (thyroid secreting hormone [TSH], necrotic) macroadenomas are hypoenhancing. A smooth "dome" at the superior border indicates displacement of the diaphragma sella by an intrasellar pituitary adenoma. The characteristic "snowman" appearance indicates an adenoma that arose primarily within the sella and expanded superiorly, with growth eventually being constricted around the "waist" by the diaphragma sellae.

Plain films of the skull can usually identify craniopharyngioma. Because these lesions characteristically expand the sella turcica, erosion of the dorsum sellae and anterior clinoids are commonly seen. Furthermore, there are commonly suprasellar calcifications that can be seen on plain films. Both CT and MRI are important in the diagnostic work-up of craniopharyngiomas. CT is useful for identifying calcifications and delineating cystic portions of the tumor. MRI, with and without gadolinium, is useful for delineating the tumor and the adjacent structures. Solid components are characteristically isointense on T1 weighted images with some heterogenicity. Cystic components are variable in their appearance on MRI because of the variable composition of the cystic fluid, but may often have the same imaging appearance as cerebrospinal fluid (CSF). Unlike pituitary adenomas, craniopharyngiomas are characterized by heterogeneous enhancement with solid nodules showing intense enhancement while other areas may not enhance at all. Figure 10.1 demonstrates the typical imaging characteristics of a pituitary macroadenoma and a craniopharyngioma. The presence of calcification is often a good clue to favor craniopharyngioma over pituitary adenoma, as is a primarily suprasellar location.

Rathke cleft cysts (RCC) appear as nonenhancing noncalcified intrasellar cysts, often with suprasellar extension. Most will appear as round

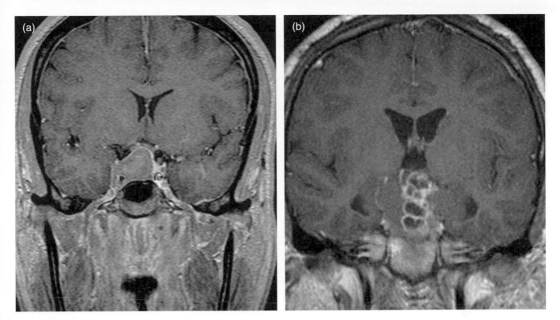

Figure 10.1. Coronal thin cut T1 weighted magnetic resonance image (MRI) with gadolinium of a pituitary macroadenoma (a) and craniopharyngioma (b). The pituitary macroadenoma is round with a smooth dome superiorly (representing an intact diaphragma sellae) and appears homogeneously hypoenhancing. By comparison, the craniopharyngioma appears irregular and heterogeneously enhancing with cystic and solid components and obvious suprasellar extension. Note the distortion of the third ventricle and resulting hydrocephalus.

lesions 5–15 mm in diameter and are hypodense on CT. On T1 weighted images, most will appear hyperintense secondary to the proteinacious content of the cysts while those with more serous fluid will appear hypointense. Similarly, intensity will be variable on T2 weighted images, but most are homogeneous throughout. The presence of an isointense or hyperintense cyst on T2 weighted images with an intracystic hypointense nodule is virtually pathognomonic for RCC. RCC rarely enhance with gadolinium. However, enhancement of a compressed rim of normal pituitary may give the appearance of rim enhancement of the cyst. The presence of calcification usually indicates craniopharyngioma as calcification of RCC is rare.

Other masses, such as choristomas, lymphocytic hypophysitis, pituitary carcinomas, abscesses, and metastases, may less frequently arise in the intrasellar region. Other relatively common lesions such as germinomas, histiocytosis, sarcoidosis, tuberculosis, meningiomas, and metastases can also arise in the suprasellar region.

Surgical approach to sellar tumors

The goals of pituitary surgery are threefold: normalization of secretion of excess hormones, alleviation of compression related to mass effect, and preservation of normal pituitary function. All of this must be accomplished while avoiding damage to critical surrounding structures. Successful resection of pituitary tumors amidst the confines of the carotid arteries, optic nerves, hypothalamus, normal pituitary gland, and cavernous sinuses can present a significant technical challenge. Moreover, the sellar region is relatively centrally located within the head, meaning any approach requires not only precise surgical technique, but also the use of relatively long instruments through a deep and narrow corridor. Suprasellar extension of pituitary macroadenomas is common and an intricate knowledge of the relevant anatomy is invaluable to safe resection of these tumors. Tumors in this region may often involve the circle of Willis, compress the floor of the third ventricle, and even extend to involve the cerebral peduncles, mesial temporal lobes, or anterior cranial fossa. The optic chiasm lies at the anterior limit of the floor of the third ventricle. Above the chiasm lie the anterior cerebral and communicating arteries, while the carotid arteries are found laterally. Preoperative localization of the chiasm is essential to ensuring adequate exposure in cases where chiasmal decompression is required.

The trans-sphenoidal route provides the safest and most efficacious route for surgical access to the sellar region. While complete removal can be achieved in most patients, subsequent craniotomy may be of additional benefit in those with substantial residual tumor, particularly within the anterior and middle cranial fossa in cases of giant adenomas. Significant predictors of successful resection include size of the tumor, degree of extension, and experience of the surgeon. Overall, the morbidity and mortality associated with the trans-sphenoidal approach is low and the common complications (diabetes insipidus and CSF fluid leakage) are usually mild and transient. The trans-sphenoidal approach is associated with high rates of gross total resection, often with corresponding improvements in function with both visual and endocrine disturbances. In experienced hands, 70–80% of those patients with compression of the optic chiasm will have some improvement in visual symptoms. Furthermore, preservation of normal pituitary function is usually possible and up to 65% may even recover lost function.

Pituitary adenomas

Prolactinomas

Prolactinomas are the most common of the functioning adenomas and account for approximately 40% of all pituitary tumors. Prolactin secreting adenomas are 10 times more common in females than males. In addition, the clinical presentation varies with gender. In females, the typical presentation is with amenorrhea and galactorrhea. Galactorrhea may be spontaneous or expressive. By contrast, males usually develop decreased libido and impotence, with galactorrhea and gynecomastia being rare. These rather nonspecific symptoms in males may result in underdiagnosis and may also account for the observation that males tend to present later and with larger tumors (40% macroadenomas) while females are more likely to present with smaller tumors (10% macroadenomas).

After establishing an initial diagnosis of hyperprolactinemia, the next step in evaluation is determination of the source including medications, hypothyroidism, ectopic secretion, and cirrhosis as well as pregnancy, which is the most common cause of secondary amenorrhea. Pregnancy should be ruled out as part of the initial work-up and potentially inciting medications should be reviewed. Medications associated with hyperprolactinemia include dopamine receptor antagonists (metoclopramide, phenothiazines), estrogens, tricyclic antidepressants, selective serotonin reuptake inhibitors (SSRIs), H2 antagonists and verapamil. In addition, the degree to which the prolactin level is elevated can be useful in determining the source. In males and non-pregnant females, normal prolactin levels are in the range 3–30 ng/mL. While most sources agree that prolactin levels higher than 150 ng/mL are diagnostic of prolactinoma, moderate elevations (30–150 ng/mL) can be more ambiguous.

EVIDENCE AT A GLANCE

HYPOTHYROIDISM AND STALK EFFECT IN HYPERPROLACTINEMIA

- Moderate elevations in prolactin may result from secondary effects of other endocrine processes.
- The production and release of prolactin from lactotrophs in the anterior pituitary is dependent on thryotropin releasing hormone (TRH) from the hypothalamus. Primary and secondary hypothyroidism can result in increased TRH in the portal circulation as a result of decreased negative feedback. Increased TRH delivery leads to increased prolactin secretion.
- Stalk effect – dopamine is produced in the hypothalamus and delivered through the

pituitary stalk to the lactotrophs. Dopamine works to inhibit prolactin secretion, which explains why dopamine agonists are useful in the medical management of prolactinomas. In addition, other pituitary tumors may compress the pituitary stalk and can prevent the delivery of dopamine, leading to increases in prolactin secretion. As a result, other pituitary tumors including nonfunctioning adenomas may manifest with signs and symptoms of hyperprolactinemia.

Because of the unpleasant effects and increased risk for development of osteoporosis in both males and females, it is recommended that all patients with symptomatic prolactinomas be treated. Prolactin-secreting tumors remain the only subtype of pituitary adenoma for which the primary treatment is medical. Nonsurgical remission and cure rates for prolactinomas approach 90% with dopamine agonists such as cabergoline and bromocriptine. These medications are effective at both reduction in prolactin levels, alleviating the symptoms of hyperprolactinemia, as well as reduction in tumor volume, with up to two-thirds of patients having at least 50% reduction in the first few months of therapy. Bromocriptine is safe to use during pregnancy and can restore fertility. Side effects of dopamine agonists include headaches, nausea, fatigue, orthostatic hypotension, depression, nightmares, and nasal congestion. While these effects normally abate after the first few weeks of treatment, some patients find them intolerable. Rapid shrinkage of large tumors has been reported to cause CSF rhinorrhea and prolonged treatment with bromocriptine may reduce the chances of a surgical cure. Cabergoline may be more effective and better tolerated than bromocriptine. Those patients who either fail or are intolerant of medical therapy and have either persistent hyperprolactinemia or mass effect may be considered for surgical resection. Surgical cure rates for medically refractory prolactinomas are in the range 28–90%, with size being the most impor-

tant determinant of outcome. Radiation therapy is a third line treatment and may provide normalization of prolactin levels in half of those treated.

Somatotroph adenomas

Excess secretion of growth hormone (GH) causes acromegaly in adults and gigantism in prepubertal children. Elevated GH is caused by a pituitary tumor in 95% of cases. GH secreting adenomas account for approximately 20% of all pituitary adenomas and are more common in males. Diagnosis of GH secreting adenomas tends to be delayed, with nearly three-quarters being macroadenomas at the time of diagnosis, often with suprasellar extension or cavernous sinus invasion. The widespread consequences of prolonged elevations in GH can result in striking cosmetic changes. The clinical features of acromegaly include the typical skeletal overgrowth abnormalities of prognathism, frontal bossing, excessive sweating, increasing hand and foot size, impaired glucose tolerance and diabetes, hypertension, cardiomegaly, macroglossia, obstructive sleep apnea, and organomegaly. Patients often present for evaluation with complaints of new nerve entrapment syndromes, such as carpal tunnel, as well as headaches. In addition, they will often report changes in shoe or glove size, or that their wedding ring no longer fits. Surprisingly, people are often unaware of the gradual transformation in their facial features, which is retrospectively obvious when comparing old photographs, such as that found on a driver's license. In particular, the diabetes, hypertension, cardiomegaly, and enhanced growth of colon polyps place these patients at significantly increased risk for morbidity and mortality. Patients with elevated GH levels have a two- to threefold increase in expected mortality.

While elevations in GH are the primary causative factor in acromegaly, initial laboratory diagnosis is established with insulin-like growth factor 1 (IGF-1) (somatomedin). Because GH secretion is pulsatile, single random measurements of GH are not typically helpful. Instead, IGF-1 provides an integrative marker of average GH secretion and fasting IGF-1 level is the diagnostic test of choice for acromegaly. An oral glucose suppression test (OGST) may also be useful for diagnosis and is often helpful in monitoring initial response to therapy. In a normal patient, administration of an oral glucose load will suppress GH production. Failure of GH suppression with OGST may indicate acromegaly, although diabetes and liver and renal disease may confound results.

Although advances have been made in medical therapy for acromegaly, surgical resection is considered first line treatment in patients with GH secreting adenomas. Trans-sphenoidal resection provides safe and effective treatment, with rapid reduction of plasma GH levels. Surgical remission can be accomplished in 50–85% of patients with GH secreting adenomas, with cure more likely in smaller tumors. The 10-year recurrence rate after initial surgical remission is less than 10%. In those patients who do develop recurrence, a second attempt at resection is reasonable as repeat surgical remission can be achieved in up to 50% of cases. In cases of failure of surgical treatment, or in patients who are not surgical candidates, medical therapy can be effective. Bromocriptine has been demonstrated to normalize GH values in approximately 50% of patients, while only 20% will experience a reduction in tumor volume. Similarly, octreotide may achieve normal plasma GH levels in 66% of patients, with 30% achieving some tumor volume reduction. Pegvisomant acts on the liver as a GH receptor antagonist and therefore does not have direct effect on the tumor. However, it is effective in treating the clinical manifestations of acromegaly as normalization of plasma IGF-1 levels can be achieved in 97% of patients. It is important to mention that pegvisomant therapy should be considered as second line and should not be used in patients with mass effect from larger tumors. Radiation therapy remains a third line treatment for somatotroph adenomas and should be considered only for recurrent or residual tumors. Finally, while many of the symptoms of acromegaly can be alleviated with treatment, some disfiguring elements may be irreversible and the risk of morbidity and mortality may remain elevated above baseline.

Cushing disease

ACTH secreting adenomas account for 10–12% of pituitary adenomas. Cushing syndrome is the characteristic constellation of symptoms that results from hypercortisolism. Overall, the most common cause of Cushing syndrome is exogenous administration of corticosteroids. The most common source of endogenous overproduction of cortisol is ACTH secreting pituitary adenomas (Cushing disease), accounting for 60–80% of cases. Cushing disease is nine times more common in women than men. Other causes of Cushing syndrome include ectopic ACTH production (most commonly from small cell carcinoma of the lung), cortisol producing adrenal adenoma or carcinoma, and hypothalamic overproduction of cortisol releasing hormone (CRH).

The clinical presentation is secondary to the effects of hypercortisolemia, characterized by weight gain, hypertension, purple striae, hyperglycemia, hyperpigmentation, amenorrhea, thin skin, osteoporosis, and cognitive and psychiatric disturbances. Hyperpigmentation may first be observed on gingival mucosa and other mucous membranes, areolae, and scars. While the stereotypical pattern of weight gain is "truncal" obesity, a generalized pattern of obesity is more common. Psychiatric disturbances include depression, dementia, emotional lability, and psychoses. Metabolic disturbances seen in Cushing disease include hypokalemic alkalosis and glucose intolerance or diabetes mellitus.

EVIDENCE AT A GLANCE

PRO-OPIOMELANOCORTIN

The hyperpigmentation seen in Cushing patients is a result of both cross-reactivity of adrenocorticotropic hormone (ACTH) with melanocyte stimulating hormone (αMSH) receptors and increased plasma levels of MSH. Pro-opiomelanocortin (POMC) is a polypeptide hormone precursor that undergoes extensive tissue-specific post-translational processing via cleavage by enzymes known as prohormone convertases yielding as many as 10 biologically active peptides involved in diverse cellular functions. The encoded protein is synthesized mainly in corticotroph cells of the anterior pituitary, producing ACTH and lipoprotein beta. In other tissues, including the hypothalamus, placenta, and epithelium, all cleavage sites may be used, giving rise to peptides with roles in pain and energy regulation, melanocyte stimulation, and immune modulation. Increased circulating levels of ACTH in patients with Cushing disease may allow cross-reactivity with αMSH receptors. In addition, ACTH, upregulation of POMC transcription, and translation results in increases in the other gene products, including αMSH, resulting in elevated circulating plasma levels. Both of these mechanisms may contribute to the hyperpigmentation seen in patients with Cushing disease.

While elevations in plasma cortisol are the hallmark of this disease, a single elevated random level is insufficient for the diagnosis. Several methods exist for establishing an initial diagnosis of hypercortisolism. Once the diagnosis of Cushing syndrome is established, the source of the excess cortisol must be ascertained. It is important to remember that the most common cause of Cushing syndrome is iatrogenic administration of corticosteroids. However, the most common cause of endogenous hypercortisolism is ACTH secreting pituitary adenoma (Cushing disease), accounting for approximately 80% of cases.

★ TIPS AND TRICKS

DIAGNOSIS OF CUSHING SYNDROME AND CUSHING DISEASE
Tests for establishing hypercortisolism

- 24-hour urine free cortisol
- 11 p.m. salivary (nadir) cortisol
- Overnight low dose dexamethasone suppression test

  ○ 1 mg dexamethasone given at 11 p.m. should suppress 8 a.m. cortisol in normal patients
  ○ a.m. Serum cortisol <1.8 μg/dL rules out Cushing syndrome

  ○ a.m. Serum cortisol 1.8–10 μg/dL – equivocal
  ○ Failure to suppress cortisol to <10 μg/dL with low dose dexamethasone indicates Cushing syndrome

Tests for establishing source of hypercortisolism

- High dose dexamethasone suppression test
  ○ 8 mg dexamethasone given at 11 p.m. should suppress 8 a.m. cortisol to less than 50% of baseline in patients with ACTH secreting pituitary adenoma (Cushing disease)
  ○ Adrenal tumors and ectopic ACTH secreting tumors will not suppress even with high dose dexamethasone
- Corticotropin releasing hormone (CRH) test
  ○ Intravenous CRH will cause even further elevation of plasma ACTH and cortisol in patients with Cushing disease
  ○ CRH will have no effect in patients with adrenal tumors or ectopic ACTH production
- Measurement of serum ACTH levels
  ○ Elevated in Cushing disease or ectopic ACTH producing tumor (small cell lung cancer)
  ○ Depressed in adrenal adenoma/ carcinoma
- Abdominal CT/MRI to look for adrenal adenoma/carcinoma
- MRI of brain to look for pituitary adenoma
- Inferior petrosal sinus sampling

EVIDENCE AT A GLANCE

INFERIOR PETROSAL SINUS SAMPLING
The test with the greatest accuracy for differentiating between ectopic adrenocorticotropic hormone (ACTH) and Cushing disease is bilateral inferior petrosal sinus sampling. The test is performed by placing catheters in both inferior petrosal sinuses and in a peripheral vein and then

obtaining serial simultaneous samples of central and peripheral plasma ACTH concentration at 2 and 0 minutes before, and 3, 5, and 10 minutes after intravenous administration of cortisol releasing hormone (CRH). Inferior petrosal sinus sampling is only useful in patients with hypercortisolism and is used to determine the source of ACTH secretion. As a result of dilution during circulation, the highest concentration of ACTH should be found in the primary venous drainage of the source tumor. As the ACTH is distributed throughout the entire blood volume, the concentration gradient rapidly dissipates. When no suspected lesion can be found, catheters can be placed in the inferior petrosal sinus, which provides the primary venous drainage for the pituitary gland (the most common site of ACTH secreting tumors). If the concentration is higher in the inferior petrosal sinus than peripheral venous blood, then the source of excess ACTH must be the pituitary gland. The results are reinforced by the administration of CRH. In patients with Cushing syndrome, the prolonged hypercortisolemia will have suppressed the normal ACTH production from the pituitary gland and therefore the gland will not respond to CRH. Similarly, an ectopic ACTH producing tumor would also not respond to CRH. Therefore an increase in venous ACTH concentration within the inferior petrosal sinus compared with the periphery with a peak ratio of 2:1 before CRH or 3:1 after CRH points towards an ACTH secreting pituitary tumor as the cause for the hypercortisolemia. In experienced hands, the diagnostic accuracy approaches 100%.

The onset of clinical features of hypercortisolism may be rapid in patients with Cushing disease. Unlike with prolactinomas and acromegaly, patients with ACTH secreting pituitary adenomas often present to medical attention early and diagnosis is frequently made when tumors are less than 5 mm in diameter. This frequently results in diagnosis of Cushing disease even in patients with no visible pituitary lesion on MRI.

In cases of "MRI negative" Cushing disease, inferior petrosal sinus sampling may be particularly helpful in establishing the diagnosis and providing enough evidence for surgical exploration.

As with GH secreting adenomas, surgical resection is indicated in patients with ACTH secreting adenomas and has an overall remission rate of 74% after initial surgery. Surgical remission is more likely in microadenomas (90%) than macroadenomas (60%). Those patients who do not experience biochemical remission in the initial postoperative period may be considered for early surgical re-exploration. For failure of repeat trans-sphenoidal resection and total hypophysectomy, bilateral adrenalectomy may be an option. While hypercortisolemia will be cured in nearly 100% of patients, lifelong replacement of glucocorticoids and mineralocorticoids will be required. In addition, up to 30% of patients undergoing bilateral adrenalectomy may develop Nelson syndrome. In an effort to decrease the occurrence of Nelson syndrome, radiosurgery or radiation therapy is recommended of the pituitary fossa prior to adrenalectomy.

Fractionated radiation and stereotactic radiosurgery are both options for surgically refractory and recurrent Cushing disease. Medical therapy including ketoconazole, metyrapone, and aminoglutethimide can be effective in reducing serum cortisol, but these are considered as fourth line therapy and rarely result in normalization.

✋ CAUTION!

ADRENAL INSUFFICIENCY
As a result of long-term suppression of the normal hypothalamic–pituitary–adrenal axis, patients with Cushing disease are at significant risk for postoperative adrenal insufficiency. Measurement of serial serum levels is essential to monitor for cortisol nadir. All patients should be discharged from the hospital with a prescription for "rescue" hydrocortisone; even those who do not "crash" in the initial postoperative period. Phone calls from patients complaining of severe headache, fatigue, or "flu-like" symptoms must be taken seriously. These

patients should be directed to return to clinic or the emergency room to assess for adrenal insufficiency.

Thyrotroph adenomas

Thyrotropin (TSH) secreting adenomas are rare, accounting for approximately 1% of pituitary adenomas. Clinically, these patients present with signs and symptoms of hyperthyroidism including palpitations, atrial fibrillation, excessive sweating, heat intolerance, weight loss, hypervigilance, and tremors. These tumors may grow to be rather large by the time of diagnosis and patients may also have symptoms of mass effect including headaches and visual disturbances. Laboratory evaluation yields elevations in circulating T3 and T4 as well as TSH (secondary hyperthyroidism). Laboratory findings of secondary hyperthyroidism may also be seen in patients with peripheral insensitivity to thyroid hormone; however, these patients do not have the clinical features of hyperthyroidism that are present in patients with TSH secreting pituitary adenomas. Primary treatment is surgical resection. However, delays in diagnosis and the invasive nature of thyrotroph adenomas results in surgical cure rates of only 50–60%. Adjuvant therapy with octreotide and radiation therapy is frequently required.

Nonfunctioning pituitary adenomas

Nonfunctioning adenomas are characterized by the absence of clinical and biochemical evidence of hormone overproduction. However, the majority will stain for pituitary hormones, with the most common being gonadotropins (40–65%). In fact, only 20–40% of all nonfunctioning adenomas are true "null-cell" tumors. While nonfunctioning adenomas account for approximately 30% of all pituitary tumors, they comprise greater than 80% of macroadenomas. Patients with macroadenomas most commonly present with symptoms of mass effect, including headache, visual field disturbances (bitemporal hemianopsia), pituitary insufficiency, and cranial nerve palsies from extension into the cavernous sinus. Up to 10% of patients with nonfunctioning macroadenomas may present with pituitary apoplexy. As with all other pituitary tumors (excluding prolactinomas) the primary treatment remains surgical. However, these tumors tend to be larger upon diagnosis and thus more likely to extend into the cavernous sinuses and suprasellar region. Accordingly, complete resection may be significantly more challenging, requiring a much wider exposure and possibly resulting in higher morbidity.

✋ CAUTION!

PITUITARY APOPLEXY

- Rapid expansion of pituitary adenoma from hemorrhage or necrosis
- Presents with sudden onset of severe headache, visual disturbance (ophthalmoplegia and bitemporal hemianopsia), and syncope
- CT and/or MRI will demonstrate hemorrhage within pituitary mass
- Treatment involves emergent administration of corticosteroids and endocrine evaluation for panhypopituitarism and diabetes insipidus
- Neurologic deficit should prompt urgent surgical exploration and decompression
- Urgent surgery (within 7 days) results in significant improvement in visual and oculomotor deficits
- Shunting may be required for hydrocephalus secondary to third ventricular compression

---

Pituitary carcinoma is rare and is defined by the appearance of metastases. These tumors affect females more often than males, and most commonly arise from prolactin or ACTH secreting pituitary adenomas. Initially, pituitary carcinomas may resemble benign pituitary adenomas. However, they are characterized by frequent local recurrences as well as craniospinal and systemic spread through both hematogenous and lymphatic channels. Long-term survival is poor.

Craniopharyngioma

Craniopharyngiomas represent 2.5–4% of intracranial tumors. Their incidence is 0.5–2.0 cases per million per year and they are slightly more common among children, where they represent roughly 50% of sellar and suprasellar tumors. They have a bimodal distribution of age at diagnosis, the first being 5–10 years old, the second being 50–65 years of age. In a study conducted in 1980–2007, 5- and 10-year survival rates were 96% and 93%, respectively.

Craniopharyngiomas are thought to be derived from the embryologic invagination of stomodeal ectoderm from the posterior pharynx that later becomes the anterior pituitary. These tumors are classified as adamantinomatous or papillary depending on their histology. The adamantinomatous type is more common in children and is characterized by palisading columnar cells that resemble ameloblasts. Papillary craniopharyngioma are more common in adults, and histologically these have a mature stratified squamous epithelium. Grossly, these tumors contain solid and cystic components and most have elements of calcification. Craniopharyngiomas may be purely cystic or solid, or mixed cystic and solid. They are benign tumors; however, their frequent recurrence and location often makes them difficult to treat and contributes to significant morbidity.

Clinical presentation

Clinically, craniopharyngiomas compress the optic apparatus, hypothalamus, infundibulum, pituitary gland, and the floor of the third ventricle causing disturbances in vision, endocrinopathies, and hydrocephalus. These are seen both in children and adults; however, there are differences in presentation. Most children will present with headache, nausea, and vomiting; typical symptoms of hydrocephalus resulting from compression of the third ventricle. Visual fields are often reduced, often profoundly; however, this is a more subtle complaint in children, often manifest as decline in school performance or insistence on sitting close to the television. Endocrine abnormalities include delayed growth or short stature with obesity brought about by hypothalamic involvement. Other common endocrin-opathies seen in the presentation of pituitary tumors are less likely, such as galactorrhea, diabetes insipidus, hypothyroidism, and hypocortisolism. There are neurobehavioral changes that are commonly associated with craniopharyngioma also associated with compression of the hypothalamus. In children, these symptoms include abulism, psychomotor retardation, and short-term memory deficits.

Adults will commonly recognize visual field deficits and present with a variety of visual disturbances including visual field defects and scotomas caused by variable compression of the optic nerves, chiasm, and tracts. Signs and symptoms of hydrocephalus are less frequent in adults than in children. Neurobehavioral changes are also prominent in adults with craniopharyngioma. Many will present with a Korsakoff-like dementia characterized by hypersomnia and confusion. Still others will present with severe depression and apathy. The most common endocrinopathy in adults is gonadal failure manifested as loss of libido in men and secondary amenorrhea in women.

Surgical aspects of therapy

In general, the primary method of treatment is surgical resection. Survival rates after gross total resection (GTR) at 10 years are greater than 85% in many series. GTR is achieved in 80–90% of attempted cases with experienced neurosurgeons. Several different surgical approaches can be used including subfrontal, trans-sylvian, and trans-sphenoidal. Surgical approach is dictated by both the anatomy of the tumor and experience of the neurosurgeon.

Radiation therapy

Given their difficult location, proximity to several critical structures and gross adherence to these structures, GTR may not be possible without causing extreme morbidity with severe impairments to quality of life. If only a subtotal resection is achieved, recurrence rate is high with a 10-year survival rate of 25%. However, subtotal resection with adjuvant radiation therapy has a 10-year survival of 80%, nearly as effective as GTR. External beam therapy is typically used with 50–60 Gy fractionated over 6 weeks. Radiation therapy alone after biopsy is thought to be inferior to total resection or subtotal resection with postoperative radiation with 5- and 10-year survival rates of 60% and 50%. Stereotactic radiosurgery for craniopharyngioma has promising but inconclusive long-term results.

Intracystic therapy

Another approach, especially for large cystic lesions in those with newly diagnosed or recurrent disease, is stereotactic or open implantation of an intracystic catheter with a subcutaneous reservoir. This catheter can be used for cyst drainage, temporary relief of pressure caused by the cyst or direct installation, or chemotherapy (e.g. bleomycin, interferon) or radioactive compounds (p32) to delay the need or obviate external beam irradiation or more extensive surgery.

Recurrent craniopharyngioma can be treated surgically. In many cases postoperative scarring or radiation-induced changes cause tumor adherence to arteries and dura precluding their re-resection. In these cases, radiation therapy is indicated.

EVIDENCE AT A GLANCE

OPTIMAL MANAGEMENT
Outcome for children and adults with craniopharyngiomas is often suboptimal. Although both gross total resections and partial resections have resulted in relatively good disease control (ranging 70–90%), dependent on series, survivors often have significant sequelae. Complications of radical surgery include the need for lifelong hormonal replacement, severe (at times, life-threatening)) obesity in up to 30% of survivors, behavioral problems, blindness, seizures, and aneurysms. Radiation therapy may also cause endocrinologic sequelae, cognitive dysfunctions, late occurring strokes, and secondary neoplasms. There is no consensus on the "optimal" treatment for large, often cystic/multicystic lesions.

Rathke cleft cysts

Rathke cleft cysts (RCC) are non-neoplastic intrasellar lesions that arise from remnants of the primitive Rathke pouch in the intermediate lobe of the pituitary gland. In this aspect, they share a common origin with craniopharyngiomas and are thought by some to exist along a single pathologic spectrum which includes both RCC and craniopharyngioma. RCC are usually asymptomatic and are most commonly found incidentally. Autopsy series indicate an incidence of small asymptomatic RCC as high as 25%. Larger RCC can present with headaches, pituitary dysfunction, and visual disturbances. RCC may be difficult to distinguish from craniopharyngioma on MRI. However, RCC typically do not calcify, the presence of which should prompt the consideration of a craniopharyngioma. Trans-sphenoidal surgery can be considered for symptomatic lesions. As with craniopharyngioma, RCC contents usually resemble motor oil, but do not typically have the cholesterol crystals that are seen with craniopharyngioma. Surgical series have shown that partial excision or fenestration and drainage are as effective as GTR and may spare the patient some of the morbidity associated with a more aggressive surgical approach.

Complications of trans-sphenoidal surgery

Trans-sphenoidal surgery is considered one of the safest fields in modern neurosurgical practice with an overall mortality of less than 1%. Mortality is usually a result of catastrophic vascular injury or meningitis. While the overall morbidity is generally low, there are several important complications that warrant discussion. Of these, postoperative CSF leakage can present a particular problem as it places the patient at risk for meningitis and may be difficult to diagnose once the patient has left hospital. While these usually arise in the immediate postoperative period, they can arise from days to weeks after the original surgery and usually present with headache and often copious clear nasal drainage. While clinical diagnosis remains paramount, confirmation of CSF rhinorrhea is accomplished by laboratory analysis of the fluid for beta tau-transferrin. Once CSF leak is confirmed, re-exploration and reclosure is the most effective technique to ensure adequate repair. While lumbar drainage has been attempted, it is our experience that its efficacy is inconsistent.

Injury to the anterior or posterior pituitary, infundibulum, and hypothalamus are additional important complications that must be monitored for. While these injuries usually occur from direct surgical insults, they can also arise from postoperative hemorrhage or ischemia. The most common of these is diabetes insipidus, with permanent loss occurring in 2–3%. Frequent postoperative monitoring of fluid and electrolyte balance will allow for early recognition and treatment, if necessary, with DDAVP. Anterior pituitary loss can also be transient or permanent, and measurement of postoperative cortisol is important to ensure continued function. Hypothalamic complications may present later and include hyperphagia, poikilothermia, and memory loss.

Visual loss can arise from direct surgical trauma including aggressive traction and cautery as well as from ischemia. This most commonly occurs while attempting to dissect tumor away from the optic chiasm and usually presents immediately postoperatively. The advantage of the endoscope is that it allows for this dissection to occur under direct visualization, thus potentially decreasing the chance of injury. Delayed visual loss can also arise and is usually the result of compression from postoperative hematoma. Early recognition and evacuation are essential to preservation and recovery of normal visual function. Additional complications include vascular injury, most commonly to the carotids, which can be catastrophic and may require internal carotid artery sacrifice. While rare, this often can result in mortality and often be avoided by using only gentle traction when attempting to dissect tumor away from vascular structures.

Selected bibliography

Barahona MJ, Sojo L, Wägner AM, Bartumeus F, Oliver B, Cano P, *et al.* (2005) Determinants of neurosurgical outcome in pituitary tumors. *J Endocrinol Invest* **28**, 787–94.

Cavalheiro S, Di Rocco C, Valenzuela S, Dastoli PA, Tamburrini G, Massimi L, *et al.* (2010) Craniopharyngiomas: intratumoral chemotherapy with interferon-alpha – a multicenter preliminary study with 60 cases. *Neurosurg Focus* **28** (4), E12.

Devin JK, Blevins LS Jr. (2006) Endocrinologic approach to the evaluation and management of the patient undergoing surgery for a pituitary tumor. In: Schmidek HH, Roberts DW (eds) *Schmidek and Sweet Operative Neurosurgical Techniques*, 5th edn. Elsevier, Philadelphia, pp. 300–20.

Greenberg MS. (2010) Pituitary tumors. In: Greenberg MS (ed.) *Handbook of Neurosurgery*, 7th edn. Thieme Publishers, New York, pp. 633–65.

Jane JA Jr, Dumont AS, Vance ML, Laws ER Jr. (2005) Pituitary adenomas and sellar lesions: multidisciplinary management. In: Schiff D, O'Neill BP (eds) *Principles of Neuro-oncology*. McGraw Hill, New York, pp. 382–413.

Linnert M, Gehl J. (2009) Bleomycin treatment of brain tumors: an evaluation. *Anticancer Drugs* **29** (3), 157–64.

Locatelli D, Massimi L, Rigante M, Custodi V, Paludetti G, Castelnuovo P, *et al.* (2010) Endoscopic endonasal transsphenoidal surgery for sellar tumors in children. *Int J Pediatr Otorhinolaryngol* **74** (11), 1298–302.

Oldfield EH, Chrousos GP, Schulte HM, Schaaf M, McKeever PE, Krudy AG, *et al.* (1985) Preoperative lateralization of ACTH secreting pituitary microadenomas by bilateral and simultaneous inferior petrosal sinus sampling. *N Engl J Med* **312**, 100–3.

Osborn AG, Hedlund GL. (2007) Sella and pituitary. In: Osborn AG (ed.) *Diagnostic Imaging: Brain*. Amirsys, Salt Lake City, pp. II 2 1–36.

Steinbok P, Hukin J. (2010) Intracystic treatments for craniopharyngioma. *Neurosurg Focus* **28** (4), E13.

Zhang YQ, Ma ZY, Wu ZB, Luo SQ, Wang ZC. (2008) Radical resection of 202 pediatric craniopharyngiomas with special reference to the surgical approaches and hypothalamic protection. *Pediatr Neurosurg* **44** (6), 435–43.

Zhao R, Deng J, Liang X, Zeng J, Chen X, Wang J. (2010) Treatment of cystic craniopharyngioma with phosphorus-32 intracavitary irradiation. *Childs Nerv Syst* **26** (5), 669–74.

11

Meningiomas

Jeffrey Raizer and Wendy J. Sherman Sojka

Department of Neurology, Northwestern University, Chicago, IL, USA

Introduction

Meningiomas represent the most common primary intracranial tumor, accounting for approximately one-third of all primary central nervous system (CNS) tumors. They can present both symptomatically and as an incidental finding on cranial imaging or at autopsy. While most meningiomas are benign, the clinician needs to know the appropriate diagnostic steps to follow in order to allow for appropriate management.

Epidemiology

The Central Brain Tumor Registry of the United States reported that meningiomas account for more than 30% of all primary brain tumors, followed by glioblastomas (20%) and astrocytomas (9.8%). The estimate for meningiomas may be low given that many remain undiagnosed and are therefore not included in the registry.

The incidence of meningiomas increases with age. While benign meningiomas are much more common in women, atypical (grade II) and anaplastic meningiomas (grade III), the more aggressive subtypes, are slightly more common in men. As meningiomas are contiguous with the meninges, they can also occur within the spinal canal, but intracranial lesions are far more common.

Pathophysiology

Histologically, meningiomas are thought to arise from arachnoidal cap cells, most commonly within the arachnoid villi, but may be found throughout the arachnoid space. Most reports involve convexity or skull base tumors, though there have been rare case reports of intraventricular or intraosseous lesions. Because of their origin from arachnoidal cap cells, they have both epithelial and mesenchymal components, making their histologic differentiation from other tumor types difficult at times.

Why arachnoidal cap cells differentiate to become meningiomas has been studied and investigators are continuing to unmask aberrant signaling pathways responsible for this transformation, hoping to further guide targeted therapies. At this point in time, the pathway most implicated in meningioma tumorigenesis involves the *NF2* gene. Loss of heterozygosity for chromosome 22q results in *NF2* gene inactivation, a gene that codes for the Merlin protein, thought to be a tumor suppressor protein. Multiple other genes, proteins, and pathways have

Neuro-oncology, First Edition. Edited by Roger J. Packer, David Schiff.
© 2012 John Wiley & Sons, Ltd. Published 2012 by John Wiley & Sons, Ltd.

been potentially implicated in meningioma tumorigenesis, but not so convincingly as *NF2*. This area requires further research.

Other pathways implicated include:

- VEGF (angiogenesis)
- Hedgehog (embryogenesis)
- Notch (activation results in chromosomal instability
- mTORC1 (tumor suppression)

Classification

Meningiomas are classified according to the World Health Organization (WHO) II system. Their classification is based upon histologic features categorizing meningiomas into three groups. Grade I meningiomas are classified as having a low risk of recurrence and nonaggressive behavior, commonly referred to as benign. Grade II and III meningiomas have a higher likelihood of recurrence and behave more aggressively. Grade II meningiomas are referred to as atypical and grade III meningiomas as malignant. Within each grade, there are further subtypes (Table 11.1). Many of these features are seen on hematoxylin and eosin staining. Meningiomas stain for epithelial membrane antigen

(EMA), and higher grade tumors have increased mitotic activity.

The Simpson classification of surgical resection (Table 11.2), first described in 1957, is still used in combination with histologic grading to stratify risk of recurrence. The Simpson system describes five grades of resection, taking into account the extent of tumor removal, as well involvement of dura, bone, and venous sinuses.

Aside from histologic grade and Simpson classification of surgical resection, the third important component in determining likelihood of

Table 11.2. Simpson classification of surgical resection.

Simpson grade	Extent of resection
Grade I	Complete tumor removal with excision of dural attachment, +/– excision of bone/sinus
Grade II	Complete tumor removal with coagulation of dural attachment
Grade III	Complete tumor removal only
Grade IV	Partial tumor removal
Grade V	Biopsy only

Table 11.1. WHO II classification of meningiomas.

WHO Grade I	WHO Grade II	WHO Grade III
• Meningothelial • Fibrous (fibroblastic) • Transitional (mixed) • Psammomatous • Angiomatous • Microcystic • Secretory • Lymphoplasmacyterich • Metaplastic	• Atypical • Clear cell • Chordoid	• Rhabdoid • Papillary • Anaplastic (malignant) • Meningiomas of any subtype or grade with high proliferation index and/or brain invasion

recurrence is proliferation index. Proliferation index can be determined using multiple immunohistochemical stains, including Ki-67 and proliferating cell nuclear antigen (PCNA) indices.

> ★ **TIPS AND TRICKS**
>
> Recurrence risk factors include:
>
> - High proliferation index
> - Partial resection
> - Histologic grading

Etiology

Ionizing radiation is the environmental risk factor most strongly linked with the incidence of meningiomas. It has been found that the risk of meningioma is related both to the number of radiation treatments, as well as to the dosage used in radiation treatments. In a recent population-based study in Britain, in a cohort of 17,980 patients surviving at least 5 years after the diagnosis of childhood cancer, incidence of subsequent development of CNS tumors was compared with doses of both radiation and chemotherapy. It was found that the risk of developing meningiomas had a strong, linear, and independent relationship with dose of radiation received to the meninges, as well as to the dose of intrathecal methotrexate received. Specifically, compared with control subjects, radiation doses of 0.01–9.99, 10.00–19.99, 20.00–29.99, 30.00–39.99, and ≥40 Gy administered to the meninges was associated with a twofold, eightfold, 52-fold, 568-fold, and 479-fold increased risk, respectively.

Hormones have a strong association with meningiomas, a relationship supported by several findings including the presence of estrogen, progesterone, and androgen receptors seen on many meningiomas. Clearly, there is a well-established increased incidence in postpubertal women, with the highest incidence ratio of 3.15 : 1 during the peak reproductive years. Additionally, some studies have indicated that meningiomas change in size during the luteal phase of the menstrual cycle, as well as during pregnancy. Oral contraceptive use has not been found to be associated with an increased incidence of meningiomas; however, the potential association with hormone replacement therapy appears to be more controversial. In a large prospective study of over 1 million postmenopausal women, there was a relative risk of 1.34 (95% confidence interval [CI] 1.03–1.75) of meningioma in women being treated with hormonal replacement therapy when compared with non-users, suggesting a slightly increased risk. Finally, there is a report of a patient with multiple meningiomas, all of which regressed after cessation of estrogen agonist therapy.

Head trauma is a controversial risk factor for the development of meningiomas. While there are some small studies supporting an association, a large cohort study of 228,055 patients hospitalized with head trauma found no association, with an incidence ratio of 1.2 (95% CI 0.8–1.7). It is thought that the suspected association between head trauma and meningioma is secondary to a detection bias given the imaging that ensues following head injury.

Debates are currently ongoing regarding exposure to electromagnetic waves from cell phone use and their correlation with meningioma formation. Multiple studies have looked at the association between cell phone use and brain tumors. Currently there is no consensus. It is thought that the follow-up time has not been long enough at this point in the history of cell phone use to assess the association accurately, given previous studies have shown that time from radiation exposure to meningioma detection averages 20–40 years.

Clinical presentation

The clinical presentation of meningiomas varies widely and depends greatly on the specific location (Table 11.3). The most common presenting symptoms include headache and altered mental status. Additionally, when meningiomas overlie the cerebrum, they can lead to focal seizures, as well as transient neurologic symptoms which may resemble transient ischemic attacks. As imaging in medicine has exponentially increased, so has the number of incidental meningiomas found in asymptomatic patients with a normal neurologic examination.

Table 11.3. Location of meningioma and site-specific symptoms. From Raizer J, Sherman W. (2011) Meningiomas. In: Gilman S. (editor-in-chief) *Medlink Neurology*. MedLink Corporation, San Diego. Available at www.medlink.com. Accessed February 5, 2011. Reprinted with permission.

Tumor location	Relative incidence (%)	Site-specific symptoms
Convexity	34.7	Headaches, seizures, motor and sensory deficits
Parasagittal	22.3	*Anterior*: chronic headaches, memory and behavior changes *Middle:* motor and sensory deficits *Posterior:* homonymous hemianopsia *All:* venous occlusion
Sphenoid ridge	17.1	*Medial:* visual loss, CN III, IV, V1, VI palsies *Lateral:* headaches, seizures, motor and sensory deficits
Lateral ventricle	5.2	Headaches, seizures, hydrocephalus
Tentorium	3.6	Ataxia, headaches, visual loss, diplopia
Cerebellar convexity	4.7	Headaches, ataxia, dizziness, facial pain, dysarthria
Tuberculum sellae	3.6	Visual loss, headaches, optic atrophy, noncongruent homonymous hemianopsia
Optic nerve sheath	2.1	Visual loss
Cerebello-pontine angle	2.1	Hearing loss, headaches, ataxia, dizziness, tinnitus, facial palsy
Olfactory groove	3.1	Anosmia, Foster Kennedy syndrome, headaches
Foramen magnum	0.52	Nuchal and occipital pain, emesis, ataxia, dysphagia, motor and sensory deficits
Clivus	0.5	Headaches, emesis, ataxia, motor and sensory deficits
Other	0.5	

★ TIPS AND TRICKS

Frontoparietal parasagittal meningiomas may present with slowly progressive spastic weakness or numbness contralaterally, then bilaterally, followed by incontinence.

Imaging

Meningiomas have characteristic findings on both computed tomography (CT) and magnetic resonance imaging (MRI). As many meningiomas are found during work-up for headaches, they are first found on CT imaging. Characteristically, on CT imaging meningiomas are isointense with brain parenchyma, many demonstrating microcalcifications. Following administration of intravenous contrast, meningiomas show homogeneous enhancement. In particular, psammomatous meningiomas may have predominant calcifications that are best appreciated on CT imaging, as opposed to MRI. Additionally, CT imaging is also useful to determine bony involvement of meningiomas, specifically hyperostosis.

Gadolinium-enhanced MRI is the modality of choice in the diagnostic work-up. On T1 sequencing, meningiomas are typically isointense compared with brain parenchyma, similar to noncontrast CT imaging. The appearance of meningiomas on T2 sequencing is more variable. However, upon administration of gadolinium, meningiomas characteristically show intense homogeneous enhancement, usually with a significant "dural tail." Findings on MRI that are suggestive of a more aggressive tumor subtype include prominent edema, heterogeneous enhancement, and irregular borders. Shown in Figure 11.1 is an example of a benign meningioma, and in Figure 11.2 a malignant meningioma on contrast-enhanced MRI.

Perfusion MRI is being investigated for potential utility in differentiating extra-axial tumors. A small case series indicated that a dural-based tumor with low perfusion should suggest an alternative diagnosis, such as a dural metastasis, as most meningiomas demonstrate increased perfusion. Additionally, intraventricular tumors with low perfusion parameters should argue against the diagnosis of meningioma. As its utility is still being determined, it is not standard of care at present, but represents an additional imaging modality that may help with diagnosis and management.

Finally, cerebral angiography may help in presurgical planning, as well as in preparation for embolization prior to surgery.

Management

In determining the appropriate course of management for a patient presenting with a meningioma, the clinician must first make the determination as to whether the patient is symptomatic or asymptomatic. In asymptomatic patients with small meningiomas, many studies have demonstrated a slow growth rate, prompting many clinicians to monitor these with serial imaging every 1–2 years, initiating treatment

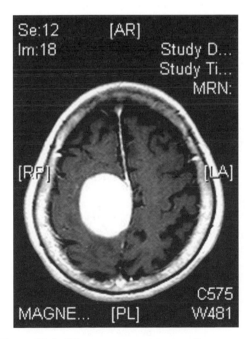

Figure 11.1. T1 post contrast magnetic resonance image (MRI) of a patient with a large grade I interhemispheric meningioma.

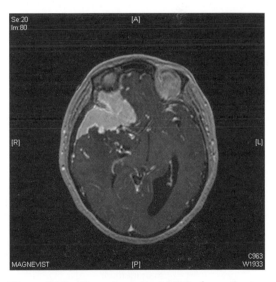

Figure 11.2. T1 post contrast MRI of a patient with a grade III right sphenoid ridge meningioma.

when there is evidence of growth or when patients become symptomatic.

Some institutions support being more aggressive in their management, even when lesions are small and asymptomatic. In a review of 22 studies, encompassing 675 patients, with median follow-up length of 4.6 years, tumors <2 cm in diameter only became symptomatic in 2% of patients. Additionally, 51% of untreated meningiomas ≤2.5 cm in diameter demonstrated no growth over the mean follow-up period of 4.6 years, with an additional 26% growing less than 10% per year. They found that the greatest risk for progression included tumors of 2–2.5 cm in initial diameter, tumor growth rate greater than 10% per year, or those tumors that were hyperintense on T2 sequencing. Tumors >2.5 cm were shown to subsequently develop new symptoms or have worsening of their pre-existing symptoms in 17% of patients. Based on this observed natural history of untreated meningiomas, though additional studies are warranted, meningiomas <2 cm in diameter without other characteristics or locations associated with increased aggressiveness may be imaged serially, monitoring for growth, development of symptoms, and encroachment upon adjacent structures. The optimal management for those tumors >2 cm in asymptomatic patients remains to be defined, but observation in most cases is likely reasonable (Figure 11.3).

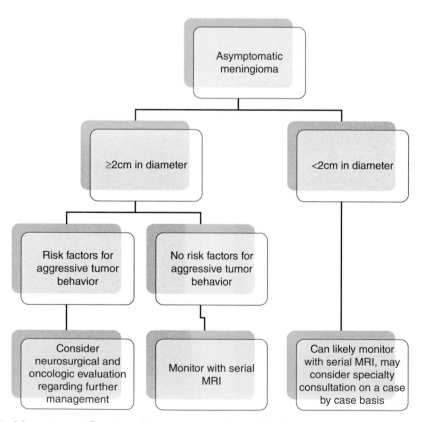

Figure 11.3. Management flowchart for asymptomatic meningiomas.

In regards to management of symptomatic WHO grade I meningiomas, surgical resection has historically been the treatment of choice, allowing confirmatory histology, relief of mass effect, and the chance of a cure in cases of total resection. This continues to be the treatment of choice for large meningiomas or those immediately adjacent to radiosensitive structures, such as structures of the optic pathway.

Stereotactic radiosurgery (SRS) has emerged as a reliable treatment modality in the management of meningiomas, with many groups demonstrating excellent control rates with good side-effect profiles. While SRS was initially used as adjuvant therapy or for recurrent disease, newer studies have indicated its use as a more definitive primary management strategy. In a large cohort of 972 patients treated with SRS, the overall control rate for benign meningiomas was 93%. After 10 years, WHO grade I tumors were controlled in 91%, demonstrating its utility in symptomatic, low risk benign meningiomas. SRS is an appealing option in that it minimizes the volume of irradiated normal brain tissue. One review advocated that SRS should be considered in patients with meningiomas involving critical neuronal or vascular structures, residual skull base tumor after surgery, and tumors where complete resection was not achieved.

Complications following SRS are uncommon, and most are transient. Most studies report a complication rate around 8%, with 3% being transient and 5% permanent. Complications seen include radiation effects seen on imaging, such as edema and necrosis, as well as cranial nerve dysfunction, depending on the location of the meningioma being irradiated, highest for parasellar or skull base tumors. Seizures have been reported following SRS, but appear to be relatively rare, with a higher incidence in those with seizures prior to treatment.

CAUTION!

Higher risk for cranial nerve dysfunction following stereotactic radiosurgery in parasellar or skull base tumors.

CAUTION!

Patients with seizure as part of their initial presentation should be continued on their anticonvulsant during surgery/radiation, as well as in the postoperative period, but not if a seizure was never documented.

Post-radiation edema has been reported in as many as 25% of patients after SRS, with risk factors for edema development including preexisting edema as well as larger tumor to brain surface area. Other risk factors identified include age >60 years, perilesional edema preceding SRS, no previous surgical resection, larger treatment volume, anterior cranial fossa location, and a higher margin dose.

★ TIPS AND TRICKS

Post-radiation edema is usually easily controlled with a short course of steroids.

Fractionated external beam radiotherapy (EBRT) is used as postoperative adjunctive therapy in the treatment of intracranial meningiomas. While prospective randomized data regarding the utility of EBRT in the management of intracranial meningiomas is lacking, retrospective studies have demonstrated improved progression-free survival when EBRT is used following subtotal resection. Additionally, EBRT is used as definitive treatment of unresectable tumors (i.e. optic nerve sheath meningiomas), as well as a method of obtaining local control in cases of anaplastic or atypical meningioma. The advantage over SRS of stereotactic fractionated EBRT is its feasibility in patients with adjacent radiosensitive normal structures who may benefit from dose-limitation.

Preoperative endovascular embolization is used is selected cases, namely tumors with angioblastic features, as well as those involving the skull base or critical vascular structures. Some studies also support its use in tumors that lie in surgically inaccessible areas, with the goal of reducing blood supply.

While most symptomatic meningiomas can be effectively treated with surgery and radiation, there is an evolving role for medical therapy, particularly when meningiomas are inoperable or in cases of recurrence when further surgery or radiotherapy is not an option. Medical modalities considered as potential therapies include chemotherapy, interferon, hormonal therapy, as well as newer targeted immunotherapies.

Chemotherapy has very limited use in meningioma management, with its primary use in cases of recurrent disease following surgery and radiotherapy. Many chemotherapies tested have had disappointing results, including temozolomide, dacarbazine, adriamycin, and ifosfamide with mesna. A small series of patients with malignant meningiomas achieved a modest benefit in survival with 3–6 cycles of cyclophosphamide, Adriamycin®, and vincristine, though patients suffered substantial toxicity following treatment.

Hydroxyurea, an oral ribonucleotide reductase inhibitor, has become standard therapy in meningiomas refractory to surgery and radiation. The mechanism by which hydroxyurea arrests meningioma cell growth is through arrest of the S phase of the cell cycle, thus inducing apoptosis. There have been debates as to whether some earlier studies truly showed slowed progression or rather reflected the natural course. A recent retrospective case series showed very limited benefit to therapy with hydroxyurea, with no radiographic response in any of 60 patients, with 35% having stable disease and 65% with progressive disease during follow-up. Combination therapy with hydroxyurea is currently under investigation.

Initial studies indicated a potential role for interferon alpha, which has been shown to inhibit meningioma cells *in vitro*. Repeated studies showed a mixed response, but given the lack of control data there is no consensus on the utility of interferon alpha in the management of meningiomas.

Hormonal receptors, first elucidated by the predominance of meningiomas in women during reproductive years, led to the use of hormonal therapy being investigated as a potential medical management option. Regarding the specific hormonal receptors, estrogen receptors are expressed in approximately 10% of meningiomas; progesterone and androgen receptors are present in approximately two-thirds of meningiomas. Additionally, progesterone receptors are most commonly found in benign meningiomas.

Estrogen receptor inhibitors, specifically tamoxifen, have not been shown to be effective in inhibition of meningioma growth. This has been explained by the presence of estrogen receptors in only 10% of meningiomas. Thus, as may have been expected, one study of 19 patients only saw a partial or minor response in three of the study participants.

On the other hand, the predominance of progesterone receptors in the meningioma population has created great interest in the potential efficacy of progesterone receptor inhibitors, namely mifepristone (RU486). Initially, some small studies demonstrated a small potential benefit, but this was refuted by a large prospective randomized multicenter study enrolling 180 patients to either daily mifepristone or placebo, which failed to show a benefit of mifepristone over placebo. It has been postulated that mifepristone may still be potentially efficacious as the majority of studies enrolled patients with meningiomas exhibiting increased proliferation index and of a higher histologic grade, as it has been shown that the incidence of progesterone receptors is markedly decreased in these meningioma subtypes. Many novel agents that target VEGF, PDGF, and other components of the MAPK pathway are being investigated with variable activity. Aside from medical therapies aimed at the tumor itself, medical therapy is also used commonly for symptoms associated with meningiomas. Anticonvulsant therapy is indicated preoperatively only if patients have had a seizure and should not be given prophylactically outside of the perioperative period. Furthermore, if patients are on anticonvulsant therapy preoperatively, the medication should be continued postoperatively if the patient initially presented with a seizure. Many physicians will monitor the patient on therapy for 6–12 months; at that point, if patients continue to be free of seizures, pending other social considerations at the physician's discretion, they can be tapered off their anticonvulsant. However, if they fail this taper, they will likely require anticonvulsant therapy throughout their lifetime.

Regarding corticosteroid therapy, corticosteroids may be required in short bursts to reduce edema following surgery or radiation. These are often not required long-term and should be tapered rapidly.

Summary

- Meningiomas are the most common intracranial tumor.
- While the overall prognosis is good, this greatly depends on the histologic subtype and location.
- Asymptomatic tumors <2 cm in diameter can often be monitored with serial imaging.
- Symptomatic tumors, tumors near critical structures, or ≥2 cm in diameter should be evaluated by a neurosurgeon for possible resection.
- Radiation may have a role depending on the extent of resection and tumor location.
- Medical therapy may be indicated in recurrent tumors, although evidence to confirm efficacy of a variety of different options is minimal.

Selected bibliography

Ahlbom A, Feychtling M, Green A, Kheifets L, Savitz DA, Swerdlow AJ; ICNIRP (International Commission for Non-Ionizing Radiation Protection) Standing Committee on Epidemiology (2009) Epidemiologic evidence on mobile phones and tumor risk: a review. *Epidemiology* **20** (5), 639–52.

Benson VS, Pirie K, Green J, Bull D, Casabonne D, Reeves GK, *et al.*; Million Women Study Collaborators (2010) Hormone replacement therapy and incidence of central nervous system tumours in the Million Women Study. *Int J Cancer* **127** (7), 1692–8.

Cai R, Barnett GH, Novak E, Chao ST, Suh JH. (2010) Principal risk of peritumoral edema after stereotactic radiosurgery for intracranial meningioma is tumor–brain contact interface area. *Neurosurgery* **66** (3), 513–22.

Central Brain Tumor Registry of the United States (CBTRUS) (2010) *CBTRUS Statistical Report: Primary brain and central nervous system tumors diagnosed in the United States in 2004–2006.* CBTRUS, Hinsdale, IL.

Chamberlain MC. (1996) Adjuvant combined modality therapy for malignant meningiomas. *J Neurosurg* **84** (5), 733–6.

Chamberlain MC, Johnston SK. (2011) Hydroxyurea for recurrent surgery and radiation refractory meningioma: a retrospective case series. *J Neurooncol* **104** (3), 765–71.

Gondi V, Tome WA, Mehta MP. (2010) Fractionated radiotherapy for intracranial meningiomas. *J Neurooncol* **99** (3), 349–56.

Goodwin JW, Crowley J, Eyre HJ, Stafford B, Jaeckle KA, Townsend JJ. (1993) A phase II evaluation of tamoxifen in unresectable or refractory meningiomas: a Southwest Oncology Group study. *J Neurooncol* **15** (1), 75 7.

Grunberg SM, Weiss MH, Russell CA, Spitz IM, Ahmadi J, Sadun A, *et al.* (2006) Long-term administration of mifepristone (RU486): clinical tolerance during extended treatment of meningioma. *Cancer Invest* **24** (8), 727–33.

Inskip PD, Mellemkjaer L, Gridley G, Olsen JH. (1998) Incidence of intracranial tumors following hospitalization for head injuries (Denmark). *Cancer Causes Control* **9** (1), 109–16.

Iwai Y, Yamanaka K, Ikeda H. (2008) Gamma Knife radiosurgery for skull base meningioma: long-term results of low-dose treatment. *J Neurosurg* **109** (5), 804–10.

Kawahara Y, Niro M, Yokoyama S, Kuratsu J. (2001) Dural congestion accompanying meningioma invasion into vessels: the dural tail sign. *Neuroradiology* **43** (6), 462–5.

Kleihues P, Cavenee WK; International Agency for Research on Cancer. (2000) *Pathology and Genetics of Tumours of the Nervous System. World Health Organization Classification of Tumours.* IARC Press, Lyon.

Kollová A, Liscák R, Novotný J Jr, Vladyka V, Simonová G, Janousková L. (2007) Gamma Knife surgery for benign meningioma. *J Neurosurg* **107** (2), 325–36.

Kondziolka D, Mathieu D, Lunsford LD, Martin JJ, Madhok R, Niranjan A, *et al.* (2008) Radiosurgery as definitive management of intracranial meningiomas. *Neurosurgery* **62** (1), 53–8; discussion 58–60.

Lamszus K. (2004) Meningioma pathology, genetics, and biology. *J Neuropathol Exp Neurol* **63** (4), 275–86.

McDermott MW. (2008) Meningiomas. In: Bernstein M, Berger MS. (Eds) *Neuro-oncology: The Essentials*, 2nd edn. Thieme, New York, pp. 307–19.

Nelson PK, Setton A, Choi IS, Ransohoff J, Berenstein A. (1994) Current status of interventional neuroradiology in the management of meningiomas. *Neurosurg Clin North Am* **5** (2), 235–59.

Ragel BT, Jensen RL. (2010) Aberrant signaling pathways in meningiomas. *J Neurooncol* **99** (3), 315–24.

Sadetzki S, Flint-Richter P, Ben-Tal T, Nass D. (2002) Radiation-induced meningioma: a descriptive study of 253 cases. *J Neurosurg* **97** (5), 1078–82.

Sheehan JP, Williams BJ, Yen CP. (2010) Stereotactic radiosurgery for WHO grade I meningiomas. *J Neurooncol* **99** (3), 407–16.

Simpson D. (1957) The recurrence of intracranial meningiomas after surgical treatment. *J Neurol Neurosurg Psychiatry* **20** (1), 22–39.

Sughrue ME, Rutkowski MJ, Aranda D, Barani IJ, McDermott MW, Parsa AT. (2010) Treatment decision making based on the published natural history and growth rate of small meningiomas. *J Neurosurg* **113** (5), 1036–42.

Taylor AJ, Little MP, Winter DL, Sugden E, Ellison DW, Stiller CA, *et al.* (2010) Population-based risks of CNS tumors in survivors of childhood cancer: the British Childhood Cancer Survivor Study. *J Clin Oncol* **28** (36), 5287–93.

Vadivelu S, Sharer L, Schulder M. (2010) Regression of multiple intracranial meningiomas after cessation of long-term progesterone agonist therapy. *J Neurosurg* **112** (5), 920–4.

Wen PY, Quant E, Drappatz J, Beroukhim R, Norden AD. (2010) Medical therapies for meningiomas. *J Neurooncol* **99** (3), 365–78.

Wiemels J, Wrensch M, Claus EB. (2010) Epidemiology and etiology of meningioma. *J Neurooncol* **99** (3), 307–14.

Zimny A, Sasiadek M. (2011) Contribution of perfusion-weighted magnetic resonance imaging in the differentiation of meningiomas and other extra-axial tumors: case reports and literature review. *J Neurooncol* **103** (3), 777–83.

12

Primary Central Nervous System Lymphomas

Jerome J. Graber[1] and Antonio M. P. Omuro[2]

[1]Department of Neurology and Oncology, Montefiore Medical Center of the Albert Einstein College of Medicine, New York, NY, USA
[2]Department of Neurology, Memorial Sloan-Kettering Cancer Center, New York, NY, USA

Introduction

Primary central nervous system lymphoma (PCNSL) is a non-Hodgkin lymphoma arising within the eyes, brain, spinal cord, and/or cerebrospinal fluid (CSF) without evidence of systemic disease outside the central nervous system (CNS). PCNSL occurs at an annual incidence of 0.46 cases per 100,000 person-years in the United States (about 1400 new cases annually) and accounts for approximately 2.4% of all primary brain tumors. The majority of cases occur in immunocompetent patients at a median age of 60 years. On pathologic examination, the vast majority of PCNSL is a diffuse large B-cell lymphoma (DLBCL) expressing the B-cell surface antigen CD20. The histologic appearance is undistinguishable from DLBCL occurring elsewhere in the body. The tumor cells display a typical angiocentric distribution and reactive T cells are common. In a minority of patients, other types of lymphoma can be found, including Burkitt, low grade, or T-cell lymphomas. Epstein–Barr nuclear antigen can be detected in tumor cells in most immunosuppressed patients. It is unknown if PCNSL originates systemically and migrates specifically to the CNS or originates directly within the CNS. Small studies have found genetic alterations in p16, p53, and CDKN2A, but the underlying cause of PCNSL in immunocompetent patients remains obscure.

Epidemiology

In patients who are immunosuppressed as a result of HIV infection, the cumulative risk of PCNSL is 2–7% over their lifetime. The median age at diagnosis is 30 years, and Epstein–Barr virus (EBV) is usually the cause in immunosuppressed patients as a result of EBV-mediated immortalization of proliferating B cells unchecked by T cells. In patients who are immunosuppressed for solid organ transplants, the risk is higher for heart, liver, and lung transplant than kidney (1–2%). EBV-related PCNSL has also rarely been reported in patients receiving immunosuppression for autoimmune diseases and in the elderly.

Presentation

The majority of PCNSL patients present with focal neurologic deficits or diffuse cognitive and behavioral changes; in some patients, particularly the elderly, symptoms are misdiagnosed as primary dementia, depression, and other psychiatric disorders. Other symptoms include headache, seizures, or visual symptoms resulting from ocular involvement. Patients with

Neuro-oncology, First Edition. Edited by Roger J. Packer, David Schiff.
© 2012 John Wiley & Sons, Ltd. Published 2012 by John Wiley & Sons, Ltd.

leptomeningeal involvement may have cranial nerve, radicular, or bladder symptoms.

Diagnosis

Magnetic resonance imaging (MRI) with gadolinium is the imaging modality of choice. In immunocompetent patients, MRI typically reveals solitary or multiple parenchymal lesions, with or without significant mass effect, which are hypointense or isointense on T1, with relatively homogeneous contrast enhancement. This pattern of contrast enhancement confers the typical "cotton" or "snowball" appearance (Figure 12.1). Lesions are usually periventricular, although they may occur anywhere within the neuraxis, including the spinal cord. Occasionally, heterogeneous patterns of contrast-enhancement and necrosis may be seen. Hypointense signal on T2-weighted MRI helps distinguish PCNSL from gliomas, which are typically hyperintense on T2. Diffusion-weighted imaging may show areas of restricted diffusion and decreased apparent diffusion coefficient corresponding to cell proliferation. Leptomeningeal involvement may be present, with various degrees of contrast enhancement with or without nodules in the cisterns, cranial nerves, and ependymal surfaces. Very rarely, patients may present with diffuse leukoencephalopathy on MRI without contrast enhancement.

The differential diagnosis is broad and includes other causes of enhancing brain lesions such as primary and metastatic brain tumors, as well as non-neoplastic diseases such as atypical and/or tumefactive demyelinating disease, other inflammatory diseases such as sarcoidosis and Behçet, and more rarely brain abscess, neurosyphilis, neurotuberculosis, fungal infection, and subacute ischemic stroke. It is important to look for history and imaging findings pointing to these alternative diagnoses, because some of these diseases may be managed without biopsy. MRI may also provide some diagnostic hints. An incomplete ring of enhancement with sparing of cortical regions may suggest tumefactive demyelinating lesions, particularly in the presence of other characteristic lesions of demyelinating disease seen on fluid attenuated inversion recovery (FLAIR) or T2 sequences. Tumefactive demyelinating lesions may also have a central vessel

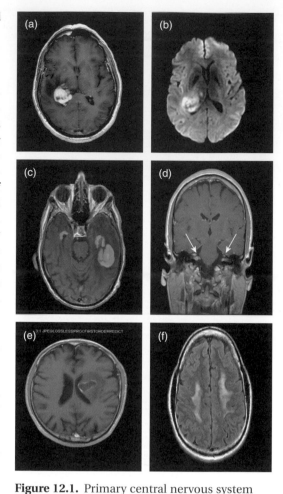

Figure 12.1. Primary central nervous system lymphoma (PCNSL) usually presents as a relatively homogeneous enhancing mass with a preferential periventricular distribution on T1 post-contrast magnetic resonance imaging (MRI) (a). Diffusion-weighted imaging shows areas of restricted diffusion (b) corresponding to cell proliferation. Lesions may be multifocal (c) and leptomeningeal involvement (d) with cranial nerve enhancement (arrows) may be present. In patients with untreated HIV infection, PCNSL may present with necrotic or hemorrhagic lesions with heterogeneous enhancement (e), mimicking toxoplasmosis abscess. After treatment with radiation or chemotherapy, patients may develop treatment-related leukoencephalopathy, seen as white matter hyperintense signal on FLAIR (f).

on MRI perfusion imaging. Predominance of a gyral pattern of enhancement is seen in subacute ischemic stroke. Rarely, PCNSL patients may present with isolated leptomeningeal involvement, and the differential includes other causes of chronic meningitis.

☆ **TIPS AND TRICKS**

Look for the following diagnostic clues that may point to an alternative diagnosis rather than PCNSL:

- Onset in young adults (think AIDS and other infectious or inflammatory diseases)
- Past history of subtle and transient neurologic deficits, including transient visual symptoms; open ring enhancement on MRI (multiple sclerosis)
- Personal or family history of autoimmune/inflammatory diseases (multiple sclerosis, Behçet, sarcoidosis)
- Sudden onset, gyral pattern of enhancement (subacute stroke)
- Sexual risk behavior, IV drug addiction (AIDS, syphilis, brain abscess)
- History of contact with tuberculosis
- Chronic fever, recent dental procedures or ears/nose/throat infections (brain abscesses)
- Presence or history of oral and genital ulcers (Behçet, syphilis) and uveitis (Behçet)
- Dental abscess (brain abscess); oral candidiasis (AIDS, immunosuppression)
- Skin rashes (Behçet, sarcoidosis, AIDS)
- Abnormalities on body CT scan (sarcoidosis, tuberculosis, fungal infections)

The differential in immunosuppressed patients is more difficult, and usually CNS toxoplasmosis or other infections are the first consideration, particularly in recently diagnosed, untreated, or refractory HIV infection. PCNSL in these patients present more often as multiple, heterogeneously enhancing lesions with areas of necrosis (Figure 12.1e). Tumors are most typically located in the cerebral hemispheres or corpus callosum in contact with the periventricular space, but less frequently lesions may occur in the deep white or gray matter, spinal cord, or leptomeningeal spaces. Hemorrhage or calcification in PCNSL is uncommon, but may be more frequent in patients with HIV. Some experts advocate treating ring enhancing lesions as toxoplasmosis in AIDS patients with positive toxoplasmosis serology and only pursuing biopsy if antitoxoplasmosis treatment is unsuccessful. However, such practice has been increasingly abandoned in the highly active antiretroviral therapy (HAART) era, as specific and early treatment may be curative, and biopsy for appropriate management is usually indicated. In HIV patients on HAART with relatively intact immunologic function, the imaging and clinical course of PCNSL may be indistinguishable from PCNSL in immunocompetent patients, with patients presenting with the typical homogeneously enhancing lesions rather than necrotic tumors.

Advanced imaging techniques may be helpful, disclosing signs of neoplastic disease, although the differential with other types of tumor may be difficult. On magnetic resonance perfusion, PCNSL is usually characterized by mildly increased relative cerebral blood volumes (rCBV). This may help in the differentiation from malignant gliomas and brain metastasis, which usually have much higher rCBV values. Infectious diseases such as CNS abscesses and toxoplasmosis tend to have lower rCBVs, but overlap may occur. Magnetic resonance spectroscopy typically shows decreased N-acetyl-aspartate and creatine with elevated choline, lactate, and lipids; however, this does not distinguish PCNSL from gliomas or metastases. Choline to creatinine peak ratios may be helpful, being lower than those found in malignant gliomas, but higher than ratios in solid metastases or infections; however, some overlap occurs. The presence of amino acid peaks suggests brain abscess rather than neoplastic disease. F-18 fluorodeoxyglucose positron emission tomography (FDG PET) shows higher metabolic levels in PCNSL than non-neoplastic diseases, although rarely some infectious and inflammatory diseases may be FDG-avid.

When PCNSL is suspected on neuroimaging, patients should be evaluated for potential sources of histologic diagnosis that could allow avoiding a neurosurgical procedure, including CSF analysis and slit lamp ophthalmologic examination. Corticosteroids can produce rapid clinical and radiographic improvement in PCNSL, but whenever possible they should be avoided prior to diagnostic confirmatory procedures in order to avoid a masking effect associated with rapid tumor lysis. In the absence of contraindication (such as significant mass effect), a lumbar puncture should be obtained. In addition to routine exams, CSF should be sent for cytology, lactate dehydrogenase (LDH) levels, EBV by polymerase chain reaction (in immunosuppressed patients), as well as fluorescence assisted cell sorting (FACS, sometimes referred to as flow cytometry) and polymerase chain reaction (PCR) for immunoglobulin gene rearrangement. CSF cytology is diagnostic when clearly positive for lymphoma cells, but often results only disclose nondiagnostic suspicious or reactive cells. FACS stains surface proteins of cells with fluorescent tags, allowing them to be identified at the single cell level; some studies have suggested superior sensitivity in the detection of lymphoma cells in the CSF in comparison to conventional cytology examination. Gene rearrangement studies may also be diagnostic in B-cell lymphomas. Normal B cells should have a varied repertoire of immunoglobulins produced by immunoglobulin gene rearrangement during development so that immunoglobulin can bind a variety of antigens. Tumor cells reproduce clonally from a single source, thus they all bear an identical rearranged immunoglobulin gene which can be identified by PCR amplification. T-cell receptor PCR can be used for patients with T-cell lymphomas. However, this technique is prone to both false negative and positive results because of relative paucity of T-cell receptor genes and occasional presence of oligoclonality in healthy individuals. While no single CSF test is universally positive, analysis for all possible signs of PCNSL can improve the diagnostic yield and may obviate the need for biopsy. Planning which tests need to be performed and sending enough fluid in the optimal condition for rapid analysis can increase the yield of lumbar puncture for diagnosis.

✋ CAUTION!

1. When PCNSL is suspected, slit lamp ophthalmologic examination and lumbar puncture (if not already done) should be promptly performed, as vitreous analysis and CSF may be diagnostic and avoid the need for brain biopsy.
2. When PCNSL is suspected, corticosteroids should be avoided prior to histologic confirmation. Corticosteroids can produce rapid tumor lysis, decreasing the chances of obtaining diagnostic CSF cytology and biopsy. If corticosteroids have been inadvertently administered prior to the diagnostic procedure, they should be discontinued prior to the procedure if possible. In cases of life-threatening cerebral edema, however, corticosteroids cannot be withheld and lumbar puncture should be avoided.

★ TIPS AND TRICKS

Staging for PCNSL should be completed promptly to avoid delays in treatment. If not done previously, the following should be obtained:

- Lumbar puncture with CSF cytology and, if possible, flow cytometry and gene rearrangement PCR studies
- Slit lamp examination (and vitrectomy if ocular lymphoma is suspected)
- Bone marrow biopsy
- CT of the chest, abdomen and pelvis (+/- whole body FDG PET scan)
- Anti-HIV testing
- LDH (may have prognostic implications)
- Repeat brain MRI with and without contrast (these tumors may grow rapidly without treatment and may also shrink rapidly with corticosteroids, so it is important to obtain an accurate baseline as close to start of treatment as possible)

Because up to 20% of PCNSL patients may have ocular involvement, slit lamp ophthalmologic examination is indicated in all patients. Primary intraocular lymphoma without brain, spine, or CSF involvement may occur, and encompasses 20% of cases of PCNSL. Of those, 60–80% of patients will eventually develop brain or CSF disease within 2 years. Ocular involvement usually presents with visual blurring or floaters, and vitrectomy may be diagnostic. Elevated vitreous levels of IL-10 may also provide a diagnostic clue but is non-specific.

If the diagnosis of PCNSL cannot be established by either CSF analysis or vitrectomy, a biopsy is indicated. Neurosurgeons and pathologists should be advised ahead of surgery when PCNSL is suspected, and the procedure of choice is usually stereotactic biopsy. Unlike gliomas and other brain tumors, attempts for complete tumor resection or tumor debulking are not indicated because PCNSL diffusely infiltrates the brain, even in normal-appearing areas on the MRI, and therefore focal therapies are not beneficial. All efforts should be made to avoid biopsies in eloquent areas of the brain, as tumors often infiltrate, rather than displace, potentially viable brain tissue that can be permanently damaged by the surgical procedure. Neurologic deficits caused by the tumor are usually reversible with chemotherapy or radiation, but many patients with PCNSL are left with permanent deficits as a result of poorly planned surgical procedures rather than disease, particularly when thalamic, internal capsule, or spinal cord lesions are biopsied.

Management

Once the diagnosis is established, a complete disease staging should be performed, including computed tomography (CT) of the chest, abdomen, and pelvis and testing for HIV infection; some authors recommend bone marrow biopsy and a body FDG PET scan. FDG PET may identify hypermetabolic occult sites of systemic lymphoma in up to 10% of patients. However, caution should be exerted as FDG PET may result in false positive findings, and lead to unnecessary diagnostic procedures for investigation of incidental FDG-avid lesions, which may inad-

vertently delay the start of treatment of PCNSL. In men, the possibility of occult testicular lymphoma should be considered, as testicular lymphoma has a predilection for CNS metastases. Patients with evidence of systemic lymphoma will require treatment for both systemic and CNS disease, because most systemic agents do not adequately penetrate the blood–brain barrier.

After initial work-up is completed, rapid initiation of treatment is recommended. Response to therapy is defined by changes in size of the enhancing areas on MRI. When present, responses to treatment are usually dramatic, with rapid decreases in size of contrast enhancement accompanied by symptomatic improvement. The goal of treatment is obtaining a complete resolution of contrast enhancement; however, interpretation of post-treatment scans can be sometimes difficult as areas of T1 hyperintensity on pre-gadolinium images may develop, mimicking persistent tumor, or small areas of contrast enhancement surrounding the original biopsy site may persist, even in patients successfully treated; close follow-up in those situations is advised. FLAIR abnormalities are usually persistent or may increase in successfully treated patients as a result of chemotherapy and radiotherapy; FLAIR sequences are thus not used for response evaluation. During treatment, careful neurologic supportive care is important.

✋ CAUTION!

1. Prophylactic use of anticonvulsants is usually not recommended. If needed, nonenzyme inducing anticonvulsants are usually preferred in patients undergoing chemotherapy. However, patients undergoing chemotherapy for PCNSL may develop renal failure, and attention should be made to adjust doses of anticonvulsants and other medicines that are renally excreted (e.g. levetiracetam) according to creatinine clearance, particularly in the elderly. These and other medications are a common cause of somnolence and delirium in PCNSL patients.

2. Patients with PCNSL and other brain tumors are prone to develop deep vein thrombosis and serious infections even before receiving chemotherapy. Measures to improve circulation and encourage mobilization should be instituted and subtle symptoms of thrombosis and infection should be assessed and explored frequently to avoid additional morbidity and mortality from these complications. *Pneumocystis* prophylaxis should always be considered, especially in patients on high dose steroids.

Chemotherapy is currently the mainstay of treatment for PCNSL. Most chemotherapies used in systemic lymphoma do not adequately penetrate the blood–brain barrier. However, studies have repeatedly demonstrated the efficacy of high dose methotrexate-based chemotherapy in PCNSL, with or without radiation. To penetrate the blood–brain barrier, methotrexate must be given at high doses (usually above $3\,g/m^2$), which can produce significant toxicity, requiring inpatient administration and monitoring. Methotrexate is renally excreted, and careful alkalinization of urine is used to avoid serious nephrotoxicity. Leucovorin, a methotrexate antidote that does not penetrate the blood–brain barrier well, is given to decrease the systemic toxicity without rescuing tumor cells. Methotrexate levels are obtained daily after the treatment administration, and patients are discharged once methotrexate has been cleared. Potential toxicities include renal, liver, and hematotoxicity, as well as leukoencephalopathy. Other cytotoxic drugs are usually administered in combination with methotrexate, including cytarabine, vincristine, procarbazine, etoposide, BCNU, and others. More recently, rituximab, a monoclonal antibody against CD20 surface protein expressed on tumor B cells, has been added to several regimens. Available studies suggest disease control rates with combination regimens are higher than methotrexate alone, although the optimal regimen remains controversial. In general, high dose methotrexate regimens achieve good response rates, with up to 80% of patients demonstrating tumor shrinkage, with a variable duration of response. Some authors advocate adding intrathecal chemotherapy with drugs such as methotrexate or cytarabine to high dose methotrexate treatments. However, such practice is controversial, especially given complications of Ommaya reservoir placement and drug administration. The authors' practice has been to restrict the use of intrathecal therapy to patients with obvious leptomeningeal disease on MRI or positive CSF cytology.

SCIENCE REVISITED

Methotrexate exerts antitumor activity through competition with folic acid for binding to the enzyme dihydrofolate reductase, impeding folate conversion to tetrahydrofolate and subsequent nucleotides, DNA, RNA, and protein, important for cell replication in S phase. Leucovorin (folinic acid) is a reduced form of folic acid that does not require reduction by dihydrofolate reductase, bypassing the pathway inhibited by methotrexate. Because leucovorin does not cross the blood–brain barrier well, it is used to rescue systemic bone marrow and gastrointestinal cells from the effects of high dose methotrexate.

CAUTION!

Patients undergoing treatment with intrathecal chemotherapy should be continuously evaluated for worsening of symptoms that could point to possible complications such as leukoencephalopathy, arachnoiditis, hydrocephalus, and infectious meningitis.

Historically, whole-brain radiotherapy had been used for PCNSL, initially as single modality, then as a consolidation treatment following methotrexate-based chemotherapy. However, treatment with standard doses of whole-brain radiotherapy (36–45 Gy) has been increasingly abandoned because of a high incidence of delayed chronic neurotoxicity, especially in the elderly. Neurotoxicity of brain radiation manifests as progressive leukoencephalopathy with frontal-subcortical dementia, abnormal gait, and urinary incontinence, sometimes mimicking normal pressure hydrocephalus. MRI shows diffuse, confluent symmetrical T2/FLAIR white matter changes with atrophy, though clinical and MRI findings often do not correlate well (Figure 12.1f). The deleterious effects of radiotherapy are thought to result from oxidative stress, demyelination, vasculopathy, and destruction of oligodendroglial and perhaps neuronal progenitor cells. Radiation injury is cumulative over time, which explains the delay in symptom onset (from a few months to several years) and the higher incidence in long-term survivors. Severity also varies from mild short-term memory deficits to profound dementia, which can be fatal. According to the regimen used and survival achieved, up to 25–30% of patients treated with conventional whole-brain radiation and chemotherapy develop significant dementia. This incidence increases to 90–100% in elderly patients over 50 years who achieve long-term survival. Cerebrovascular events are also another possible complication of radiation. In spite of all these adverse effects, whole-brain irradiation remains one of the most effective modalities for improving tumor control. Radiotherapy remains largely used in patients intolerant or unresponsive to chemotherapy and at relapse. There is also a relative consensus currently that newly diagnosed elderly patients should avoid radiotherapy and be treated with chemotherapy only. However, the use of radiotherapy in newly diagnosed young patients remains controversial. Chemotherapy-only treatments result in increased relapse rates, but patients can usually be salvaged with additional chemotherapy and radiation. However, the impact of such relapses and salvage therapies on cognitive function, and how that compares with cognitive function from radiotherapy given upfront, remains to be determined. Current studies are testing whether reduced dose whole-brain radiation can be as effective and less toxic as conventional doses. Other consolidation treatment options to replace radiotherapy are being explored, including high dose chemotherapy with stem cell transplant. It is also noteworthy that, because of the diffusely infiltrative nature of

PCNSL, focal radiotherapy and stereotactic radiosurgery are not generally indicated in this disease.

CAUTION!

Radiation therapy produces significant responses in the majority of patients with PCNSL. However, risk of neurotoxicity is high, particularly in the elderly. Patients present with a progressive leukoencephalopathy with subcortical dementia, shuffling gait, and urinary incontinence months to years later mimicking disease recurrence. Diffuse white matter abnormalities are seen on MRI, though MRI findings do not always correlate with clinical dementia. Leukoencephalopathy is less common but can occur with methotrexate chemotherapy alone, especially when given intrathecally.

EVIDENCE AT A GLANCE

Changes in PCNSL treatment over time:

- 1980s: Whole brain radiation found to produce responses in PCNSL, but high relapse rates and poor survival
- 1990s: First studies suggesting survival benefit of adding high-dose methotrexate to radiotherapy
- 1998: Recognition of high rate of neurotoxicity in survivors of PCNSL, especially those older than 60 years
- 2000s: Studies of high dose chemotherapy with stem cell transplant demonstrate efficacy in recurrent PCNSL. Studies of chemotherapy-only regimens in the elderly show similar progression-free survival and overall survival when compared with chemotherapy with whole-brain radiotherapy
- 2009: Combination chemotherapy with methotrexate and cytarabine demonstrated to be superior to single-agent methotrexate in a randomized trial, validating the use of polychemotherapy regimens over single-agent treatments.

- 2010: A randomized phase 3 study suggests that deferring radiotherapy after chemotherapy decreases progression-free survival but not overall survival

The ideal treatment regimen for primary intraocular lymphoma also remains to be determined. Ocular irradiation remains the most commonly used treatment, but there is a risk of radiotherapy-related retinopathy. Intraocular chemotherapy with drugs such as methotrexate, cytarabine, and rituximab may also produce responses, but the long-term efficacy remains undetermined. It is also unclear whether the addition of IV high dose methotrexate reduces the risk of brain and CSF recurrence in patients with ocular PCNSL.

Prognosis

Prognosis is highly variable in PCNSL. The likelihood of survival depends on several factors and one-quarter of patients will achieve long-term survival (>5 years). Age and Karnofsky performance status (KPS) are the most important prognostic factors and have been confirmed in multiple studies. A KPS of 70 is defined as patients unable to work but able to support their activities of daily living. These two factors form the basis for the Memorial Sloan-Kettering Cancer Center (MSKCC) prognostic score, which classifies patients by recursive partitioning analysis (RPA). Class 1 RPA includes patients younger than 50 years who have a median progression-free survival of 2 years. Class 2 RPA corresponds to patients older than 50 years but with a KPS ≥70. These patients have a median progression-free survival of 1.8 years. Class 3 RPA patients are older than 50 years, have a KPS <70, and have a median progression-free survival of only 0.6 years. The presence of Bcl-6 protein in tumor cells may also favorably predict responsiveness to chemotherapy and overall prognosis. Initial radiologic response to corticosteroids may also indicate a better prognosis. During treatment, increasing apparent diffusion coefficient values may also correlate with response to treatment. Some studies have also suggested that patients treated in referral centers tend to fare better than patients in smaller centers. Thus, referring PCNSL patients to experienced centers and participation in clinical trials should be encouraged, as therapy is not without potentially serious side effects, is difficult to manage, and a number of important questions remain unanswered.

Treatment for immunosuppressed PCNSL patients is similar to immunocompetent patients, although chemotherapy administration may be more difficult. Reversing the cause of immunosuppression, if possible, helps improve outcomes. In HIV-related PCNSL, institution of retroviral therapy to restore immune function is essential, and agents should be chosen that will be compatible with chemotherapy (especially in regard to renal function with methotrexate). The use of radiotherapy may add to long-term cognitive dysfunction seen in HIV infected patients. In patients who are immunosuppressed because of autoimmune disease or after solid organ transplant, reversal of immunosuppression may improve outcomes, but this is a complex decision that should be made in cooperation with their medical team. Rituximab is an interesting drug to consider adding to the chemotherapy regimens in these patients because of its immunosuppressant properties. Antiviral therapies against EBV do not appear beneficial.

For rare types of PCNSL other than DLBCL, treatment and prognosis vary and data are limited by the extreme rarity of cases. T-cell lymphomas are treated similarly, but may be associated with a better prognosis than DLBCL. Low grade marginal zone lymphomas usually present as slow-growing dural-based masses mimicking meningiomas. These tumors are thought to lie outside the blood–brain barrier and therefore do not technically correspond to PCNSL, although brain parenchyma and CSF invasion may occasionally occur. When no CNS invasion is detected, these patients may achieve long-term disease control with focal radiotherapy at reduced doses. Intravascular lymphomas are especially challenging to diagnose, as they present with intermittent neurologic deficits that can mimic multiple sclerosis, CNS vasculitis, or stroke. The prognosis in those patients is poor.

Select bibliography

Abrey LE, Ben-Porat L, Panageas KS, Yahalom J, Berkey B, Curran W, *et al.* (2006) Primary central nervous system lymphoma: the Memorial Sloan-Kettering Cancer Center prognostic model. *J Clin Oncol* **24**, 5711–5.

Abrey LE, Yahalom J, DeAngelis LM. (2000) Treatment for primary CNS lymphoma: the next step. *J Clin Oncol* **18**, 3144–50.

Batchelor T, Carson K, O'Neill A, Grossman SA, Alavi J, New P, *et al.* (2003) Treatment of primary CNS lymphoma with methotrexate and deferred radiotherapy: a report of NABTT 96-07. *J Clin Oncol* **21**, 1044–9.

DeAngelis LM, Seiferheld W, Schold SC, Fisher B, Schultz CJ; Radiation Therapy Oncology Group study 93-10. (2002) Combination chemotherapy and radiotherapy for primary central nervous system lymphoma. *J Clin Oncol* **20**, 4643–8.

Ferreri AJ, Reni M, Foppoli M, Martelli M, Pangalis GA, Frezzato M, *et al.* (2009) High-dose cytarabine plus high-dose methotrexate versus high-dose methotrexate alone in patients with primary CNS lymphoma: a randomized, phase II trial. *Lancet* **374**, 1512–20.

Graber JJ, Omuro A. (2011) Pharmacotherapy in primary CNS lymphoma: progress beyond methotrexate? *CNS Drugs* **25**, 447–57.

Hoang-Xuan K, Chinot OL, Taillandier L. (2003) Treatment of primary central nervous system lymphoma in the elderly. *Semin Oncol* **30**, 53–7.

Illerhaus G, Marks R, Ihorst G, Guttenberger R, Osterlag C, Derigs G, *et al.* (2006) High-dose chemotherapy with autologous stem-cell transplantation and hyperfractionated radiotherapy as first-line treatment of primary CNS lymphoma. *J Clin Oncol* **24**, 3865–70.

Küker W, Nägele T, Korfel A, Heckl S, Thiel E, Bamberg M, *et al.* (2005) Primary central nervous system lymphomas (PCNSL): MRI features at presentation in 100 patients. *J Neurooncol* **72**, 169–77.

Nelson DF, Martz KL, Bonner H, Nelson JS, Newall J, Kerman HD, *et al.* (1992) Non-Hodgkin's lymphoma of the brain: can high dose, large volume radiation therapy improve survival? Report on a prospective trial by the Radiation Therapy Oncology Group (RTOG): RTOG 8315. *Int J Radiat Oncol Biol Phys* **23**, 9–17.

Omuro A, Taillandier L, Chinot O, Sierra Del Rio M, Carnin C, Barrie M, *et al.* (2011) Primary CNS lymphoma in patients younger than 60: can whole-brain radiotherapy be deferred? *J Neurooncol* **104**, 323–30.

Omuro AM, Leite CC, Mokhtari K, Delattre JY. (2006) Pitfalls in the diagnosis of brain tumours. *Lancet Neurol* **5**, 937–48.

Pels H, Schmidt-Wolf IGH, Glasmacher A, Schulz H, Engert A, Diehl V, *et al.* (2003) Primary central nervous system lymphoma: results of a pilot and phase II study of systemic and intraventricular chemotherapy with deferred radiotherapy. *J Clin Oncol* **21**, 4489–95.

Soussain C, Hoang-Xuan K, Taillandier L, Fourme E, Choquet S, Witz F, *et al.* (2008) Intensive chemotherapy followed by hematopoietic stem-cell rescue for refractory and recurrent primary CNS and intraocular lymphoma: Societe Francaise de Greffe de Moelle Osseuse-Therapie Cellulaire. *J Clin Oncol* **26**, 2512–8.

Thiel E, Korfel A, Martus P, Griesinger F, Rauch M, Röth A, *et al.* (2010) High-dose methotrexate with or without whole brain radiotherapy for primary CNS lymphoma (G PCNSL-SG-1): a phase 3, randomised, non-inferiority trial. *Lancet Oncol* **11**, 1036–47.

13

Intradural Spinal Cord Tumors

Ben Shofty[1], Akiva Korn[2], Zvi Lidar[3] and Shlomi Constantini[1]

[1]Department of Pediatric Neurosurgery, The Gilbert Israeli Neurofibromatosis Center (GINFC), Dana Children's Hospital, Tel Aviv Medical Center, Tel Aviv, Israel
[2]Department of Pediatric Neurosurgery, Dana Children's Hospital, Tel Aviv Medical Center, Tel Aviv, Israel
[3]Spine Unit, Department of Neurosurgery, Tel Aviv Medical Center, Tel Aviv, Israel

Introduction

Intradural spinal cord tumors (SCT) compose a heterogeneous group of neoplasms. Over the past four decades, the overall mortality and morbidity caused by these tumors has been dramatically reduced. The advantages of early diagnosis via modern imaging and modern neurosurgical tools such as intraoperative electrophysiologic monitoring, the surgical microscope, and the ultrasonic aspirator have led to an improvement in surgical morbidity and in general prognosis.

This chapter focuses on common intradural primary SCT.

Epidemiology

There are few population-based data available on primary SCT. Many of the existing statistics are not current, often obtained from old surgical series. Intradural spinal tumors as a whole are believed to occur with an incidence that is in the range 0.7–1.1 cases per 100,000 persons. Intramedullary spinal cord tumors (IMSCT) comprise approximately 2–4% of all central nervous system (CNS) tumors. The most common types of intramedullary tumors are ependymo-mas, astrocytomas, and hemangioblastomas. The most common types of extramedullary tumors are meningiomas and nerve sheath tumors.

In the adult population, it has been estimated that IMSCT constitute 20% of all primary SCT. Ependymomas are the most common type of IMSCT (40–60%), with a mean presentation age of 35–40 years.

In the pediatric population, it has been estimated that approximately 36% of SCT are intramedullary, 24% are extramedullary, and 24% are extradural (and not included in this chapter). Astrocytomas are the most common type of intramedullary tumors, accounting for around 60% of all pediatric IMSCT, with a mean presentation age of 5–10 years.

Presentation

Reported clinical manifestations of SCT have changed since the beginning of the MRI era as a result of earlier diagnosis. Yet, even today, the primary physician, neurologist, and orthopedist must have a high index of suspicion towards primary sensory complains such as dys-

Neuro-oncology, First Edition. Edited by Roger J. Packer, David Schiff.

esthesias and localized back pain, in order to make an early diagnosis before permanent damage occurs.

In the pediatric age group, it is common for parents to become aware of a problem before any objective signs are apparent in the neurologic examination. In many of these patients the onset of symptoms is attributed to an apparently trivial injury. Occasionally, parents describe exacerbations and remissions. For both children and adults, the most common early symptom is local pain along the spinal axis that is usually most acute in the bony segment directly over the tumor. Typically, pain is worse in the recumbent position because venous congestion further distends the dural tube and results in characteristic night pains. Other symptoms include motor disturbances, radicular pain (occurring in about 10% of patients, usually limited to one or two dermatomes), paresthesias, painful dysesthesia (hot or cold painful sensations), and, rarely, sphincter dysfunction. Weakness of the lower limbs is usually first manifested as an alteration in normal gait. This is often very subtle and may only be evident, at first, to a watchful parent who notes more frequent falling and/or walking on heels or toes. In young children there is often a history of being a "late walker," and in very young children (under 3 years) there is often history of motor regression.

Different SCT subtypes may present with slightly different clinical pictures. For rare malignant astrocytomas, clinical presentation will include a more rapid decline in gait and pain of increasing intensity. Cervical ependymomas characteristically present with bilateral and symmetric dysesthesias.

As expected, anatomical location of the tumor correlates to clinical presentation. Cervical tumors may present with torticollis. Scoliosis is the most common early sign of an intramedullary thoracic cord tumor. Sphincter laxity is considered a very late sign except for tumors that originate in the conus or cauda equine area. Higher tumors, even with cystic components extending into the conus, less commonly present with sphincter abnormality.

Hydrocephalus, because of protein secretion into the cerebrospinal fluid (CSF), is a common presentation of IMSCT in infants.

Imaging

> ## ☆ TIPS & TRICKS
>
> **WHEN TO OBTAIN AN MRI IN A PATIENT WITH SCOLIOSIS**
>
> - Documented rapid progression
> - Atypical curve
> - Age: early onset <8 years
> - Any neurologic and/or urologic sign
> - Vertebral and midline anomalies
> - Pain (especially at night) (bone scan)
> - As screening in dysraphic children

Once an SCT is suspected, spinal magnetic resonance imaging (MRI) is the imaging method of choice. The only exceptions are in patients with contraindications to MRI, or severe scoliosis (for whom it may be difficult to obtain the important mid-sagittal images). In these cases, computed tomography (CT) myelography may be of help. The MRI protocol should always be carefully planned according to the clinical symptoms and neurologic signs, in conjunction with a neuroradiologist. It should consist of unenhanced T1 and T2-weighted images and contrast-enhanced T1-weighted images. Gadolinium may enhance the solid component of the tumor and help delineate it from surrounding edema. Ependymomas, meningiomas, and nerve sheath tumors contrast-enhance brightly following gadolinium injection. Astrocytomas have a variable enhancement pattern and may give the cord a lumpy appearance. These images should be acquired in both sagittal and axial planes. In pediatric patients, anesthesia is sometimes needed. Table 13.1 describes the radiologic characteristics, recommended treatment method, and overall prognosis of the different SCT.

Plain films and CT are not sensitive enough to effectively evaluate patients with suspected intradural, and especially intramedullary lesions. Secondary bony changes, such as pedicle erosion or foraminal widening, are better demonstrated with CT. However, plain films are better for diagnosis of instability and quantification of scoliotic and kyphotic deformities. Bladder ultrasound

Table 13.1. Tumor characteristics, treatment recommendations, and average prognosis.

Tumor	MR appearance	Typical location	Treatment	Prognosis
Extramedullary				
Meningioma	T1-hypo T2-hyper Contrast enhancing	Thoracic region Dural based	CR	Generally good Beware of anteriorly located tumors
Schwannoma and neurofibroma	Solid T1-iso T2-hyper Contrast enhancing	Sometimes dumbbell-shaped Extending towards the foramen	Resection	Generally good
Ependymoma of cauda equina (myxopapillary)	Expansile T2-hyper Contrast enhancing	Filum/conus/ cauda	Resection	Very good Beware of infiltration into the conus
Intramedullary				
Ependymoma	Expansile T2-hyper Contrast enhancing Cyst and/or syrinx	Cervical	Resection RT reserved for special cases	Very good
Astrocytoma	Widening T2-hyper Heterogeneous enhancement Cyst and/or syrinx	Cervical/ thoracic	Aggressive resection	Good
Malignant glioma	T2-hyper Contrast enhancing	Cervical/ thoracic	Resection RT/CT	Poor
Hemangioblastoma	Syringobulbia Syringomyelia Highly vascular	Cervical/ thoracic	Resection	Good

CR, complete resection; CT, chemotherapy; MR, magnetic resonance; RT, radiotherapy; T1-hypo, T1 hypointense; T2-hyper, T2 hyperintense.

with an examination following emptying is an important base line before surgery.

Tumor subtypes

Extramedullary spinal cord tumors

The most common primary extramedullary spinal cord tumors (EMSCT) are derived from sheath cells covering the spinal nerve roots (neurofibromas and schwannomas) or the endothelial lining of the meninges (meningiomas). Myxopapillary ependymomas are glial EMSCT arising from the conus medullaris or the filum terminale. Other tumor types such as hemangiopericytomas, lipomas, paragangliomas, and epidermoid/dermoid cysts are less common.

EMSCT generally cause chronic, slowly progressive compression of the cord. Symptomatology is caused by the displacement of the cord and adjacent nerve roots, and by secondary venous engorgement. Most patients will be symptomatic at the time of diagnosis; symptom onset can precede diagnosis by months to years. Because of the chronic, slow course of these tumors, the cord often looks atrophic, yet neurologic function may be preserved. The most common clinical presentation of all EMSCT is with back pain that may be indistinguishable from non-neoplastic causes. This pain is often described as aching, pressing, and dull, and is usually stronger at night. Radicular pain is uncommon with meningiomas but is common with nerve sheath tumors. Paresthesias and numbness are common symptoms, and hypoesthesia or anesthesia at and below the level of the tumor is often evident on clinical examination. Patterns of sensory deficit such as posterior cord syndrome can suggest tumor localization. Upper motor neuron injury in the form of spastic paraparesis is common too, and is usually first evident upon climbing stairs and trying to use proximal muscle groups. High cervical tumors may cause quadriparesis. When the tumor or the associated cyst extends rostrally into the brainstem, low cranial nerve involvement, dysphagia, and respiratory disturbances can occur.

Spinal meningiomas

More than 90% of meningiomas are intradural and more than 95% are benign tumors arising from the endothelium that lines the leptomeningeal spaces (arachnoid cap cells). These tumors occur mostly in older patients (peak incidence in the fifth and sixth decades). When occurring in younger patients, spinal meningiomas are associated with a poorer prognosis, a more aggressive course, and often co-morbidity with neurofibromatosis type 2. Most meningiomas affect females (80%), possibly because of the high percentage of meningiomas in which progesterone receptors are expressed, and arise in the thoracic region (80%). Less common is involvement of the cervical (15%) or lumbar (5%) regions. They

are usually solitary lesions; multiple spinal meningiomas (2% of patients) are associated with neurofibromatosis type 2. Intradural meningiomas are usually located laterally or posteriorly to the spinal cord; anterior location is less common.

Meningothelial and psammomatous meningiomas are the most common histologic subtypes of spinal meningiomas. Intradural clear cell meningiomas are less common and are associated with a worse prognosis. Atypical or anaplastic spinal meningiomas are rare. On MRI, spinal meningiomas appear hypointense to isointense on T1 and hyperintense on T2. With gadolinium contrast they often display homogeneous enhancement. However, calcifications are common and may preclude gadolinium enhancement.

Management

Spinal meningiomas are managed by surgery. This surgery is often considered to be the most rewarding procedure in neurosurgery. Even with the technical challenges of anteriorly located tumors, gross total removal (GTR) (defined as over 99%) of meningiomas is attainable in more than 90% of patients. Tumor recurrence rate is between 3% and 7%. Radiotherapy could be considered after subtotal removal (STR) or recurrence, but is seldom needed. Neurologic morbidity of the surgical procedure is directly related to preoperative neurologic status. Patients with little or no disability are at little risk of sustaining an injury, while patients with more advanced neurologic dysfunction have a greater risk of impairment. With modern use of electrophysiologic monitoring, perioperative complications are usually limited to wound healing and CSF fistulas. Long-term recovery is usually excellent. Anteriorly located spinal meningiomas require a very lateral approach, with special care to avoid injury to the pyramidal tracts and to the anterior spinal artery. These cases may be more challenging, carrying a potential risk of spinal cord damage. The use of the ultrasonic aspirator to internally debulk the tumor allows better manipulation of the capsule, and careful microsurgical separation from the spinal cord without the need for cord retraction.

Peripheral nerve tumors (neurofibromas, schwannomas)

Nerve sheath tumors (NST) are World Health Organization (WHO) grade I tumors. They usually present as solitary lesions, typically in the fourth or fifth decade of life. Earlier presentation, or multiple lesions, are usually associated with genetic syndromes such as neurofibromatosis types 1 and 2, and schwannomatosis. These syndromes are associated with multiple neurofibromas, spinal meningiomas, and schwannomas, respectively. Schwannomas are more common than neurofibromas. Approximately 60–80% of NST arise from nerve roots before leaving the dural sac, usually affecting the lumbosacral region. Anatomically, schwannomas tend to arise from the dorsal nerve root, whereas neurofibromas are more commonly on the ventral root. Other than this difference, schwannomas and neurofibromas are indistinguishable on MRI. NST have an isointense signal on T1 and a hyperintense signal on T2. Their characteristic pattern on fluid-sensitive sequences has been described as "target lesion." Tumor enhancement varies, ranging from homogeneous to a peripheral ring-like enhancement. Schwannoma pathology usually contains neoplastic Schwann cells, while neurofibromas more frequently invade the nerve root and contain Schwann cells, nerve fibers, and fibroblasts.

Management

NST management depends on the patient's clinical presentation and radiologic follow-up. A clinically and radiologically stable tumor needs only close follow-up with MRI and physical examination. During follow-up, or at presentation, if the tumor causes additional symptoms, or displays imaging progression, surgical intervention is warranted. GTR is the definitive treatment of such lesions, resulting in only 5% recurrence rate. To achieve total resection, the ventral or dorsal roots are commonly sacrificed. However, this is usually not associated with pronounced postoperative motor or sensory deficit. Resection of schwannomas is usually safer because of their typical location on the dorsal root and the fact that they are less invasive than neurofibromas. STR may be preferable if the tumor is attached to the spinal cord, if the origin of the tumor is an important ventral rootlet, or if the tumor exhibits extradural components closely associated with vital structures.

Ependymomas of the conus medullaris

These tumors are usually extradural myxopapillary ependymomas, which account for approximately 40–50% of spinal ependymomas. They are more common in adults. Patients usually present with a long history of back pain, lower sensorimotor deficit, and sphincter dysfunction.

On MRI they are often seen as well-circumscribed masses with hypointense signal on T1 and hyperintense signal on T2 (Figure 13.1). Gadolinium enhancement is usually homogeneous.

Management

Complete resection is the treatment of choice, and is generally feasible if nerve roots are not entrapped by the tumor. STR is reserved for cases with severe encasement of cauda equine nerve roots, especially low sacral S2–S4 innervation. Focal fractionated radiotherapy seems to contribute to long-term tumor control. Recurrence following complete resection is less rare than previously thought, and is associated with poor outcome.

Intramedullary spinal cord tumors

Presentation

IMSCT usually present with myelopathic symptoms of insidious onset. Localized pain and upper extremity paresthesias are the initial symptoms in 50–90% of adult patients with cervical lesions. Thoracic lesions may present with lower limb sensory losses and with upper motor neuron signs. Radicular pain is usually associated with IMSCT of the cauda equine area. Sphincter dysfunction is present in up to 40% of adult patients. In the pediatric population, pain is less often a presenting symptom, but is present in approximately 50% of patients. Symptoms usually last months, or even years prior to diagnosis.

Intramedullary tumors are diagnosed and followed using MRI. They are recognized by focal involvement. In rare instances, holocord involvement is seen, with the solid bulk accompanied by caudal and rostral cysts (especially in pediatric

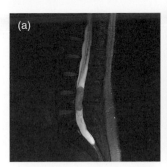
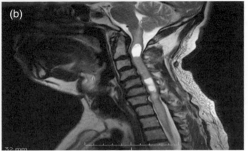

Figure 13.1. (a) Extramedullary ependymoma of the cauda equina region. A magnetic resonance imaging (MRI) scan of a 37-year-old man who presented a 2-year history of intermittent back pain and urinary hesitancy. The sagittal T2 image demonstrates a large caudal myxopapillary ependymoma. (b) Intramedullary ependymoma. An MRI of a 60-year-old patient who presented with a year of progressive neck pain that was stronger at night and was accompanied by upper limb dysesthesia. The patient was "diagnosed" with carpel tunnel syndrome. CT was interpreted as normal. On sagittal T2 images a large intramedullary ependymoma (C3–C6) is noted accompanied by rostral and caudal cysts. Note the signal changes in the medulla oblongata.

patients). The spinal cord expansion is associated with T2 and fluid attenuated inversion recovery (FLAIR) hyperintensity, T1 hypointensity or isointensity, viable contrast enhancement, and occasional tumor-associated cyst or syrinx.

Glial tumors

While IMSCT comprise only about 20% of all adult SCTs, at least 35–50% of pediatric SCTs are intramedullary. The vast majority of IMSCT are members of the glioma family. Among 436 patients of all ages with IMSCT operated upon by Fred Epstein between 1985 and 1999:

- 37% presented with ependymomas
- 29% presented with astrocytomas
- 14% presented with gangliogliomas
- 7% presented with mixed gliomas
- 14% presented with other lesions, such as hemangioblastomas, primitive neuroectodermal tumors (PNET), lipomas, and ganglioneurocytomas.

Of these 436 patients, 49% were in the pediatric age range. Astrocytomas and gangliogliomas were especially prevalent in the younger age groups, while ependymomas were more frequently observed in the older groups. Intramedullary ependymomas almost never appear in the

first decade. Note that within the spectrum of low grade glial tumors, significant differences are found in reported series in the rates of different tumor subtypes such as low grade astrocytomas, juvenile pilocytic astrocytomas, gangliogliomas, oligodendrogliomas, and others. Intramedullary metastatic tumors account for approximately 1–3% of lesions, and non-neoplastic processes, such as multiple sclerosis, can account for up to 4%.

Intramedullary ependymomas

Ependymomas are the most common IMSCT in the adult population, representing 40–60% of adult IMSCT, while constituting only 16–35% of IMSCT in the pediatric population. Categorization of ependymomas, both spinal and cranial, is based upon histologic properties. Classic (WHO grade II and III) cellular ependymomas arise from the spinal canal and usually occupy the cervical and thoracic regions. Myxopapillary (WHO grade I) ependymomas arise from the filum terminale, occupy the conus medullaris almost exclusively, and are usually extradural. Most ependymomas are WHO low grade tumors (class I and II). Malignant subtype anaplastic ependymomas are rarely encountered in the spine.

On MRI, these tumors appear hypointense on T1 and hyperintense in T2 weighted images.

Ependymomas display homogeneous enhancement. Although usually not encapsulated, there is often a clear plane evident between the tumor and the cord. Cysts, syrinx, and hemorrhage may also be evident.

Management

Management of ependymomas is aggressive resection in most cases. Complete resection, with the aid of intraoperative electrophysiologic monitoring, yields local control in 90–100% of patients. In partial resections of grade II and III tumors, the addition of adjuvant radiotherapy may be warranted. It is important to remember that adjuvant radiotherapy may make future surgical intervention more difficult and increases postoperative neurologic morbidity. The role of adjuvant chemotherapy is unclear at this time. Spinal intramedullary ependymomas generally have a good prognosis, with an average progression-free survival (PFS) of 82 months and an average overall survival of 180 months.

Low grade astrocytomas

In the adult population, approximately 40% of IMSCT are astrocytomas, out of which 75% are low grade (WHO grade II) fibrillary astrocytomas. Peak incidence is in the third decade. In the pediatric population, astrocytomas are the most common spinal tumor. On MRI they appear as a fusiform expansion of the cord, sometimes including a cystic component (Figure 13.2). Syrinx is seen in approximately 40% of patients and edema is often present. This tumor is hypointense or isointense on T1 images, and hyperintense on T2 and FLAIR, displaying partial enhancement. It is very difficult to differentiate astrocytomas from ependymomas based on MRI alone.

Management

Management of intramedullary astrocytomas is based on maximal safe resection followed by observation or radiation treatment, depending on the extent of the resection, the presence of progressive tumor, and the age of the patient. Because of the infiltrative nature of these tumors, complete resection is highly dependent on the surgeon's experience, mostly to identify a change

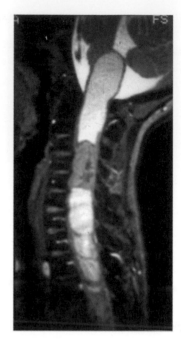

Figure 13.2. Intramedullary astrocytoma. An MRI of a 10-year-old boy who presented with drooling and neck pain. The low grade astrocytoma spans C3–C6.

in color (interface) between the tumor and the normal white matter around it.

Because there is no clear evidence that radiation or chemotherapy have a significant impact on the outcome for patients presenting with IMSCT, especially astrocytomas, surgery is the first step in management. If a pediatric patient with a low grade IMSCT astrocytoma is treated with radical excision, long-term PFS generally ensues without the need for adjuvant treatment. In many cases, pediatric intramedullary tumors are a "surgical disease."

Long-term follow-up has demonstrated that PFS rates are similar between those treated with GTR and those with STR. This finding, surprising at the time, has led to the recommendation of less aggressive resection if the surgeon feels that function may be jeopardized. Such concerns are supported by a change in evoked potentials during surgery or a lesion with a poor interface between tumor and normal tissue, especially in patients who come to surgery with significant neurologic compromise at diagnosis. For those tumors that do recur, the option of another operation is often superior to the alternatives. Studies have demonstrated that second operations do not carry a higher risk for morbidity. Properly excised, pediatric low grade intramedullary astrocytomas have a 5-year PFS rate of 80–100%, and the overall prognosis is good. In selected cases, chemotherapy with carboplatin and vincristine has been shown to be effective in children with recurrent disease. Focal radiotherapy can also be used in select cases.

In the pediatric population, adjuvant oncologic treatment is usually reserved for those with multifocal disease, or children who are at a very high risk of developing plegia following a second, or even third, operation. The standard low intensity chemotherapy used for low grade astrocytomas in the brain has been shown to be effective in selective cases of intramedullary astrocytomas, especially in infants. In children younger than 5 years, radiation should be avoided because of the detrimental effects on the immature CNS. Susceptibility to the destructive effects of radiation on the spinal cord increases with the extent of cord irradiation as well as with the total dose. Therapeutic irradiation in substantial doses over extensive segments of spinal cord may result in myelitis. In addition, irradiation subsequent to spinal surgery predisposes to kyphosis and subluxation. Finally, irradiation may trigger development of a second malignant tumor.

Malignant spinal gliomas

High grade gliomas of the spinal cord represent approximately 25% of intramedullary gliomas in adults and less than 10% in the pediatric population. These tumors are associated with poor prognosis and almost 100% recurrence. On MRI they display malignant characteristics such as heterogeneous enhancement caused by the presence of intramural cysts, necrosis, and surrounding edema. High grade astroglial IMSCT, especially glioblastomas, invariably progress.

Management

The optimal treatment for this entity has yet to be determined. Despite aggressive adjuvant therapy, patients with malignant IMSCT have a postoperative median survival of up to 12 months. This is usually because of progressive infiltration of the tumor within the cord and through its pial banks, resulting in paraplegia, quadriplegia, and, eventually, death. A patient with a high grade spinal astrocytoma has an average life expectancy of 15 months.

Hemangioblastomas

Hemangioblastomas are the third most common IMSCT, and can be associated with von Hippel–Lindau (VHL) syndrome. Some 10–30% of hemangioblastoma patients have VHL while the rest are sporadic. Sporadic hemangioblastomas have a peak incidence in the third or fourth decades, with male predominance. Hemangioblastomas usually arise from the dorsal region of the cord, and patients usually present with proprioceptive sensory complaints. These complaints are usually slow to progress, except for the rare cases presenting with subarachnoid or intramedullary hemorrhage.

On MRI these tumors appear homogeneous and brightly enhancing, with a highly vascular nodule (Figure 13.3). Surrounding edema,

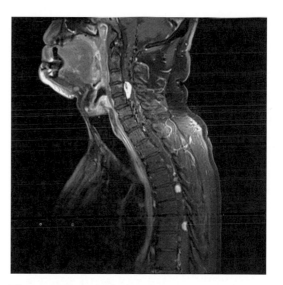

Figure 13.3. An MRI showing hemangioblastoma in a 50-year old male with von Hippel–Lindau syndrome. This man presented with progressive nightly back pain and lower limb pain, together with gait disturbances. On a sagittal T1 sequence with gadolinium, several highly enhancing hemangioblastomas were noted on C3, T5, and T7.

associated with dorsal and rostral cysts, maybe pathognomonic for intramedullary hemangioblastomas. Spinal angiography might demonstrate feeding and draining vessels, and might be of use in surgical planning. Hemangioblastomas can be differentiated from ependymoma by the tumor hypervascularity and the vascular abnormalities evident on MRI. Hemangioblastomas can be differentiated from spinal arteriovenous malformation by the associated syrinx and enhancement. In patients with VHL, serial imaging should be utilized, as new lesions are known to appear.

Management

Complete resection is the primary treatment for symptomatic hemangioblastomas. The margins are often well defined, so that the tumor can often be fully resected and a cure can potentially be achieved. Intraoperative bleeding from the tumor may severely impede the procedure and lead to subtotal resection. If possible, hemangioblastomas should be removed in one piece, dissecting the capsule between the tumor and normal cord; this is very different from the removal method recommended for astrocytomas, which optimally are resected from inside out. The use of preoperative embolization for intramedullary spinal hemangioblastomas is controversial. Data regarding the use of radiotherapy and chemotherapy are almost nonexistent. Recently, in several small series, antiangiogenic factors (SU5416, bevacizumab) have demonstrated positive clinical and radiologic responses.

Complications of spinal tumor surgery

☆ TIPS & TRICKS

PRINCIPLES OF INTRAOPERATIVE NEUROPHYSIOLOGY IN IMSCT SURGERY
Intraoperative neurophysiologic assessment of the spinal cord has become the standard of care for safe IMSCT resection in leading institutions. The goal of intraoperative neurophysiologic assessment is threefold:

1 To monitor, in real time, the functional integrity of the motor and sensory systems and to detect iatrogenic injury at early, reversible stages, thus aiding in maximizing the extent of resection and allowing appropriate immediate intervention before long-term deficits are incurred
2 To map the spinal cord dorsal columns in order to delineate a physiologic midline or "safe entry" zone along the midline raphe of the spinal cord's dorsal columns for safe access to the tumor
3 To localize the corticospinal tract within the tumor cavity in order to delineate "danger zones" to avoid

✋ CAUTION!

COMPLICATIONS OF SCT SURGERY

- Motor/sensory deficits
- Impaired position sense
- Infection
- CSF leak
- Kyphoscoliosis
- Cord tethering
- Postoperative cyst formation

Surgery for radical removal of IMSCT entails significant risks in inexperienced hands. Surgical morbidity is also highly dependent on preoperative clinical status. In experienced hands, the incidence of significant postoperative motor deficit in an intact patient is less than 5%. In a patient with a significant pre-existing (preoperative) deficit, the morbidity is higher. Early diagnosis, an advantage under any circumstances, is especially important with IMSCT, as functional outcome in nonambulatory patients is usually suboptimal. Patients with malignant tumors are also at a relatively higher risk of surgical injury. Patients with severe preoperative disability and extensive noncystic tumors are more likely to deteriorate after surgery.

Impaired position sense, even in the presence of normal motor function, is a serious functional disability that mandates extensive rehabilitative physical therapy. This potential complication should be stressed in the preoperative discussion with patients and parents. However, the risk of injury to the posterior columns is significantly less when operating on an astrocytoma in a child than in an adult. Other postoperative complications include those related to ineffective wound healing and perioperative CSF fistulae.

Scoliosis and kyphosis commonly evolve after surgery. In some cases of kyphosis, the deformity is of a sufficient magnitude to cause spinal cord compression and progressive myelopathy. In these patients, recurrent tumor should always be considered before the spinal deformity is identified as being responsible for neurologic dysfunction. It is imperative that the type of spinal deformity be clarified because treatment and prognosis are obviously very different. Scoliosis usually does not cause spinal cord compression, although it may exacerbate a pre-existing neurologic disability. It is essential that a pediatric orthopedic surgeon experienced in the care of kyphosis and scoliosis follow all children closely. Surgical indications for spinal fusion should be considered more urgent in this group of patients than in those with idiopathic deformities.

Cord tethering may become symptomatic only many years following surgery. This usually can be demonstrated on MRI with a dorsal position of the remaining cord, in a deteriorating patient with no other apparent reason.

Selected bibliography

Alter M. (1975) Statistical aspects of spinal cord tumours. In: Vinken PJ, Bruyn GH (eds) *Handbook of Clinical Neurology*, Amsterdam: North-Holland, pp. 1–22.

Clayton PE, Shalet SM. (1991) The evolution of spinal growth after irradiation. *Clin Oncol (R Coll Radiol)* **3** (4), 220–2.

Cohen AR, Wisoff JH, Allen JC, Epstein F. (1989) Malignant astrocytomas of the spinal cord. *J Neurosurg* **70** (1), 50–4.

Constantini S, Houten J, Miller DC, Freed D, Ozek MM, Rorke LB, *et al.* (1996) Intramedullary spinal cord tumors in children under the age of 3 years. *J Neurosurg* **85** (6), 1036–43.

Constantini S, Miller DC, Allen JC, Rorke LB, Freed D, Epstein FJ. (2000) Radical excision of intramedullary spinal cord tumors: surgical morbidity and long-term follow-up evaluation in 164 children and young adults. *J Neurosurg* **93** (2 Suppl), 183–93.

Constantini S, Siomin V, Epstein FJ. (2006) Surgical management of intramedullary spinal cord tumors. In: Fessler RG (ed.) *Atlas of Neurosurgical Techniques: Spine and Peripheral Nerves.* Thieme Medical Publishers, New York.

Duffner PK, Horowitz ME, Krischer JP, Friedman HS, Burger PC, Cohen ME, *et al.* (1993) Postoperative chemotherapy and delayed radiation in children less than three years of age with malignant brain tumors. *N Engl J Med* **328** (24), 1725–31.

Goh KYC, Constantini S, Epstein FJ. (2000) Surgical management of intramedullary spinal cord tumors, In: Schmidek HH, Sweet WH (eds) *Schmidek & Sweet's Operative Neurosurgical Techniques*, 4th edn. W.B. Saunders Company, Philadelphia.

Hsu W, Pradilla G, Constantini S, Jallo GI. (2009) Surgical considerations of spinal ependymomas in the pediatric population. *Childs Nerv Syst* **25** (10), 1253–9.

McGirt MJ, Constantini S, Jallo GI. (2008) Correlation of a preoperative grading scale with progressive spinal deformity following surgery for intramedullary spinal cord tumors in children. *J Neurosurg Pediatr* **2** (4), 277–81.

Packer RJ, Ater J, Allen J, Phillips P, Geyer R, Nicholson HS, *et al.* (1997) Carboplatin and vincristine chemotherapy for children with newly diagnosed progressive low-grade gliomas. *J Neurosurg* **86** (5), 747–54.

Russell DS, Rubinstein LJ. (1989) *Pathology of Tumours of the Nervous System.* Williams & Wilkins, Baltimore.

Slooff JL, Kernohan JW, MacCarty CS. (1964) *Primary Intramedullary Tumors of the Spinal Cord and Filum Terminale.* W.B. Saunders, Philadelphia.

Yao KC, McGirt MJ, Chaichana KL, Constantini S, Jallo GI. (2007) Risk factors for progressive spinal deformity following resection of intramedullary spinal cord tumors in children: an analysis of 161 consecutive cases. *J Neurosurg* **107** (6 Suppl), 463–8.

Part III

Pediatric Brain Tumors

14

Gliomas in Childhood

Bruce H. Cohen

Children's Hospital Medical Center of Akron, Northeast Ohio Medical University, Akron, OH, USA

Introduction

About 50% of pediatric brain tumors are gliomas, with an equal distribution of low grade gliomas (LGG) and high grade gliomas. The high grade brainstem glioma and high grade supratentorial glioma each account for 20% of pediatric gliomas, with the remaining 5% occurring in the cerebellum. High grade gliomas are classified, as in adults, as anaplastic astrocytomas (AA) and glioblastoma (GB) (Plate 14.9, see plate section opposite p. 52).

Gliomas are among the most diverse group of brain tumors affecting children, and as a whole these tumors in children span a wider range of pathologic subtypes and prognosis than any other neoplasm. This clinical diversity is matched by the wide array of genetic alterations and how mutations may affect tumorigenesis. Response to therapy is yet to be discovered.

Biology

The molecular features of pediatric high grade gliomas differ from those arising in adults. Childhood primary malignant gliomas usually lack epidermal growth factor receptor (EGFR) amplification and pTEN deletions found in adult primary glioblastoma multiforme. Both tumor types may exhibit TP53 mutations, especially in tumors that arise in older children. Pediatric high grade gliomas resemble adult secondary glioblastoma multiforme genetically. However, adult secondary tumors usually have a high frequency of mutation of the *IDH1* and *IDH2* genes, while pediatric high grade gliomas do not. Integrated molecular genetic profiling of pediatric gliomas demonstrates focal amplification of platelet-derived growth factor receptor A (PDGFRA), which is not commonly seen in high grade gliomas in adults.

Recently, results from biopsy studies of children with newly diagnosed disease and autopsy studies have begun to unravel the molecular changes associated with pediatric diffuse intrinsic gliomas. A subgroup of diffuse intrinsic pontine gliomas show gains in PDGFRA and PDGFR-alpha expression. In addition, low level gains of PARP-1 have been identified. EGFR amplification is rarely seen in these pediatric brainstem tumors. Unlike gliomas in adults, O[6]-methylguanine-DNA methyltransferase (MGMT) expression does not seem to be a mechanism of drug-induced resistance.

There is recent improved understanding of the genetic substrate of pediatric LGG. Routine karyotyping has not been helpful. The gene *BRAF*, an

Neuro-oncology, First Edition. Edited by Roger J. Packer, David Schiff.
© 2012 John Wiley & Sons, Ltd. Published 2012 by John Wiley & Sons, Ltd.

identified oncogene linked to melanoma and some carcinomas, is located within 7q34 and functions to upregulate the RAS/RAR/MEK pathway. The 7q34 region duplication is found in 66% of sporadic juvenile pilocytic astrocytomas (JPA) (80% of cerebellar JPA, 62% of brainstem and visual pathway, but only 14% of hemispheric JPA) but not identified in either NF1-associated JPA or other pediatric LGG. These tumors demonstrate an abnormal gain of function in the MAP kinase signaling pathway, and it is hoped that treatments can be targeted to affect this pathway.

High grade gliomas

Brainstem gliomas

Brainstem gliomas (BSG) account for 10–20% of childhood brain tumors. Until the advent of magnetic resonance imaging (MRI), it was difficult to diagnose these tumors with absolute certainty. Therefore, the true natural history of these tumors, and their response to therapy, could not be defined until the later part of the 1980s when the use of MRI became widespread.

Clinical presentation

Presenting signs and symptoms relate to the specific location and invasion of the tumor within the brainstem, the rate of growth, and whether cerebrospinal fluid (CSF) dynamics are disturbed. For most brainstem gliomas there is a triad of specific cranial nerve involvement, long-tract signs, and ataxia. The CSF dynamics may be disturbed from tumor invasion causing headache, vomiting, irritability, limited upgaze, and abnormal motor tone. The neoplasms involving the tectal plate present with macrocrania caused by evolving hydrocephalus. Those neoplasms with an exophytic component, especially the cervicomedullary gliomas, may have a protracted course of gait disturbance with or without vomiting, and late cranial nerve dysfunction.

Imaging and pathology

MRI will lead to a firm diagnosis in most circumstances. Computed tomography (CT) is of limited value, and can sometimes fail to show any abnormalities. In the infiltrating BSG, CT can show a non-enhancing low density area in the pontine region, with obliteration of the surrounding cisterns. Lower grade neoplasms tend to be iso-dense or hyperdense on CT, with varying degrees of cystic changes or contrast enhancement. If the clinical diagnosis or CT findings suggest the possibility of a brainstem glioma, an MRI is necessary. The high grade infiltrating BSG will appear as a mass or masses with decreased signal intensity on T1-weighted images and increased signal intensity on fluid attenuated inversion recovery (FLAIR) and T2-weighted images. These masses expand the majority of the pons and can extend into adjoining regions. These may not enhance, although there can be small portions of the tumor that may enhance with contrast. Less malignant tumors tend to have a more focal appearance and enhance, with the lowest grade neoplasms showing confluent enhancement patterns (Figure 14.1).

> ### ★ TIPS AND TRICKS
>
> In general, the infiltrating tumors in the midbrain and diencephalon are less aggressive and have a higher rate of survival following radiotherapy than the tumors involving the pons.

Diffuse infiltrating pontine glioma

This tumor most commonly occurs between 5 and 10 years of age and is very uncommon before 2 years of age. The location of the tumor is defined by its name, but on occasions this tumor can have an exophytic component. The diagnosis of this neoplasm is made by the distinctive MRI characteristics described and surgical confirmation of a diagnosis is seldom necessary. Early leptomeningeal spread of the tumor may occur so a complete spinal MRI at the time of initial diagnosis is recommended. Symptoms usually improve with dexamethasone. A CSF diversion procedure is necessary in about one-third of patients because of symptomatic hydrocephalus.

Standard treatment is involved-field radiotherapy, with a dose of 5500–5960 cGy, given in 180–200 cGy daily fractions. There is a survival advantage to those children treated with more than 5000 cGy, but higher dosages that include

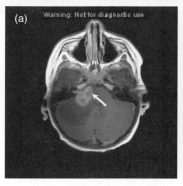 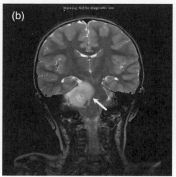 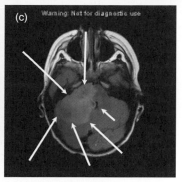

Figure 14.1. Pontine glioma. (a) Axial T1 with gadolinium demonstrating enhancing mass arising from the lateral pons. (b) Coronal T2 demonstrating bright mass involving brainstem structures and the cerebellar tracts, causing right to left shift of midbrain. (c) Axial FLAIR image showing the hyperintense mass arising from the pons and extending through the cerebellar peduncles into the cerebellum (long arrows), compressing the fourth ventricle (short arrow). Radiographic images courtesy of Dr Shankar Ganapathy.

b.i.d. fractionation to total doses of 7800 cGy do not seem to affect event-free or overall survival. Within weeks of initiating radiotherapy, most children demonstrate clinical improvement, with some showing complete resolution of their symptoms along with improvement in the MRI findings. The mean time to progression is about 6 months, with most patients surviving only 9–13 months after diagnosis. About 10% of children are alive in a relapse-free state at 18 months after initial diagnosis. Salvage therapy after initial relapse is seldom effective.

> ✋ **CAUTION!**
>
> There is no role for Gamma Knife® or other hypofractionation techniques because of the risk of radiation necrosis.

Chemotherapy trials used to treat these tumors have been uniformly disappointing. The Children's Cancer Group conducted a study using two different intensive-dose chemotherapy arms prior to giving hyperfractionated radiotherapy (7200 cGy in 100 cGy b.i.d. fractions). The event-free survival at 1 year was 17% and at 2 years was 6%, and children who responded to chemotherapy tended to have a longer survival, but the overall response rate, event-free survival, and overall survival was unchanged from historical controls. Other studies using standard dose radiotherapy and a variety of different radiosensitizers did not improve survival.

Trials of temozolomide (TMZ) when given in standard dosing or metronomic dosing along with radiotherapy does not appear to improve survival. At recurrence, bevacizumab plus irinotecan was not efficacious. A recent publication reported potential efficacy using oral gefitinib at a dose of 250 mg/m²/day along with standard radiotherapy, with gefitinib continuing for up to 13 monthly courses.

The most intensive chemotherapy regimen has employed high dose chemotherapy with autologous bone marrow rescue, which failed to improve survival, although there were occasional patients who did benefit.

Dorsal exophytic brainstem tumors

This distinct subset comprise 20% of brainstem tumors and most have a benign histology with slow growth. They may obstruct CSF flow but tend not to invade the parenchyma. These may present early in life, and are followed expectantly without intervention but often are not diagnosed until the teenage years when macrocrania or upgaze paresis occurs. The MRI characteristic is low intensity on T1 and high intensity on FLAIR and T2-weighted images, tends to have sharp

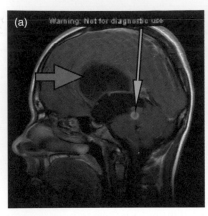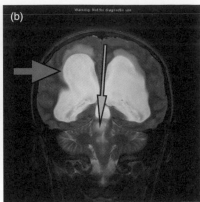

Figure 14.2. Tectal glioma. Hydrocephalus (block arrows) is demonstrated on the sagittal T1 with gadolinium image (a) and coronal FLAIR images (b). The tumor demonstrates enhancement with contrast (a) and increased signal on the FLAIR image (thin arrow). Radiographic images courtesy of Dr Shanker Ganapathy.

borders and enhance intensely with contrast (Figure 14.2). Treatment may include CSF diversion but seldom requires surgical removal. Standard radiotherapy is effective but withheld until a point when surgery is not an option.

Focal intrinsic and cervicomedullary gliomas

These less common neoplasms are often pilocytic astrocytomas and amenable to surgical debulking. In the case of the focal intrinsic brainstem tumor, surgery may cause increased morbidity and involved field radiotherapy is a reasonable treatment option.

Consideration for patients with neurofibromatosis type 1

Although most gliomas in the setting of neurofibromatosis type 1 (NF1) localize to the visual pathway, there is a propensity for brainstem tumors as well. It is difficult to differentiate between the spongiform changes involving the cerebellum and brainstem structures (as well as the deep gray masses) and a glioma on the basis of MRI alone. Often found on surveillance imaging, the T2 and FLAIR hyperintense areas can have mass effect, yet show no signs of growth over years. Patients demonstrating growth with progressive neurologic dysfunction may require a biopsy or surgical resection to guide therapy. In general, children with NF1 bearing a brainstem

glioma have a better prognosis than other children with a typical pontine glioma.

> ☆ **TIPS AND TRICKS**
>
> Lack of radiographic progression and stability in the neurologic examination differentiate non-neoplastic spongiform changes from clinically active infiltrating glioma in children with NF1.

Nonbrainstem high grade glioma

Clinical presentation

High grade gliomas involving nonbrainstem structures occur at any age in childhood, including infancy. Because the sutures in children do not fuse until after the second or third year, the clinical presentation in babies often occurs because of abnormal head growth, sometimes with mild or slowly evolving neurologic signs. Long-standing hydrocephalus may result in stretching or vascular injury to the optic apparatus and leads to slowly evolving optic disk pallor and slowly constricting visual fields. However, focal neurologic signs and seizures may be the presenting signs, even in infants. The clinical presentation in children outside of the infant age range is similar to that of adults; seizures, focal neurologic signs, and headaches. In one study the neurologic examination was abnormal in 94% at the time of diagnosis. High grade gliomas located near CSF pathways and within the posterior fossa may disseminate early in the course of the disease.

Surgical considerations

Complete or near-complete gross total resection can improve overall survival; therefore, aggressive surgery is recommended for tumors amenable to resection. In a study of 131 children with AA and GB located in the cerebrum (63%), deep and midline structures (28%), and posterior fossa (8%); results of surgery were stratified as gross total or near total (>90% of the mass removed) versus subtotal or less (<90% of the mass removed). Following surgery the children were treated with radiotherapy followed by eight cycles of chemotherapy (vincristine, CCNU, and prednisone) or two cycles of 8-in-1 chemotherapy followed by radiotherapy and then an additional eight cycles of 8-in-1 chemotherapy. Patients having the more complete surgical resection had a 5-year progression-free survival of 35% versus 17%, which held true regardless of histology.

★ TIPS AND TRICKS

A gross total surgical resection may be the most important factor in determining survival in children with high grade glioma.

Radiotherapy

Standard daily fractionation radiotherapy is considered a standard of high grade glioma treatment in children. The use of conformal fields has become a standard practice in the past 10 years. In a historical study, children with AA treated with surgery and radiation therapy had a 29% 5-year survival and a 26% 10-year survival. Children with malignant hemispheric glioma during 1957–1980 treated with 54–60 Gy had a 60% 5-year survival rate compared with a 14% survival in those treated with 35–50 Gy. This study also showed that children with midline high grade gliomas fared poorly (0% 5-year survival) when compared with those with hemispheric or cerebellar tumors (44% 5-year survival). The patients with grade III astrocytomas (now known

as AA) had survival rates of 74% at 1 year, 56% at 2 years, 36% at 5 years, and 32% at 10 years, which is better than seen in adult series. However, children with GB had survival rates of 44%, 26%, 4%, and 0% at 1, 2, 5, and 10 years, similar to that seen in adults. In patients treated similarly, other studies reported a 5–10% 5-year overall survival and a 24% 1-year overall survival. Tumors that have disseminated at the time of diagnosis have a very poor prognosis, but nevertheless will require craniospinal irradiation for palliation of symptoms. Prophylactic craniospinal irradiation is suggested if the tumor involves CSF pathways or is located in the posterior fossa, even if leptomeningeal dissemination is not proven. Spinal irradiation will affect hematopoetic function and therefore the ability to deliver cytotoxic chemotherapy. Regardless of the presence of tumor dissemination, local disease recurrence remains the biggest challenge with high grade glioma.

Chemotherapy

The beneficial role of chemotherapy was first demonstrated in a Children's Cancer Group (CCG) study where patients underwent initial maximal surgical resection and involved field radiotherapy. Following radiotherapy, patients were randomized to no further treatment or to receive eight cycles of CCNU, vincristine, and prednisone. The overall survival at 3 years was 19% in those with GB and 60% in those with AA. The children receiving chemotherapy had a 5-year progression-free survival of 46%, compared to 18% in those not treated with chemotherapy ($P = 0.026$). The use of preirradiation chemotherapy was explored in a later CCG study. Following maximal surgical resection, patients were randomized to radiation followed by chemotherapy (CCNU, vincristine, and prednisone) or two cycles of preradiation 8-in-1 chemotherapy followed by radiotherapy and then eight additional cycles of 8-in-1 chemotherapy. There was no difference in outcome between the two treatment arms of this study, with a progression-free survival and overall survival at 5 years of 33% and 36%, respectively.

In adults, TMZ has become a standard therapy that is given daily along with radiotherapy followed by six or more monthly cycles of treatment consisting of typically five daily doses each cycle.

TMZ has been explored in a multicenter phase II trial in the setting of recurrent high grade astrocytoma in childhood. Patients were treated with 5 days of TMZ at a dosage of 200 mg/m²/day and repeated every 28 days. The response rate was 12% in those 25 children with supratentorial and cerebellar grade III or IV astrocytomas and 6% in 18 children with intrinsic brainstem glioma. Even if stable disease was taken into consideration, the partial response and stable disease rates were 22%. In a more recent study of 15 children with recurrent high grade glioma (including seven with oligodendroglioma features) treated with TMZ (200 mg/m²/day for 5 days, in 28-day cycles), the reported overall response rate was 20%, with a median progression-free survival of 2.0 months (range 3 weeks to 34+ months) and a progression-free survival of 20% at 6 months.

The most recent and robust study investigating the role of TMZ as an effective therapy, and whether activity is influenced by the expression of the *MGMT* gene was conducted by the Children's Oncology Group. A total of 177 patients with malignant glioma were treated with surgical resection followed by radiotherapy with concomitant TMZ, then with standard courses of TMZ. In the 90 patients (31 with AA, 55 with GB, and 4 others) the 3-year event-free survival rate was 13% in AA and 7% in GB. The 2-year event-free survival rate was 17% in those without *MGMT* overexpression and 5% in those with *MGMT* overexpression (*P* = 0.045). The study report con-cluded there was no evidence that this course of treatment provided an advantage over CCG-945, but did demonstrate that *MGMT* overexpression negatively affected survival.

The role of high dose chemotherapy followed by autologous bone marrow rescue or peripheral stem cell support has been explored in several trials with variable results. Similarly, biologic agents, including Avastin®, a vascular endothelial growth factor inhibitor and platelet and epidermal growth factor inhibitors have been undertaken without clearcut benefit. The role of the biologic therapies are under investigation.

Low grade glioma

Visual pathway glioma

The visual pathway gliomas represents the most common midline glial neoplasm. The location tends to segregate between orbital or intracranial, which can extend posteriorly through the chiasm, along the visual tracts to the medial geniculate body and even within the optic radiations. Generally, the tumors that originate in the orbit tend not to extend into the chiasm, although they can expand the orbital canal. Some of these tumors appear to originate in the chiasm itself, and can extend both anteriorly and posteriorly. Depending on the series, 20–40% involve the prechiasmatic structures alone, with 60–80% involving the optic nerves, chiasm, and posterior structures (Figure 14.3).

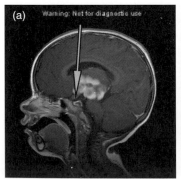 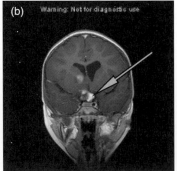 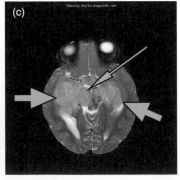

Figure 14.3. Chiasmatic glioma. (a – sagittal T1 with gadolinium) and (b – coronal T1 with gadolinium) images demonstrate the nonuniform enhancement and origin of the tumor within the optic chiasm (arrows), as well as the extensive size of the neoplasm. (c) The axial FLAIR image demonstrates extension into the midbrain (thin arrow) and optic radiations (block arrows). Radiographic images courtesy of Dr Shanker Ganapathy.

About half of all children diagnosed with visual pathway gliomas will have NF1. Children with NF1 have a 5–21% chance of developing these tumors. The discovery of a visual pathway tumor are often on surveillance imaging of children with NF1, and thus often discovered in isolation of any clinical symptoms or signs. About 80% of these children never demonstrate radiographic progression or clinical signs of the tumor, suggesting that the radiographic finding alone, especially for small tumors, does not warrant therapy. The velocity of tumor growth is highly variable even in those children who have radiographic progression. The tumors occurring in NF1 tend to be more extensive and have a more variable growth pattern.

The clinical presentation for the prechiasmatic glioma is proptosis, unilateral visual loss with optic nerve pallor, and an afferent pupillary defect. For those children with intracranial tumors, which most often involve the chiasm with intracranial unilateral or bilateral optic nerve involvement, the presentation will include slowly evolving visual loss, loss of visual fields, optic nerve pallor, complex patterns of afferent pupillary defects, and sometimes an endocrinopathy that may include growth hormone failure, failure to achieve sexual maturity, or precocious puberty.

The imaging findings are characteristic and usually diagnostic, therefore a biopsy is generally not necessary. Unless there are signs of progressive neurologic dysfunction or demonstration of tumor growth, treatment is withheld. This is a difficult process in child too young to participate in a visual examination. Because of the high risk in children with NF1, an annual ophthalmologic examination and growth assessment are suggested as screening methods.

The role of surgery is limited to tumors involving the orbit, which have caused visual loss with proptosis. Amputation of the nerve in the orbit will generally result in a cure. Surgery is also helpful as an adjunct to therapy for bulky tumors involving midline structures, usually for the purpose of either re-establishing CSF flow through the ventricular system or for removing tumor bulk. The role of biopsy is limited to those lesions where the histology is not certain.

For the tumors involving the chiasm and post-chiasm structures there has been a shift from radiotherapy to chemotherapy as the initial intervention. The most studied regimen of carboplatin with vincristine has become the mainstay of initial therapy for optic pathway and/or hypothalamic gliomas, which results in tumor stability or reduction in the size of the mass with a 3-year progression-free survival of 68%. This therapy allows for radiotherapy to be deferred, if necessary, until the patient is older. About 40% of all children develop an anaphylactic type reaction to carboplatin. This risk increases with exposure to the drug, so alternative therapies are often necessary.

As the carboplatin–vincristine regimen was being studied, another combination of agents was also shown to be effective in this tumor: 6-thioguanine, procarbazine, lomustine (CCNU), dibromodulcitol, and vincristine demonstrated a 3-year progression-free survival of 45%. The use of actinomycin and vincristine, vinblastine, or the combination of 6-thioguanine, procarbazine, lomustine, and vincristine chemotherapy (TPCV) have shown efficacy. Alkylating agents such as lomustine and procarbazine should be avoided in patients with NF1 because of the oncogenic risk.

The natural history of LGG of all intracranial locations, with the intent to postpone irradiation in younger children by using carboplatinum and vincristine in nonsurgical cases, has been studied in a cohort of 1044 children, aged 1–15.4 years (median age of 5.1 years). A total of 109 (10.4%) had NF1 trait and 83 of these (76%) had an optic pathway tumor. Fifty-five children were treated with chemotherapy and 10 with radiotherapy. The overall survival rate was 96% after a median time of 5.25 years, but the progression-free survival rate was only 24% at 5 years. The 5-year progression-free survival rates were similar in the chemotherapy group (73%) and radiotherapy group (78%).

Following relapse in LGG, treatment may include surgery, often to debulk the neoplasm or drain cysts that may have formed. In most circumstances, when children have been treated with chemotherapy they will be treated with another chemotherapy regimen. This cycle of treating patients with several different chemotherapy regimens will be repeated until the patient is free of progressive disease or a point when the decision is made to treat with radiotherapy. Alternatively, some physicians recommend treatment with radiotherapy at the time of diagnosis (usually in selected older patients with well-defined and nonbulky disease) or after the first one or two failed attempts at chemotherapy.

It is not known if the response to chemotherapy results in improved vision. A review of 85 studies identified eight publications with sufficient details to address this question. These included three single-arm trials (one multi-institutional and two single institution trials) and five retrospective series, but no randomized trials. Of the 174 children reported in these studies, 25 (14.4%) had an improvement in vision after chemotherapy, with the response rate ranging 0–45.5%. Vision was stable in 82 children (47.1%, range 27–100%). No study documented the duration of the visual response.

The role of radiotherapy is generally reserved for those patients who have no remaining surgical or chemotherapeutic options because of the concern for neuropsychologic injury or oncogenesis. Conventional radiotherapy in doses of 45–54 Gy has been shown to improve survival in uncontrolled studies of this tumor in children and adults. Radiotherapy allows for a 10-year progression-free survival of 65–90%. Unfortunately, those treated with radiotherapy often suffer the consequences of an endocrinopathy, cerebrovascular disease, and neurocognitive deficits that may not become apparent for many years or even decades after the treatment.

Juvenile pilocytic astrocytoma of the cerebellum

This tumor accounts for 10% of all childhood brain tumors, generally occurring between ages 5 and 15 years. About 80% of these tumors are cystic and the classic presentation is that of a large cyst with a mural nodule. The more solid tumors contain microcystic features (Plate 14.10, see plate section opposite p. 52). Patients present with signs of increased intracranial pressure (headache, emesis, personality change), local meningeal irritation or pressure (head tilt), or ataxia. Late in the course patients may present with spells of loss of consciousness and extensor posturing, the so-called "cerebellar fits" caused by transient increases in posterior fossa pressure but early access to neuroimaging in the evaluation of headache and other neurologic signs has made this presentation rare. The tumor cyst is dark on T1 MRI and bright on FLAIR and T2 MRI. The tumor, which may only appear as a small mural nodule within the cyst, will enhance with contrast. Treatment for these lesions is surgical, with the intent of a gross total resection of the mural nodule or mass as well as the cyst wall. Some tumors can extend into the brainstem, and are therefore less amenable to complete surgical resection. Following a gross total resection these tumors seldom reoccur, with survival approaching 100% at 5 years in many series. If the tumor does recur, which is more common after a subtotal resection, then further attempts at gross total resection are recommended with a curative intent if surgical morbidity can be avoided. The role of radiotherapy in the modern management era is not clear and should be avoided unless other therapies have failed, or the tumor has transformed into a histologically high grade neoplasm (Figure 14.4).

Other low grade glial tumors

The ganglioglioma (grade II) is commonly located in the temporal lobe and often presents with seizures (Plate 14.11, see plate section opposite p. 52). The primary treatment for this disease is surgical resection and there is no role for radiotherapy in the primary treatment of this neoplasm. If both the tumor and surrounding epileptogenic zone is resected an excellent outcome is expected

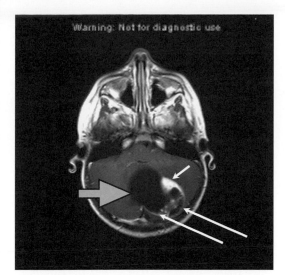

Warning: Not for diagnostic use

Figure 14.4. Cerebellar juvenile pilocytic astrocytoma. Axial T1 with gadolinium image demonstrates the mural nodule (short arrow), neoplastic cyst wall (long arrows) and cyst formation. The compressed fourth ventricle appears as a horizontal dark oval immediately ventral to the cyst at the 12 o'clock position. Radiographic images courtesy of Dr Shanker Ganapathy.

both in terms of long-term remission (and cure) for the seizures and tumor. The pilomyxoid astrocytoma is a grade II neoplasm and is most often located in the hypothalamic region. These may be bulky tumors that tend to occur in toddlers and present with the hypothalamic syndrome (cognitively normal children with a failure-to-thrive picture that includes weight and growth failure). Treatment includes combinations of surgery and chemotherapy. The pleomorphic xanthoastrocytoma is another grade II tumor that presents in the cortex, most often in the temporal lobe, and is generally approached initially with surgery, and if necessary chemotherapy. Oligodendrogliomas are very rare in childhood. Finally, the subependymal giant cell astrocytoma is a tumor found in the intraventricular region in patients with tuberous sclerosis complex. These tumors are usually very slow growing and seldom require intervention. When treatment is needed, both surgery and rapamycin chemotherapy are reasonable.

Outcome in low grade glial tumors

The outcome of 361 patients with LGG, which includes 240 5-year survivors, was reported. Patients with NF1 made up 11.6% of this group. Tumor location included hypothalamic/chiasmatic (32%), cerebellar (25%), brainstem/spinal cord (18%), cerebral (16%), and thalamic (8%). A complete surgical resection was obtained in 44%, incomplete in 48%, and 9% did not have surgery. Patients had a variety of therapies, including surgery alone in 60%. At 20 years, the overall survival was 82% and progression-free survival was 51%. The progression-free survival at 20 years was 86% in those having a gross total resection, 42% in those with less than gross total resection, and 27% in those without having surgery. At 15 years the incidence of hypothyroidism was 33%, growth hormone deficiency was 29%, and adrenocorticotropic hormone (ACTH) deficiency was 26%, all of which were more common in those children with tumors in the hypothalamic and chiasmatic region. The incidence of at least one seizure was 38% at 15 years. Neurocognitive outcome demonstrated that 34% had an IQ of <85, although those tested were more likely to have received radiotherapy or had otherwise complicated courses.

✋ CAUTION!

Long-term clinical evaluation is necessary for most long-term survivors of childhood glioma.

Conclusions

Pediatric gliomas represent a vast array of disorders with a spectrum of outcomes. Challenges including finding more effective therapy for both the high and low grade tumors and limiting treatment morbidity in the large number of survivors of the low grade cohort. For survivors, long-term management is necessary, not only for tumor surveillance but for the long-term sequelae to endocrine and neuropsychologic function, with attention to the subsequent emotional issues that often occur.

Selected bibliography

Albers AC, Gutmann DH. (2009) Gliomas in patients with neurofibromatosis type 1. *Expert Rev Neurother* **9** (4), 535–9. (Review)

Armstrong GT, Conklin HM, Huang S, Srivastava D, Sanford R, Ellison DW, *et al.* (2010) Survival and long-term health and cognitive outcomes after low-grade glioma. *Neuro-Oncology* **12** (11), 1173–86.

Bestak M. (2001) Epidemiology of brain tumors. In: Keating RF, Goodrich JT, Packer RJ (eds) *Tumors of the Pediatric Central Nervous System.* Thieme, New York, pp. 14–21.

Cohen BH, Garvin J. (2002) Brain tumors. In: Rudolph CD, Rudolph AM, Hostetter MK, Lister G, Siegel NJ (eds), *Rudolph's Pediatrics*, 21th edn. Appleton & Lange, Stamford, pp. 2207–18.

Cohen KJ, Pollack IF, Zhou T, Buxton A, Holmes EJ, Burger PC, *et al.* (2011) Temozolomide in the treatment of high-grade gliomas in children: a report from the Children's Oncology Group. *Neuro Oncol* **13** (3), 317–23.

Cohen ME, Duffner PK. (1984) Principles of clinical diagnosis. In: Cohen ME, Duffner PK (eds) *Brain Tumors in Children: Principles of Diagnosis and Treatment.* Raven Press, New York, pp. 9–21.

Fangusaro J. (2009) Pediatric high-grade gliomas and diffuse intrinsic pontine gliomas. *J Child Neurol* **24** (11), 1409–17. (Review)

Finlay J, Boyett J, Yates A, Wisoff JH, Milstein JM, Geyer JR, *et al.* (1995) Randomized phase III trial in childhood high-grade astrocytomas comparing vincristine, lomustine and prednisone with eight-drug-in-one-day regimen. *J Clin Oncol* **13**, 112–23.

Jacob K, Albrecht S, Sollier C, Faury D, Sader E, Montpetit A, *et al.* (2009) Duplication of 7q34 is specific to juvenile pilocytic astrocytomas and a hallmark of cerebellar and optic pathway tumours. *Br J Cancer* **101** (4), 722–33.

Listernick R, Ferner RE, Liu GT, Gutmann DH. (2007) Optic pathway gliomas in neurofibromatosis-1: controversies and recommendations. *Ann Neurol* **61** (3), 189–98.

Moreno L, Bautista F, Ashley S, Duncan C, Zacharoulis S. (2010) Does chemotherapy affect the visual outcome in children with optic pathway glioma? A systematic review of the evidence. *Eur J Cancer* **46** (12), 2253–9.

Packer RJ. (1999) Brain tumors in children. *Arch Neurol* **56** (4), 1999.

Packer RJ, Ater J, Allen J, Phillips P, Geyer R, Nicholson HS, *et al.* (1997) Carboplatin and vincristine chemotherapy for children with newly diagnosed progressive low-grade gliomas. *J Neurosurg* **86** (5), 747–54.

Packer RJ, Vezina G, Nicholson HS, Chadduck WM. (1999) Childhood and adolescent gliomas. In: Berger MS, Wilson CB (eds) *The Gliomas.* W.B. Saunders, Philadelphia, pp. 689–701.

Sievert AJ, Fisher MJ. (2009) Pediatric low-grade gliomas. *J Child Neurol* **24** (11), 1397–408. (Review)

Wisoff JH, Boyett JM, Berger MS, Brant C, Li H, Yates AJ, *et al.* (1998) Current neurosurgical management and the impact of the extent of resection in the treatment of malignant gliomas of childhood: a report of the Children's Cancer Group trial no. CCG-945 [see comment]. *J Neurosurg* **89** (1), 52–9.

15

Embryonal Tumors

Roger J. Packer

Center for Neuroscience and Behavioral Medicine, Brain Tumor Institute, Gilbert Neurofibromatosis Institute, Children's National, Washington, DC, USA

Introduction

Embryonal tumors are the most common form of malignant brain tumor of childhood. They can also arise in adults, predominantly in those less than 40 years of age. Embryonal tumors represent a heterogeneous group of lesions that are histologically characterized by a component of undifferentiated round cells, but may often demonstrate divergent patterns of histologic differentiation, are malignant, and share the tendency to disseminate the neuraxis early in illness or at the time of relapse. Until recently, diagnosis was based predominantly on presumed site of origin of the tumor coupled with light microscopy and immunohistochemical features. Molecular testing is increasingly being utilized for diagnosis and will likely significantly alter classification and treatment approaches.

Table 15.1 lists the present World Health Organization (WHO) classification of embryonal tumors. Pineoblastomas, which share histologic features with the embryonal tumors, are classified separately within the pineal categorization, but are historically treated as an embryonal tumor.

Clinical presentation and diagnosis

Given the heterogeneity of embryonal tumors and their growth patterns, presentation is highly dependent on location of the tumor, modified, to some extent, by the age of the patient. Diagnosis early in the course of illness can be quite difficult in the very young. Embryonal tumors may manifest with symptoms referable to the site of the lesion, such as unsteadiness and cranial neuropathies for posterior fossa lesions, and seizures and/or motor dysfunction in patients with cortical masses. However, tumors, especially those arising in the region of the fourth ventricle (medulloblastoma) or the third ventricle (pineoblastomas), are as likely or more likely to present with headaches, nausea, vomiting, unsteadiness, and alterations of level of consciousness resulting from obstruction of cerebrospinal fluid flow and secondary hydrocephalus. Although as a group, approximately 20–25% of patients with embryonal tumors will be disseminated along the neuraxis at the time of diagnosis, symptoms referable to leptomeningeal tumor spread are usually subtle or absent.

Medulloblastoma is one of five major tumor types arising in the posterior fossa in childhood. Age of onset, duration of symptoms prior to diagnosis, and the neurologic deficits present early in illness can often provide important clues to the type of tumor present (Table 15.2).

Diagnosis is usually readily made on computed tomography; however, magnetic resonance imaging (MRI) is the neuroimaging technique of choice, as it is more sensitive in determining the extent of the tumor at the

Neuro-oncology, First Edition. Edited by Roger J. Packer, David Schiff.

primary site, as well as providing important information concerning the degree of tumor dissemination (Figure 15.1). Other neuroimaging techniques such as magnetic resonance diffusion imaging and spectroscopy can be helpful in differentiation of medulloblastoma from other posterior fossa tumors, but are not usually required for diagnosis. Positron emission tomography (PET) scanning has not had a major role in tumor diagnosis or staging.

Table 15.1. World Health Organization (WHO) classification of medulloblastoma and other embryonal tumors (2007).

Medulloblastoma
Desmoplastic/nodular medulloblastoma
Medulloblastoma with extensive nodularity
Anaplastic medulloblastoma
Large cell medulloblastoma
CNS primitive neuroectodermal tumor
CNS neuroblastoma
CNS ganglioneuroblastoma
Medulloepithelioma
Ependymoblastoma
Atypical teratoid/rhabdoid tumor
Pineoblastoma (listed in WHO as a pineal region tumor)

Aspects of general management

The majority of treatment approaches used for embryonal tumors are derivations of schemas developed for medulloblastomas. Because all embryonal tumors share the tendency to disseminate to the nervous system, staging is usually employed for all embryonal tumors and is a key component of risk stratification. Staging schemas usually include determination of the amount of residual tumor after operation and the degree of tumor dissemination, based both on MRI of the entire neuraxis (preferably performed preoperatively) and, if deemed safe, lumbar cerebrospinal fluid analysis. These studies have found MRI of the neuraxis and lumbar cerebrospinal fluid

Table 15.2. Clinical presentation of posterior fossa tumors in children.

Tumor type	Incidence in posterior fossa	Peak age	Symptoms duration prior to diagnosis	Common symptoms/signs
Medulloblastoma	30–40%	3–5 years 7–10 years	1–3 months	Early headache Nausea Vomiting Papilledema Truncal ataxia
Cerebellar astrocytoma	30–40%	6–10 years	2–5 months	Early appendicular dysmetria Gait disturbance Later, nausea, vomiting, headache
Ependymoma	10%	5–9 years Early age peak (<2 years)	2–5 months (variable)	VIth, VIIth, VIIIth neuropathies Ataxia Headaches Nausea/vomiting
Brainstem glioma	10–20%	5–15 years	1–6 months (variable)	Cranial neuropathy Ataxia Hemiparesis (crossed)
Atypical teratoid/ rhabdoid	2–5%; (?15–20%) of all infantile	Less than 2 years	1–4 months	Cranial neuropathy (VIth, VIIth) Swallowing difficulties Vomiting, ataxia

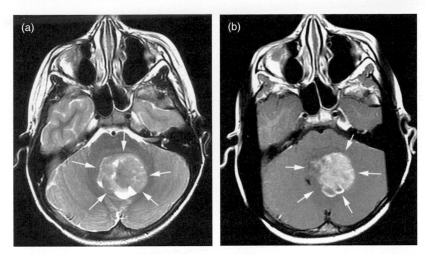

Figure 15.1. Medulloblastoma filling the fourth ventricle (a) without and (b) after gadolinium. (a) T1 weighted; (b) T2 weighted post gadolinium.

analysis to be complementary in determination of extent of disease.

Specific tumor types

Medulloblastoma

Medulloblastoma is the most common embryonal tumor and comprises approximately 20% of all childhood brain tumors, 40% of all malignant childhood brain tumors, and approximately 2% of adult brain tumors. The tumor in childhood has a bimodal distribution, peaking at 3–5 years of age, and then again between 7 and 10 years of age. Up to 20% occur in children less than 3 years of age. As is the case for all embryonal tumors, the etiology of the majority of medulloblastoma is unknown. However, several familial syndromes have been associated with an increased risk of developing medulloblastoma.

> **SCIENCE REVISTED**
>
> Cancer predisposition syndromes underlie a minority of childhood medulloblastoma. Syndromes include: Gorlin (nevoid basal cell carcinoma) syndrome characterized early in life by features including calcification of the falx, bifid/fused ribs and mandibular cysts (basal cell carcinomas occur later in life), and is associated with desmoplastic (sonic hedgehog driven) medulloblastomas; Turcot (familial polyposis) characterized by colorectal tumors and is associated with medulloblastomas driven by the WNT pathway; and Li–Fraumeni (multiple familial cancers) syndrome.

By definition, all medulloblastomas must arise in the posterior fossa. The tumor is histologically characterized by large areas of small round cells with deeply basophilic nuclei of variable sizes and shapes, little discernible cytoplasm, and abundant mitoses. However, it has been recognized for decades that this tumor may also display areas of apparent cellular differentiation. In addition, some tumors are relatively homogeneous, while others are "anaplastic." Still another subgroup of medulloblastomas have prominent desmoplasia. Anaplasia and desmoplasia (especially nodular) have been shown to be prognostic in certain settings or age groups.

Molecular genetic studies have demonstrated that medulloblastomas are likely genetically comprised of different tumor types with varying degrees of aggressivity and possibly differing responses to treatment. It is still unclear how many distinct tumor types exist, although it is now fairly well accepted that the following subgroups exist:

1 WNT-driven pathway tumors, immunohisto-chemically characterized by nuclear beta-catenin immunostaining and monosomy 6 occurring predominantly in older children.
2 Sonic hedgehog-driven tumors identified by polyclonal antibody staining, and a 9q loss and/or 9p gain, often histologically manifest by desmoplasia (especially extensive nodularity in infants) occurring both in very young children (carrying "excellent" prognosis) and in older children and adults.
3 Tumors with MYC or MYCN amplification, comprising 5–10% of medulloblastomas occurring across all age groups and carrying a "poorer" prognosis.
4 The remaining 60–65% of tumors, which have been split by some authors into different subsets and carrying an intermediate prognosis.

This rapid expansion in the understanding of the molecular genetics of medulloblastoma has yet to result in major therapeutic alterations. These molecular findings are now being incorporated into risk stratification schema, although no one stratification schema has yet to be accepted (Table 15.3).

Clinical presentation

The presentation of medulloblastoma, as noted in Table 15.2, is usually from early obstruction of the fourth ventricle, with associated hydrocepha-

lus, headaches, vomiting, nausea, and ataxia. Unsteadiness is usually truncal and quite marked. Cranial neuropathies, other than VIth nerve palsies and/or paresis are relatively infrequent, although upbeat and lateral nystagmus is common. Approximately 20% of patients will have no or little hydrocephalus at diagnosis and primarily cerebellar deficits. Presentation can be acute, caused by hemorrhage into the tumor, and may include the sudden onset of coma. As in all infants, diagnosis can be difficult and early symptoms can include failure to thrive and loss or slowing of gain of motor milestones – associated with vomiting, crossed eyes, and "sun-setting" (downward deviation) of the eyes. Because tumors in adults tend to have a predilection for the cerebellopontine angle region, the tempo of the illness may be slower, with VIth and VIIth nerve paresis, appendicular dysmetria, associated with nonspecific headaches, early in the course of illness, until the tumor fills the fourth ventricle and causes more classic symptoms.

Management

The initial step in the management of all patients with medulloblastoma is surgery to both confirm diagnosis and to remove the majority of the tumor, if possible. In patients with nondisseminated disease, the extent of surgical resection has been correlated with better outcome, as patients after total or near-total resections have been

Table 15.3. Risk stratification of medulloblastoma in children older than 3 years.

	Good risk	Average risk	High risk (any factor)
Extent of disease	Localized	Localized	Disseminated
Degree of resection	Total/near-total	Total/near-total	Subtotal (>1.5 cm^2 residual)
Histology/ immunohistochemistry	Nuclear Beta-catenin staining	Classic	Anaplastic
Molecular findings	Monosomy 6 (isolated)	Non-specific No MYC/MYCN amplification	MYC/MYCN amplification
Associated features	Usually older patients	All age groups	All age groups
Progression-free survival at 5 years	90%	70–80%	30–60%

shown to experience a higher event-free and overall survival rate. Over the past two decades, an increasing incidence of the postoperative posterior fossa mutism syndrome has been reported, believed to be secondary to surgery-associated disruption of cerebellar pathway to the thalamus and cerebrocortex, with many patients having significant permanent sequelae. Extent of resection has not been clearly associated with improved outcome in patients with disseminated disease.

☙ CAUTION!

Posterior fossa mutism syndrome, also known as the cerebellar mutism syndrome, is manifest by the delayed onset of mutism (6–48 hours post-surgery), emotional lability/irritability, truncal hypotonia, supranuclear palsies, and ataxia/dysmetria. It has much in common with cerebellar affective disorder. For diagnosis, there should be no clinical or radiographic evidence of direct brainstem damage. Recovery is variable in tempo and is incomplete in at least 50%; those affected are at higher risk of neurocognitive sequelae.

Following surgery, children greater than 3 years of age (and in some series greater than 4 or 5 years of age) have been stratified into two risk groups. Newer data suggest that future stratification schemas incorporating biologic data will separate patients into three or more risk groups. Those patients with so-called "average risk" disease (those with neoplastic, nondisseminated, and totally or near-totally resected tumors) are treated with craniospinal and local boost radiotherapy (total dose 5400–5960 cGy) and chemotherapy. Although 3600 cGy of craniospinal radiotherapy was historically utilized for patients with nondisseminated disease, recent studies have demonstrated that a reduced dose of craniospinal radiation therapy (2400 cGy) is as effective, if coupled with chemotherapy during and after radiotherapy. Preradiation chemotherapy following surgery has not been shown to be as effective as the immediate institution of postoperative radiotherapy.

A variety of multiagent chemotherapeutic regimens have been utilized, with similar rates of disease control. Most of these regimens have been cisplatin-based multiagent drug combinations, and have also included drugs such as vincristine, CCNU, and cyclophosphamide.

☙ CAUTION!

Ototoxicity is frequently dose limiting in patients of all ages. Older children and adults may have difficulty in tolerating vincristine because of excessive peripheral neuropathy.

Higher dose adjuvant regimens following radiation therapy have also been utilized supported by peripheral stem cell rescue with similar, but not clearly better, survival rates. Such regimens have the advantage of truncating treatment and decreasing cisplatin exposure, but have more potential for bone marrow toxicity and sepsis. After treatment with total or near-total resection, radiotherapy, and chemotherapy, 80% or more of children with "average-risk" medulloblastoma can be expected to be alive and free of disease 5 years following diagnosis, many of whom are likely cured.

For patients with "high risk" disease, similar treatment approaches are usually undertaken, although survival rates are lower, in the range (dependent on series) 50–65% 5 years from diagnosis. For the majority of high risk patients, the craniospinal dose has remained at 3600 cGy and chemotherapeutic approaches have utilized more aggressive regimens, including using chemotherapy concomitant with radiation therapy (carboplatin) or using higher doses of chemotherapy following completion of radiation therapy. Once again, the use of chemotherapy before radiation therapy has not been shown to improve the likelihood of long-term disease control.

⚛ SCIENCE REVISITED

Progress in the therapeutic approach to patients with medulloblastoma has been facilitated by the performance of large, and often randomized, prospective trials performed in children on both the national and international level.

Adult management

The optimal therapeutic regimen for adults with medulloblastoma is far from clearcut. In general, adults tolerate poorly the chemotherapy used in children and it is often difficult to deliver similar amounts of chemotherapy (especially cisplatin and vincristine) to patients over 21 years of age. Vincristine is less well tolerated in adolescents and in adults, often with dose-limiting peripheral neuropathy. Cisplatin has been noted to more likely cause large-fiber neuropathy in adults than children. For this reason, there has been hesitancy in reducing the amount of craniospinal radiation therapy from 3600 cGy and there is no consensus on which chemotherapeutic regimen is more effective and can be tolerated in adults with this disease. Survival figures in adult series are usually in the range of 50–65% at 5 years, dependent on the stage of disease and type of treatment given.

Infant management

The management of infants with medulloblastoma is far from optimal. A subset of very young children have desmoplastic tumors, especially those with extensive nodularity (thought to be driven by sonic hedgehog aberrant signaling), have an extremely good prognosis (70–80% survival) after treatment with chemotherapy alone. There is significant hesitancy to utilize craniospinal radiation therapy in very young children because of concerns over long-term neurologic sequelae. Chemotherapy is usually utilized as the initial treatment after surgery for children younger than 3 years and in some series for children younger than 4 or 5 years of age. A variety of different chemotherapeutic approaches have been utilized and have become increasingly intensified by the addition of drugs such as methotrexate (both intravenously at high dose or intrathecally) which may be neurotoxic, or the use of higher doses of chemotherapy supported by autologous bone marrow or peripheral stem cell rescue. There is a sense that the more intensive regimens have been somewhat more effective, although some of the improvements in survival may be more apparent than real, as some subsets of highly virulent embryonal tumors such as the atypical teratoid or rhabdoid tumor have been recently recognized and removed from medulloblastoma studies and other studies seem to produce a high (? over) representation of the better prognosis desmoplastic infantile tumors. Survival rates for infants with classic (nondesmoplastic) medulloblastoma treated with chemotherapy alone are in the range of 20–40% and studies are underway to attempt to intensify chemotherapy even further or to introduce focal radiation therapy early in the course of treatment. Infants with disseminated disease at diagnosis have a particularly poor outcome, independent of treatment.

Sequelae

Of major concern in all subgroups of patients with medulloblastoma, and for that matter in all embryonal tumors, are the sequelae of treatment. Although radiation therapy has been recognized as a major cause of long-term neurologic sequelae, other factors also add to the likelihood of long-term neurologic compromise including presurgical neurologic impairment, neurologic (usually brainstem) damage caused during surgery, posterior fossa mutism, side effects of chemotherapy (especially cisplatin-induced ototoxicity), and still to be determined, likely genetically driven host vulnerabilities. Children who have received craniospinal radiation therapy, especially those between 3 and 7 years of age, are likely to develop significant intellectual decline within 3 years of treatment. Even with a reduction of the dose of craniospinal radiation therapy from 3600 to 2400 cGy, a 10 to 15 point IQ drop within 3 years of treatment is common. The presence of posterior fossa mutism or chemotherapy-induced ototoxicity intensifies such intellectual compromise. Other long-term sequelae such as seizures, vertigo, other motoric dysfunction, psychologic difficulties, and specific learning disabilities are also common. Dependent on the dose of craniospinal radiation therapy and the age of the patient, significant hormonal deficits may also be present, especially growth hormone deficiency. All of these considerations have led to studies attempting to reduce the dose of craniospinal radiation therapy even further (as low as 1800 cGy in average risk patients); reducing the total dose of cisplatin; or using different forms of radiotherapy, such as proton beam, to decrease radiation scatter to other organs. In addition to the above sequelae, secondary tumors, including malignant gliomas, usually peaking 5–15 years following completion of therapy, and meningiomas usually beginning to become evident 8–10 years after completion of radiotherapy, have been increasingly reported. It is hoped that a better understanding of the molecular underpinnings of medulloblastomas will lead to the development of more personalized, biologically based, safer treatments in the near future.

Atypical teratoid/rhabdoid tumors

Atypical teratoid/rhabdoid tumors (AT/RT) were first clearly described as a distinct entity in 1987. The exact incidence of these tumors in unclear, but they probably comprise 15–20% of all embryonal tumors occurring in children younger than 2 years of age. The median age at diagnosis has been between 1 and 2 years of age, although this tumor has now been recognized in older children and even in young adults. Diagnosis of AT/RT is strongly suggested by histologic and immunohistochemical features. These tumors are comprised of areas resembling other primitive neuroectodermal tumors, such as medulloblastoma, intermixed with other areas containing larger rhabdoid cells. Immunohistochemical analysis has demonstrated that in the regions of rhabdoid cells there is epithelial membrane antigen, vimentin, and smooth muscle actin expression. Cytogenetically, tumors demonstrate a deletion of chromosome 22 in the region which contains the *INI1/hSNF5* (*SMARCB1*) gene, a tumor suppressor gene. Although initially these tumors were thought to be predominantly sporadic, germline mutations are increasingly being diagnosed.

Clinical presentation and diagnosis

AT/RT present similarly to other embryonal tumors. Dependent on series, 20–50% of AT/RT arise in the cerebellopontine angle, and up to 50% occur supratentorially. Leptomeningeal dissemination, at the time of diagnosis, is present in 20–25% of patients. Neuroimaging does not clearly differentiate AT/RT from other primitive neuroectodermal tumors; however, these tumors do tend to enhance readily with gadolinium, are likely to be in the cerebellopontine angle if infratentorial, and often contain hemorrhagic or necrotic foci.

Management

The management of AT/RT is extremely problematic. The smaller subgroup of patients who are older, especially those older than 3 years of age, and treated with immediate craniospinal radiation therapy and adjuvant chemotherapy, have a better prognosis; especially after total or near-total resection. Survival rates of more than 50% have been reported in this subset. Outcome for children younger than 3 years, especially less than 1 year of age with AT/RT, is quite poor. Overall, fewer than 20% of infants survive. As is the case with medulloblastoma, most series have suggested better outcomes in all age groups, if total tumor resection can be performed. Because of the cerebellopontine angle location (? origin) of many AT/RT and involvement of multiple cranial nerves at diagnosis, total resection is often impossible. Radiotherapy is used as in most medulloblastoma therapeutic approaches, with the caveat that most would recommend earlier intervention with focal radiation therapy in patients with nondisseminated disease, usually after a short course of induction chemotherapy.

The chemotherapeutic approaches that have been applied to AT/RT have varied. Some have utilized the same "intensified" chemotherapies used in infants and young children with medulloblastoma and others have recommended a more hybrid approach utilizing drug regimens that include the agents used for infantile medulloblastoma, coupled with drugs that are employed in sarcoma regimens.

CNS primitive neuroectodermal tumors

CNS primitive neuroectodermal tumors are a confusing subgrouping of embryonal tumors. Those that have arisen in the cortical or subcortical regions of brain, in the past, have been classified as supratentorial primitive neuroectodermal tumors, cerebral or central neuroblastomas, cerebral medulloblastomas, and/or pineoblastomas. They account in total for 2% or less of childhood brain tumors and usually arise in the first decade of life, especially in infancy.

Clinical presentation

Vomiting, nausea, and headaches are the most common initial symptoms resulting from cerebrospinal fluid obstruction or local mass effect. Dependent on location of tumor origin in the nervous system, other more focal neurologic deficits may be present. This is especially true for supratentorial primitive neuroectodermal tumors which can present with hemiparesis and/or seizures. In infancy, these tumors are notoriously difficult to diagnose and may be extremely large at the time of diagnosis. Diagnosis is usually readily made on neuroimaging, as these lesions are classically heterogenic with two-thirds demonstrating some type of cystic or necrotic foci. Interestingly, in supratentorial tumors, peritumoral edema may be mild or absent.

Management

As is the case with other embryonal tumors, surgical resection is a significant component of treatment and prognosis may be improved after gross total resection even in those tumors arising in the pineal region. Tumors are staged like medulloblastomas, but because of the supratentorial location of these lesions, cerebrospinal fluid cytological examination is often contraindicated.

Radiation therapy is a major component of treatment. Given the age of the majority of patients and cortical location of the tumors, there is a reluctance to utilize craniospinal large volume local boost radiotherapy in the very young. For localized tumors, one approach has been to use aggressive chemotherapy followed by focal radiotherapy to the tumor site, utilizing conformal techniques to minimize the amount of radiotherapy to the surrounding cortex. The chemotherapeutic regimens have been similar to those utilized for medulloblastoma. Overall, prognosis has varied significantly between series. Survival rates of over 50% at 5 years have been noted in older children with supratentorial primitive neuroectodermal tumors after treatment with craniospinal and local boost radiotherapy and chemotherapy. Survival is better in those "totally" resected. However, survival rates are not nearly as favorable in younger children.

Other central nervous system embryonal tumors

Data on which to determine the optimal management of other embryonal tumors are lacking. These tumors tend to be rare and most reports either have included them into series of patients treated for infantile medulloblastoma or as case series of patients treated in a variety of different ways. Even the existence of some of these tumor types as a distinct entity has been questioned. Central neuroblastoma is an old term and most patients are now considered to have supratentorial primitive neuroectodermal tumors.

Medulloepitheliomas are rare and are characterized by a histologic appearance that mimics the embryonal neural tube. Prognosis is quite poor. The majority of patients die of their disease within 1 year of diagnosis. Survival has been noted primarily in those amenable to a gross total resection followed by some form of aggressive adjuvant therapy, which usually includes radiation therapy and chemotherapy. The few long-term survivors usually have significant neurologic and neurocognitive sequelae.

The existence of ependymoblastomas as a distinct entity has been recently challenged. Molecular genetic evidence suggests that this tumor might be better grouped as an embryonal tumor with abundant neuropil and true rosettes. In older series, ependymoblastomas were noted predominantly in the first 2 years of life, clinically tended to present explosively with focal neurologic deficits and symptoms of increased intracranial pressure, and were large lesions with significant surrounding contrast enhancement and edema. In some series, ependymoblastomas were often grouped into studies evaluating ependymomas as a variant of malignant ependymoma, making recommendations even more difficult. Outcome has been noted to be quite poor, with few patients surviving.

Selected bibliography

Albright AL, Wisoff JH, Zeltzer PM, Boyett JM, Rorke JM, Stanley P. (1996) Effects of medulloblastoma resections on outcome in children: a report from the Children's Cancer Group. *Neurosurgery* **38** (2), 265–71.

Chintagumpala M, Hassall T, Palmer S, Ashley D, Wallace D, Kasow K, et al. (2009) A pilot study of risk-adapted radiotherapy and chemotherapy in patients with supratentorial PNET. Neuro Oncol 11 (1), 33–40,.

Cohen BH, Zeltzer PM, Boyett JM, Geyer JR, Allen JC, Finlay JL, et al. (1995) Prognostic factors and treatment results for supratentorial primitive neuroectodermal tumors in children using radiation and chemotherapy: a Children's Cancer Group randomized trial. J Clin Oncol 13 (7), 1687–96.

Duffner PK, Horowitz ME, Krischer JP, Friedman HS, Burger PC, Cohen ME, et al. (1993) Postoperative chemotherapy and delayed radiation in children less than three years of age with malignant brain tumors. N Engl J Med 328 (24), 1725–31.

Eberhart CG, Kratz J, Wang Y, Summers K, Stearns D, Cohen K, et al. (2004) Histopathological and molecular prognostic markers in medulloblastoma: c-myc, N-myc, TrkC, and anaplasia. J Neuropathol Exp Neurol 63 (5), 441–9.

Gajjar A, Chintagumpala M, Ashley D, Kellie S, Kun LE, Merchant TE, et al. (2006) Risk-adapted craniospinal radiotherapy followed by high-dose chemotherapy and stem-cell rescue in children with newly diagnosed medulloblastoma (St. Jude Medulloblastoma-96): long-term results from a prospective, multicentre trial. Lancet Oncol 7 (10), 813–20.

Geyer JR, Sposto R, Jennings M, Boyett JM, Axtell RA, Breiger D, et al. (2005) Multiagent chemotherapy and deferred radiotherapy in infants with malignant brain tumors: a report from the Children's Cancer Group. J Clin Oncol 23 (30), 7621–31.

Giangaspero F, Wellek S, Masuoka J, Gessi M, Kleihues P, Ohgaki H. (2006) Stratification of medulloblastoma on the basis of histopathological grading. Acta Neuropathol 112 (1), 5–12.

Grill J, Sainte-Rose C, Jouvet A, Gentet JC, Lejars O, Frappaz D, et al. (2005) Treatment of medulloblastoma with postoperative chemotherapy alone: an SFOP prospective trial in young children. Lancet Oncol 6 (8), 573–80.

Judkins AR, Ellison DW. (2010) Ependymoblastoma: dear, damned, distracting diagnosis, farewell! Brain Pathol 20 (1), 133–9.

Kool M, Koster J, Bunt J, Hassett NE, Lakeman A, van Sluis P, et al. (2008) Integrated genomics identifies five medulloblastoma subtypes with distinct genetic profiles, pathway signatures and clinicopathological features. PLoS One 3 (8), e3088.

Louis DN, Ohgaki H, Wiestler OD, Cavenee WK, Burger PC, Jouvet A, et al. (eds) (2007) WHO Classification of Tumours of the Central Nervous System, 4th edn. IARC Press, Lyon, France.

Merchant TE, Kun LE, Krasin MJ, Wallace D, Chintagumpala MM, Woo SY, et al. (2008) Multi-institution prospective trial of reduced-dose craniospinal irradiation (23.4 Gy) followed by conformal posterior fossa (36 Gy) and primary site irradiation (55.8 Gy) and dose-intensive chemotherapy for average-risk medulloblastoma. Int J Radiat Oncol Biol Phys 70 (3), 782–7.

Packer RJ, Gajjar A, Vezina G, Rorke-Adams L, Burger PC, Robertson PL, et al. (2006) Phase III study of craniospinal radiation therapy followed by adjuvant chemotherapy for newly diagnosed average-risk medulloblastoma. J Clin Oncol 24 (25), 4202–8.

Pfister S, Remke M, Benner A, Mendrzyk F, Toedt G, Felsberg J, et al. (2009) Outcome prediction in pediatric medulloblastoma based on DNA copy-number aberrations of chromosomes 6q and 17q and the MYC and MYCN loci. J Clin Oncol 27 (10), 1627–36.

Pomeroy SL, Tamayo P, Gaasenbeek M, Sturla LM, Angelo M, McLaughlin ME, et al. (2002) Prediction of central nervous system embryonal tumour outcome based on gene expression. Nature 415, 436–42.

Reddy AT, Janss AJ, Phillips PC, Weiss HL, Packer RJ. (2000) Outcome for children with supratentorial primitive neuroectodermal tumors treated with surgery, radiation, and chemotherapy. Cancer 88 (9), 2189–93.

Robertson PL, Muraszko KM, Holmes EJ, Sposto R, Packer RJ, Gajar A, et al. (2006) Incidence and severity of postoperative cerebellar mutism syndrome in children with medulloblastoma: a prospective study by the Children's Oncology Group. J Neurosurg 105 (6), 444–51.

Rutkowski S, Bode U, Deinlein F, Ottensmeier H, Warmuth-Metz M, Soerensen N, et al. (2005) Treatment of early childhood medulloblastoma by postoperative chemotherapy alone. *N Engl J Med* **352** (10), 978–86.

Taylor RE, Bailey CC, Robinson K, Weston CL, Ellison D, Ironside J, *et al.* (2003) Results of a randomized study of preradiation chemotherapy versus radiotherapy alone for nonmetastatic medulloblastoma: The International Society of Paediatric Oncology/United Kingdom Children's Cancer Study Group PNE-3 Study. *J Clin Oncol* **21** (8), 1581–91.

Thomas PR, Deutsch M, Kepner JL, Bovett JM, Krischer J, Aronin P, *et al.* (2000) Low-stage medulloblastoma: final analysis of trial comparing standard-dose with reduced-dose neuroaxis irradiation. *J Clin Oncol* **18** (16), 3004–11.

von Hoff K, Hartmann W, von Bueren AO, Gerber NU, Grotzer MA, Pietsch T, *et al.* (2010) Large cell/anaplastic medulloblastoma: outcome according to myc status, histopathological, and clinical risk factors. *Pediatr Blood Cancer* **54** (3), 369–76.

Wells EM, Khademian ZP, Walsh KS, Vezina G, Sposto R, Keating RF, *et al.* (2010) Postoperative cerebellar mutism syndrome following treatment of medulloblastoma: neuroradiographic features and origin. *J Neurosurg Pediatr* **5** (4), 329–34.

Zeltzer PM, Boyett JM, Finlay JL, Albright AL, Rorke LB, Milstein JM, *et al.* (1999) Metastasis stage, adjuvant treatment, and residual tumor are prognostic factors for medulloblastoma in children: conclusions from the Children's Cancer Group 921 randomized phase III study. *J Clin Oncol* **17** (3), 832–45.

16

Infantile Brain Tumors

Alyssa T. Reddy

University of Alabama at Birmingham Departments of Pediatrics, Neurology and Surgery, Children's of Alabama, Birmingham, AL, USA

Introduction

The treatment of brain tumors is nowhere more vexing than in infants and very young children. As a group, those less than 36 months of age, referred to here as "infants," have to deal with the impact of both disease and treatment on the delicate developing nervous system. This patient population is considered extremely vulnerable to the side effects of treatment, particularly radiation therapy. At the same time, infants often have large, highly aggressive tumors which have grown quickly in and around critical structures. Many of the tumors require a multimodal approach to cure. Lessons from the last three decades have taught us that treatment of infantile brain tumors must be based on histology and even histologic subtype as well as extent of disease and age of the patient. Prior to the mid-1980s, surgery and radiation were traditional treatments for malignant infantile brain tumors and mimicked treatment in older children. Poor outcomes and severe neurotoxicity led to the use of chemotherapy in this population and the delay or avoidance of radiation therapy. In 1986, the Pediatric Oncology Group (POG) conducted the first cooperative group study in which infants with malignant brain tumors were treated with prolonged post-operative chemotherapy in order to avoid or delay radiation. The Children's Cancer Group (CCG) and European consortiums quickly made this shift with varying combinations of cytotoxic drugs. These studies demonstrated that chemotherapy had a role in some but not all infantile brain tumors and the neuro-oncology community began to tease out disease-specific treatment protocols. This chapter discusses the spectrum of brain tumors in infants, current treatment strategies, and ongoing challenges to improve long-term outcome. The balance of disease control and treatment toxicity has driven paradigms in the treatment of brain tumors in very young children.

Epidemiology

Approximately 25% of childhood brain tumors are diagnosed in children younger than 36 months of age and over half of these in the first 24 months of life. The overall location of brain tumors in infants differs from the posterior fossa predominance in older children. In the first year of life, the supratentorial location is more common, with 70% of infantile patients having tumors in this location. However, medulloblastoma, which by definition occurs in the posterior fossa, is the most common type of malignant tumor.

Infantile brain tumors are not histologically distinct from those tumors occurring in older children. Similar to older children, the common malignant brain tumors are medulloblastoma, followed by ependymoma, and high grade glioma. Cortical primitive neuroectodermal tumors (PNET) and pineoblastoma as well as other more rare entities also occur. There are two histologic types that occur predominantly in very young children: atypical teratoid rhabdoid tumor (ATRT) and choroid carcinoma; these are rare overall but combined represent 20–40% of malignant infantile brain tumors. Low grade glial neoplasms are not uncommon but, because they are not grouped with malignant tumors in studies, their true incidence is not clear. Because of the congenital nature of many of both the benign and malignant tumors of infancy, histologic classification can be difficult.

Initial presentation and evaluation

Infants with brain tumors, both slow and fast growing, often present with hydrocephalus and macrocephaly. Because young children have open sutures, a rapidly enlarging head size should alert the practitioner to evaluate the patient for a brain mass as this may be the only symptom at presentation. The pliable young skull allows for compensation of hydrocephalus and tumors are often quite large before clinical symptoms are overtly apparent. Infants are non-verbal, making picking up of subtle symptoms difficult. Fussiness, loss of milestones, and failure to thrive can all be associated signs and symptoms. Just as with older children, patients may present with cranial nerve palsies, vision loss, hemiparesis, or seizures, depending on tumor location.

All infants with brain tumors should undergo magnetic resonance imaging (MRI) with and without gadolinium prior to surgical resection unless emergent surgery is necessary. If a malignant tumor is suspected, patients should also have their spines imaged prior to surgery to look for evidence of disseminated disease. It is also often helpful to have serum electrolyte tests, particularly sodium, as either diabetes insipidus or

cerebral salt wasting can occur. Postoperatively, further work-up is dictated by tumor type and is discussed throughout the chapter.

Medulloblastoma

Medulloblastoma is the most common malignant tumor in infants as it is in older children. Because it is a posterior fossa tumor, patients typically present with symptoms of hydrocephalus, balance difficulty, cranial nerve palsies, particularly VIth and VIIth, and fussiness. MRI typically shows a large heterogeneously enhancing mass. Patients should always be evaluated for leptomeningeal and spinal dissemination at diagnosis as this occurs in up to 25% of cases (Figure 16.1).

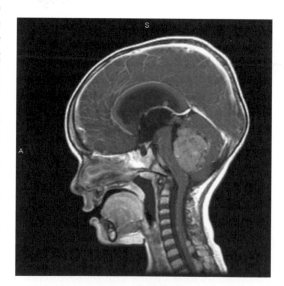

Figure 16.1. Disseminated medulloblastoma: sagittal post-gadolinium magnetic resonance image (MRI) demonstrates large posterior fossa tumor with disseminated disease in brain and spine of a 2-year-old with medulloblastoma.

Management

The recognition that medulloblastoma is sensitive to chemotherapy has led to a key role of multiagent therapy in infant treatment protocols for the disease. Both the POG and Children's Oncology Group (COG), as well as European consortiums, have conducted large prospective trials for patients younger than 3 years of age with medulloblastoma. These cooperative group studies in the 1980s and 1990s demonstrated excellent initial response rates to chemotherapy with varying regimens. Combinations of drugs that include such agents as carboplatin or cisplatin, cyclophosphamide, etoposide, vincristine, ifosfamide, and methotrexate have been used. In these studies, patients were typically given multiagent chemotherapy after surgery and radiation was either delayed or avoided completely. Unfortunately, the responses were not always durable and overall disappointing survival rates of 21–50% have been reported. A COG study that incorporated chemotherapy and conformal posterior fossa irradiation demonstrated a 3-year event-free survival rate of 50%. More recently, there have been intensified regimens that utilize high dose chemotherapy followed by stem cell rescue in an attempt to improve survival. The COG has demonstrated that this approach is feasible in their recent study 99703 where patients were given three cycles of induction therapy followed by triple tandem transplant with thiotepa and carboplatin. Some survival advantage appears to have been gained from this more aggressive approach. The Head Start protocols and German HIT studies report improved survival with intensive regimen multiagent chemotherapy that includes methotrexate. A key finding of the German study was the prognostic significance of desmoplastic histology. Survival rates for patients with desmoplastic medulloblastoma was more than double those with classic histology, regardless of initial staging, with a 5-year progression-free survival of 85%. On the Head Start study patients with disseminated medulloblastoma treated with high dose therapy had a 3-year progression-free survival of 49%. Similar encouraging results were reported for patients with nondisseminated desmoplastic medulloblastoma, who had a 5-year progression-free survival of 68% when treated with high dose chemotherapy.

What can be gleaned from these studies is that survival seems to be improved by complete surgical resection and lack of dissemination. There is also emerging evidence that histologic subtype has prognostic significance. Infants with desmoplastic medulloblastoma appear to have improved survival while those with classic or anaplastic histology appear to have poorer survival. Regardless of risk factors, patients who relapse tend to do so early, within the first few months of treatment, and late failures are rate.

The current COG study is attempting to evaluate further the role of methotrexate in induction therapy followed by high dose chemotherapy during consolidation for patients with high risk disease. Obtaining biologic specimens for further histologic subtype and correlation with outcome is a key part of the study.

Infants with medulloblastoma should be staged into high, low, or average risk categories like their older counterparts. Care should be given to degree of resection, extent of disease, and histologic subtype. Although no standard of care currently exists for these patients, consideration should be given to entering them on a treatment protocol if they are eligible. For survivors of medulloblastoma, the potential long-term side effects are well known. Infants who have survived medulloblastoma need close monitoring of neurocognitive, physical, and social development as well as endocrinologic function, hearing, and vision. They should be evaluated early and often with a multidisciplinary approach to assure the best outcome possible.

✋ CAUTION!

Patients with desmoplastic medulloblastoma appear to have significantly increased rates of survival and may require less intensive therapy than those with nondesmoplastic tumors. Care should be given to identify the histologic subtype.

Primitive neuroectodermal tumors

Medulloblastoma is considered a PNET of the cerebellum but PNET occurs throughout the nervous system. As the name implies, supratentorial PNET (SPNET) occurs above the tentorium cerebri, the most common of which is the pineoblastoma. The tumors also rarely occur in the cortex and spinal cord. These tumors are high grade malignancies and carry risk of cerebrospinal fluid (CSF) dissemination similar to medulloblastoma. Because they are relatively rare, these tumors typically have been lumped into treatment trials with medulloblastoma and more recently with high risk medulloblastoma. From a histologic standpoint this would intuitively seem to make sense although many studies have indicated that outcome for these patients may be even worse than those with high risk medulloblastoma.

Management

The POG and CCG infant protocols in the 1990s reported dismal results for patients with pineoblastoma treated with conventional chemotherapy and radiation, with early relapses and no long-term survivors. A marginal improvement of 17% 5-year event-free survival was seen with the more chemo-intensive CCG protocol but survival was still poor compared with medulloblastoma. Other studies have demonstrated better survival for those with cortical PNET especially when complete resection can be achieved. More recently, protocols have attempted to improve survival rates with more intensive chemotherapy to including high dose treatment with stem cell rescue. Because of small patient numbers in any one study, however, it is hard to demonstrate a clear survival advantage with one regimen or approach.

Infants with PNET must be fully staged with MRI of brain and spine and CSF cytology unless medically contraindicated. Tumor tissue should be collected, not only for diagnosis, but also for submission into a national tumor bank so that further studies can be carried out on this rare entity. Again, no clear standard of care exists and consideration should be given to treating patients on a treatment trial. Currently, treatment trials for PNET are looking at the role of intensive chemotherapy with and without methotrexate, high dose therapy with stem cell rescue, and focused radiation. The degree of surgical resection is also assessed.

Ependymoma

Ependymoma in infants typically arises in the posterior fossa, specifically in and around the fourth ventricle. It can invade the cerebellopontine angle and cause cranial nerve palsies. In 20% or less of cases it is located supratentorially. Although patients should be fully staged at diagnosis with MRI imaging of brain and spine as well as CSF cytology, dissemination at diagnosis is rare. Histologically, ependymoma is classified as either classic, sometimes referred to as differentiated, or anaplastic. The clinical significance of this distinction is not clear but some studies have suggested that patients with anaplastic tumors do less well.

Management

A complete surgical resection has a bearing on survival and appears to be the most important prognostic indicator. Aggressive surgery, even if it imparts a deficit, is often justified if no tumor is left behind. Radiation therapy also has an important role in survival for patients with ependymoma. In a series of 78 patients between the ages of 2 and 3 years treated with conformal irradiation, the 5-year event-free and overall survival rates were 68% and 80%, respectively. Survival rates fall to about half of those with subtotal or partial resection. Earlier attempts by cooperative group infant brain tumor studies to treat ependymoma without radiation were not as successful. Although responses were seen, 4-year progression and overall survival rates for those treated with surgery followed by chemotherapy hovered between 20–26% and 35–60%. This has led to a willingness on the part of the neurooncology community to treat patients younger than 3 years with conformal or intensity modulated radiotherapy.

Newer conformal or intensity modulated radiation techniques allow for an increased dose to the primary site while reducing the dose of radiation to the surrounding normal brain tissue. At least one study has shown no decline in learning in young children treated with conformal therapy. The current COG trial provides conformal radiation to those as young as 12 months. If this approach is successful in curing most very young patients with ependymoma, careful analysis of the long-term side effects should follow. The question of whether children less than 12 months should be treated with radiation therapy will be raised. Current studies also continue to attempt to define the role of chemotherapy and second look surgery.

Glioma

Both low and high grade gliomas occur in young children. Low grade glioma may well be the most common brain tumor in infants but their true incidence is hard to gauge because some of the tumors are surgical cases only. High grade glioma, a grouping that includes glioblastoma multiforme, anaplastic astrocytoma, and malignant glioma, is the third most common malignant brain tumor in infants. All of these tumors are considered World Health Organization (WHO) grade IV malignancies. Infants with pilocytic astrocytoma often have bulky midline tumors that affect vision and endocrine function causing failure to thrive like "diencephalic syndrome."

Management

Most patients with low grade glioma will have prolonged survival, making decisions regarding any therapeutic intervention and its potential short and long-term morbidity very important. Patients with low grade glioma should be treated with surgery when feasible and with adjuvant therapy for unresectable and progressive tumors as outlined in other chapters. Radiation should be avoided or at least delayed for those who are deemed to require treatment. The regimen of carboplatin and vincristine is considered current first line treatment although other regimens are known to be active. The addition of biologic agents such as mTOR (rapamcyin) and VEGF (bevacizumab) inhibitors is being investigated clinically and offer new promise for targeted and potentially less toxic treatment.

Infants with high grade glioma may do better than older children and adults. Several studies have demonstrated that infants less than 2 years of age have about a 50% 3- to 5-year progression-free survival when treated with surgery and chemotherapy. Those with hemispheric tumors and complete surgical resection have a trend toward improved survival and some have advo-

cated the use of focal radiation to treat high grade glioma. It remains a mystery as to why infants with high grade glioma have better survival rates than older children. There may be inherent biologic differences in the tumor that somehow make it either less aggressive or more susceptible to treatment. Again, the collection of tissue for tumor banking and biologic studies may help answer this question.

✋ CAUTION!

Infants with high grade glioma have better survival rates than older children and adults with the same disease. Although the reason for this is unknown, both practitioners and families need to be made aware of this when making treatment decisions.

Atypical teratoid rhabdoid tumor

Atypical teratoid rhabdoid tumor (ATRT) is a rare, highly malignant central nervous system tumor. It is primarily a disease of young children, usually younger than 2 years of age. ATRT was first identified by Lefkowitz *et al.* as a unique tumor type in 1987. Prior to that time, patients with ATRT were often misdiagnosed as having medulloblastoma or another primitive neuroectodermal tumor because approximately two-thirds have components that resemble neuroectodermal tumors. Pathologic diagnosis is now assisted with the availability of a special antibody stain to the INI-1 gene product which is altered in most ATRT. If the *INI1* gene is altered, the tumor cells do not stain for the normal gene product. The WHO began classifying ATRT as an embryonal grade IV neoplasm in 1993. Based on prior cooperative group studies, approximately 10% of children younger than 36 months of age with malignant brain tumors have ATRT. In a more recent study, ATRT was as common as medulloblastoma in infants.

Because ATRT is a highly malignant, rapidly growing tumor, patients typically have a fairly short history of progressive symptoms which can be measured in days to weeks. As is the case with other brain tumors, patients with ATRT present with signs and symptoms that reflect the location of the tumor. About half of ATRT patients have posterior fossa tumors and present with symptoms related to hydrocephalus. They may also develop ataxia or regression of motor skills. Cranial nerve palsies, particularly VI and VII, are not uncommon. Patients with supratentorial tumors may present with signs and symptoms of hydrocephalus if it is present, enlarging head size, hemiparesis, seizures, or visual changes, depending of the location of the tumor. Imaging characteristics are also helpful but nonspecific for ATRT. On T1-weighted MRI, the tumor mass is typically isointense with frequent hyperintense foci secondary to intratumoral hemorrhage. The tumor does take up contrast intensely but in a heterogeneous pattern. Although clinical and radiographic findings can suggest ATRT, the diagnosis is made pathologically.

Histologically, ATRT contains sheets of rhabdoid cells against a background of primitive neuroectodermal, mesenchymal, or epithelial cells. Some tumors are composed entirely of rhabdoid cells, whereas others show a combination of rhabdoid cells and areas resembling PNET or medulloblastoma. Pediatricians and neuropathologists have become increasingly aware of ATRT, but accurate diagnosis may still be difficult. Immunohistochemical features help to identify the disease but vary depending on the cellular composition of the tumor. These are rapidly growing tumors that can have MIB-1 labeling indices of 50–100%. Molecular studies are able to identify ATRT. Work by Biegel *et al.* has identified a candidate tumor suppressor gene, *INI1*, which is abnormal in the majority (85%) of ATRT. *INI1* is a component of a SWI and SNF ATP-dependent chromatin remodeling complex. The exact function of the *INI1* gene product is unknown, but it is likely that a mutation results in altered transcriptional regulation of downstream targets. In addition to somatic mutations, germline mutations in *INI1* have been reported in some ATRT patients who may be predisposed to renal or other malignancies. Patients with germline mutations have a lower median age at diagnosis and a poorer prognosis. *INI1* gene mutations have also been found in patients with renal and extrarenal rhabdoid malignancies. Immunohistochemical staining for *INI1* appears to be a useful tool in distinguishing ATRT from PNET, medulloblastoma, and other CNS tumors. Most centers now routinely stain primitive central nervous tumors for *INI1* as part of their evaluation.

Management

The earliest reported prognosis for patients with ATRT was extremely grim. There are case series reports of long-term survivors; they tend to be older patients who have had both radiation and chemotherapy. Recent reports conclude that progression-free survival is improved with intensive multimodal therapy that includes intense systemic and intrathecal chemotherapy in addition to radiation, or intensive chemotherapy that includes stem cell transplant.

Surgery is typically the first step in treatment for patients with ATRT. Although no prospective data exist regarding the impact of surgical resection on outcome, retrospective data available from the ATRT registry suggests that patients who have had a gross total resection have a longer median survival. It has been estimated, however, that less than one-third of patients have tumors that are amenable to complete resection. This may be because the tumor often invades vital structures, such as cranial nerves at the cerebellopontine angle, and young patients often have large and invasive tumors at the time of diagnosis. That being said, the goal of surgery should be to remove as much tumor as is deemed safely possible by the surgeon as this may prolong survival. Treatment with chemotherapy may improve the surgeon's ability to resect large vascular tumors and consideration should be given to second look surgery in cases where complete resection is not possible at the time of diagnosis. Surgery also provides important tumor tissue for diagnostic and research purposes.

For infants with ATRT, chemotherapy is often the main initial form of postsurgical adjuvant therapy. A variety of chemotherapeutic approaches have been utilized, with only a few reported patients being treated on any one protocol. Some of these patients have also been treated with radiation, adding further complexity to evaluating the efficacy of chemotherapy. The outcome for children treated with surgery and standard chemotherapy regimens only is

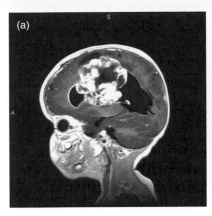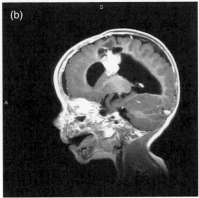

Figure 16.2. Atypical teratoid rhabdoid tumor (ATRT) response. (a) Sagittal post-gadolinium MRI demonstrates large ATRT in an 8-month-old that was extremely vascular and unresectable. (b) MRI demonstrates excellent response to induction chemotherapy; tumor resection was possible prior to further treatment.

extremely poor. Prolonged survival and improved outcome have been reported for those treated with more intensive regimens, some of which include intrathecal or high dose chemotherapy and stem cell rescue. Initial chemotherapy may also have a role in reducing tumor vascularity and making a large tumor more amenable to surgical resection (Figure 16.2).

Radiation therapy appears to have an impact on survival for patients with ATRT. Of the 42 patients in the ATRT registry, 13 patients (31%) received radiation therapy in addition to chemotherapy as part of their primary therapy. Their median survival was 48 months, while the median survival of all patients on the registry was 17 months. Of the 14 long-term survivors in the registry, seven received radiation as part of their primary therapy including four patients who were less than 36 months at diagnosis. It is unclear whether craniospinal irradiation is necessary. Although there is unease in treating young children with irradiation because of the potential long-term side effects, recent advances in radiation therapy technology, primarily using conformal treatment methods, appear to decrease the morbidity associated with radiation. One study that treated patients younger than 36 months with posterior fossa ependymoma showed no change in IQ tested serially from diagnosis to 48 months after treatment. Although

long-term sequelae need to be monitored in survivors, the potential benefits of at least focal irradiation appear to outweigh the risks.

The COG is currently conducting the first consortium-based prospective clinical trial specific for ATRT. This study builds on a prior infant brain tumor treatment regimen, CCG99703, which incorporates intensive chemotherapy with triple tandem stem cell transplant. Patients are treated with multiagent induction chemotherapy, which includes systemic methotrexate, followed by stem cell transplant. Involved radiation is given between induction and maintenance chemotherapy or after the completion of therapy, depending on the age of the patient. Tumor tissue submission is mandatory on this study which may reveal prognostic indicators and provide tissue for continued biology studies.

★ **TIPS AND TRICKS**

All malignant brains tumors in infants should be stained for *INI1*. Atypical teratoid rhabdoid tumor (ATRT) tumors cells do not pick up the stain because of their genetic alteration of the *INI1* gene and therefore are readily identified from other primitive tumors types. Choroid plexus carcinoma, however, can also have alteration in *INI1*.

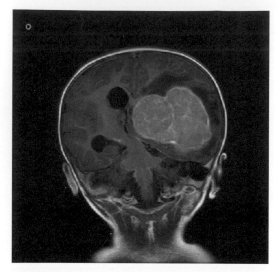

Figure 16.3. Choroid plexus carcinoma: coronal post-gadolinium MRI demonstrates choroid plexus carcinoma arising in the left lateral ventricle; the tumor is producing cerebrospinal fluid (CSF) and creating significant mass effect.

Choroid plexus tumors

Tumors of the choroid plexus represent about 3% of pediatric brain tumor and 10–20% of those presenting in the first year of life. Most patients are diagnosed before the age of 2 years. The tumors arise in areas where choroid plexus is normally found, primarily the lateral and fourth ventricles (Figure 16.3). Most patients present with signs and symptoms of hydrocephalus and increasing head size in those with open sutures. The tumors themselves can produce CSF and exacerbate the hydrocephalus. Patients may also have cranial nerve palsies, hemiparesis, or seizures. There are two histologic types: choroid plexus papilloma and choroid plexus carcinoma. Papilloma is four times more common than carcinoma. An intermediate form of atypical choroid plexus papilloma has been described.

Management

Choroid plexus papilloma is a relatively benign tumor that histologically resembles non-neoplastic choroid plexus but with elongated and crowded cells. Long-term survival is excellent with complete surgical resection. Second look surgery is indicated for patients with resid-ual disease. There is no proven benefit for adjuvant therapy in choroid plexus papilloma although focused radiation may be helpful if a complete resection is not possible. Patients with choroid plexus papilloma often have long-term sequelae from their tumor and hydrocephalus including developmental delay, seizures, and behavioral problems.

Choroid plexus carcinoma is a highly malignant tumor and patients have much poorer survival than those with papilloma. This tumor has frank signs of malignancy with nuclear pleomorphism and frequent mitoses as well as other finds of a rapidly growing neoplasm. This tumor can rarely seed throughout the neuraxis and both brain and spine should be imaged with MRI at the time of diagnosis. Lumbar CSF should also be examined for tumor cells. Although complete resection may improve survival, it is often made difficult either by tumor invasion or the vascular nature of the tumor. At initial surgery, the surgeon must be prepared for the possibility of significant blood loss as the tumor often takes its blood supply from the vascular pedicule. Tumor embolization and radiosurgery have been used to reduce blood supply. In a tumor that cannot be resected because of bleeding, chemotherapy may reduce the vascular supply enough so that after a few cycles of treatment, the tumor can be resected. The likelihood of survival is best after "gross-total" resection.

The role of adjuvant chemotherapy or radiation is unclear. Long-term survivors have been reported treated with either or both but the vast majority of patients with carcinoma die from their disease. Interestingly, many of these tumors have a mutation in the *INI1* gene that is aberrant in ATRT. Perhaps biologic therapy will eventually hold the key in finding more effective treatment for choroid plexus carcinoma.

Summary

The treatment of infants with brain tumors is a major challenge for the neuro-oncology community. Significant strides have been made toward predicting better outcome for certain disease such as desmoplastic medulloblastoma and completely resected ependymoma. A better understanding of tumor biology for all disease types is necessary, not only to stratify risk, but also eventually to lead to less toxic therapies. As patients with high and low risk disease are stratified for treatment, those with poor prognoses are being subjected to increasingly intense regimens that have significant potential short and long-term sequelae. We must continue to look for ways to limit toxicity and improve not only survival but quality of life for infants with brain tumors.

Selected bibliography

Biegel JA, Zhou JY, Rorke LB, Stenstrom C, Wainwright LM, Fogelgren B. (1999) Germ-line and acquired mutations of INI1 in atypical teratoid and rhabdoid tumors. *Cancer Res* **59**, 74–9.

Burger PC, Yu IT, Tihan T, Friedman HS, Strother DR, Kepner JL, *et al.* (1998) Atypical teratoid/rhabdoid tumor of the central nervous system: a highly malignant tumor of infancy and childhood frequently mistaken for medulloblastoma: a Pediatric Oncology Group study. *Am J Surg Pathol* **22** (9), 1083–92.

Dhall G, Grodman H, Ji L, Sands S, Gardner S, Dunkel IJ, *et al.* (2008) Outcome of children less than three years old at diagnosis with non-metastatic medulloblastoma treated with chemotherapy on the "Head Start" I and II protocols. *Pediatr Blood Cancer* **50** (6), 1169–75.

Duffner PK, Horowitz ME, Krischer JP, Friedman HS, Burger PC, Cohen ME, *et al.* (1993) Postoperative chemotherapy and delayed radiation in children less than three years of age with malignant brain tumors. *N Engl J Med* **328** (24), 1725–31.

Duffner PK, Krischer JP, Burger PC, Cohen ME, Backstrom JW, Horowitz ME, *et al.* (1996) Treatment of infants with malignant gliomas: the Pediatric Oncology Group experience. *J Neurooncol* **28** (2–3), 245–56.

Geyer JR, Sposto R, Jennings M, Boyett JM, Axtell RA, Breiger D, *et al.* (2005) Multiagent chemotherapy and deferred radiotherapy in infants with malignant brain tumors: a report from the Children's Cancer Group. *J Clin Oncol* **23** (30), 7621–31.

Grill J, Sainte-Rose C, Jouvet A, Gentet JC, Lejars O, Frappaz D, *et al.* (2005) Treatment of medulloblastoma with postoperative chemotherapy alone: an SFOP prospective trial in young children. *Lancet Oncol* **6** (8), 573–80.

Hilden JM, Meerbaum S, Burger P, Finlay J, Janss A, Scheithauer BW, *et al.* (2004) Central nervous system atypical teratoid/rhabdoid tumor: results of therapy in children enrolled in a registry. *J Clin Oncol* **22** (14), 2877–84.

Jakacki RI, Zeltzer PM, Boyett JM, Albright AL, Allen JC, Geyer JR, *et al.* (1995) Survival and prognostic factors following radiation and/or chemotherapy for primitive neuroectodermal tumors of the pineal region in infants and children: a report of the Children's Cancer Group. *J Clin Onco* **13** (6), 1377–83.

Lefkowitz IB, Rorke LB, Packer RJ, *et al.* (1987) Atypical teratoid tumor of infancy: definition of an entity. *Ann Neurol* **22**, 448–9.

Kleihues P, Cavenee WK. (1997) *Pathology and Genetic of Tumours of the Nervous System.* International Agency for Research on Cancer, Lyon.

Merchant TE, Li C, Xiong X, Kun LE, Boop FA, Sanford RA. (2009) Conformal radiotherapy after surgery for paediatric ependymoma: a prospective study. *Lancet Oncol* **10** (3), 258–66.

Packer RJ, Biegel JA, Blaney S, Finlay J, Geyer JR, Heideman R, *et al.* (2002) Atypical teratoid/rhabdoid tumor of the central nervous system: report on workshop. *J Pediatr Hematol Oncol* **24** (5), 337–42.

Rickert CH, Paulus W. (2001) Epidemiology of central nervous system tumors in childhood and adolescence based on the new WHO classification. *Childs Nerve Syst* **17** (9), 503–11.

Rutkowski S, Bode U, Deinlein F, Ottensmeier H, Warmuth-Metz M, Soerensen N, *et al.* (2005) Treatment of early childhood medulloblastoma by postoperative chemotherapy alone. *N Engl J Med* **352** (10), 978–86.

Sanders RP, Kocak M, Burger PC, Merchant TE, Gajjar A, Broniscer A. (2007) High-grade astrocytoma in very young children. *Pediatr Blood Cancer* **49** (7), 888–93.

Part IV

Effects of Systemic Cancer and Treatment on the Nervous System

17

Intracranial Metastases

Mary R. Welch and Thomas J. Kaley

Department of Neurology, Memorial Sloan-Kettering Cancer Center, New York, NY, USA

Epidemiology

With an incidence in excess of 100,000 cases per year in the United States, brain metastases comprise the most common intracranial tumor in adults. They outnumber primary brain tumors by a factor of 10 and, in autopsy studies, affect nearly 25% of patients who die of cancer. As our means of diagnosis improve and patients survive longer with cancer, these numbers are on the rise.

Table 17.1 lists the frequency of brain metastases by site of origin. While the majority arise from lung cancer, breast cancer, and melanoma, any primary systemic cancer can spread to the central nervous system (CNS). Consequently, one should always consider metastatic disease in the differential diagnosis of a brain lesion in a cancer patient.

As shown in Table 17.2, the likelihood of developing brain metastases and multiplicity of lesions generally correlates with tumor histology. The multiplicity of lesions has important clinical implications. For patients with a single intracranial tumor – roughly half according to retrospective data – the goal should be complete local control with resection or stereotactic radiosurgery (SRS). By contrast, patients with three or more lesions typically require whole-brain radiotherapy (WBRT). At the extreme end of the spectrum, among patients with small cell lung carcinoma (SCLC), there is good evidence supporting the use of prophylactic whole-brain cranial irradiation to increase both survival and quality of life.

Pathogenesis

Before they present as metastases within the brain, tumor cells must successfully navigate a complex series of steps:

1 Escape from the primary tumor
2 Access to the arterial circulation
3 Arrest and extravasation within the brain
4 Survival and growth within the CNS microenvironment.

While it is beyond the scope of this chapter to address each of these in detail, a few points bear mentioning.

The work of James Ewing and Charles Paget has provided a useful conceptual framework for understanding the biologic features of brain metastases. In 1928, Ewing proposed that once tumor cells reach the arterial circulation, their distribution should be based on blood flow. This mechanical hypothesis has much to support it. Metastases frequently do occur at the gray–white junction and in watershed areas of the brain

Neuro-oncology, First Edition. Edited by Roger J. Packer, David Schiff.

Table 17.1. Primary tumors in 215 patients with brain metastases at MSKCC.

Primary tumor type	MSKCC Study	
	No. of patients	Percent
NSCLC	73	34.8%
Breast	39	18.6%
SCLC	12	5.7%
Genitourinary	15	7.1%
Melanoma	20	9.5%
Gynecologic	10	4.8%
Gastrointestinal	14	6.6%
Unknown	5	2.3%
Miscellaneous	27	12.9%

MSKCC, Memorial Sloan-Kettering Cancer Center; NSCLC, non-small cell lung carcinoma; SCLC, small cell lung carcinoma.

Table 17.2. Correlations exist among tumor histology, risk of brain metastases, and likelihood of multiple lesions.

Histology	Risk of brain metastases	Risk of having two or more intracranial metastases
SCLC	Up to 80%	57%
Melanoma	Up to 75%	51%
NSCLC	25–30%	50%
Breast	10–20%	51%
Renal	5–10%	44%
Testicular	8–15%	45%
Prostate	1%	18%
Choriocarcinoma	10–15%	

NSCLC, non-small cell lung carcinoma; SCLC, small cell lung carcinoma.

where tumor emboli are effectively trapped in narrowing arterioles. Moreover, the usual distribution of brain metastases does reflect intracranial blood flow with supratentorial predominance.

However, blood supply does not account for the propensity of certain cancers to metastasize to specific organs. To explain this observation, oncologists have supplemented Ewing's ideas with the soil and seed hypothesis. As conceived by Paget over 100 years ago, this theory proposes that certain features of a particular organ (the soil) make it a more favorable environment for the growth of certain cancers (the seed).

Pathology

The pathologic features of brain metastases are as varied as the primary tumors from which they originate. Though on gross inspection most appear well demarcated, microscopically they often expand within the Virchow–Robin spaces, destroying neuroglial tissue and invading the parenchyma. It is this infiltrative quality that contributes to local recurrence and may justify the use of postoperative radiation.

By histology and immunohistochemistry, brain metastases mimic their primary of origin. However, biologic differences may exist. For example, mutation in the epidermal growth factor receptor (EGFR) found in some lung cancers may not be found in coexistent brain metastases of the same patient. As clinicians increasingly turn to molecularly targeted therapy including those that specifically target cellular components such as EGFR, these differences will come to have greater significance.

Presentation

As with any expanding intracranial mass, brain metastases produce symptoms in one of two ways: either indirectly by raising intracranial pressure or by direct displacement of adjacent neural structures. Table 17.3 outlines the most common presenting signs and symptoms.

Generalized symptoms such as headache or cognitive changes tend to arise gradually over time and persist. Alternatively, a patient may develop plateau waves – acute, transient symptoms secondary to sudden rises in intracranial pressure. These classically present when a patient assumes a standing position. Brief episodes of altered consciousness or headache are the usual manifestations, though other, more varied symptoms have been described and differentiating plateau waves from seizure activity can present a diagnostic challenge. Both phenomena may last 5–20 minutes and resolve spontaneously. However, plateau waves do not have a characteristic post-ictal component. In patients suspected of plateau waves, measuring opening pressure or a trial of steroids may provide clarification.

Table 17.3. Common presenting signs and symptoms of brain metastases.

Symptoms	Signs
Headache	Impaired cognition
Focal weakness	Hemiparesis
Seizures	Hemisensory loss
Speech difficulty	Papilledema
Visual disturbance	Gait ataxia
Sensory disturbance	Visual field cut

Reproduced from DeAngelis LM, Posner JB. (1995) Neurological Complications of Cancer, 2nd edn. Oxford University Press, New York. By permission of Oxford University Press, Inc.

Focal signs are also common on presentation. Weakness is most frequently noted, but other localizable deficits including a visual field cut, sensory loss, or aphasia may lead the neurologist to suspect brain metastases, particularly in a patient with a pre-existing cancer diagnosis. These signs typically evolve insidiously over a period of days to weeks, reflecting the gradual displacement of brain tissue by a growing tumor or its associated edema. A certain number of patients, however (less than 10% according to Memorial Sloan-Kettering Cancer Center's experience), will present acutely with sudden, stroke-like onset of a deficit without intratumoral hemorrhage. The pathogenesis of such pseudovascular syndromes remains to be fully elucidated.

Seizures, whether focal or secondarily generalized, may develop at any point in the patient with brain metastases. Based on the American Academy of Neurology (AAN) practice parameter, one can estimate that about 10–40% will present with such an event and another 10–40% will experience them at some point in their disease course. Not surprisingly, seizures tend to occur more frequently in patients with more than one lesion and thus are over-represented among patients with melanoma and SCLC.

Regardless of how a particular brain metastasis presents, treatment – typically with corticosteroids followed by more definitive measures – often produces a dramatic therapeutic effect with substantial improvement or even complete resolution of neurologic deficits. However, anticonvulsants should not be used reflexively, but only prescribed to patients who have experienced a seizure.

Diagnostics

Contrast-enhanced MRI is the study of choice in the work-up of patients with suspected brain metastases. In general, intraparenchymal involvement appears as one or more well-circumscribed lesions with mild T1 hypointensity and T2 hyperintensity. Larger metastases are typically outlined by a ring of enhancement which delineates tumor from surrounding vasogenic edema. The latter, which may be larger than the metastasis itself, is best appreciated on T2 imaging as an area of increased signal intensity.

☚ CAUTION!

Though CT scan may have a role in the acute presentation of brain metastases to look for evidence of hemorrhage or hydrocephalus, it cannot be relied upon to determine the number and characteristics of lesions.

Differential diagnosis

Among patients with a history of cancer who present with a single intracranial lesion, 90% will have brain metastases. By contrast, in a patient without a diagnosis of malignancy, the probability that an intracranial lesion reflects a metastasis is less than 15%. In cases like these where a brain lesion is the presenting manifestation of cancer, additional work-up must include a search for a primary tumor. Traditionally, this involves a computed tomography (CT) scan of the chest, abdomen, and pelvis. Alternatively, as body positron emission tomography (PET) scanning has become more widely available, physicians increasingly rely on this type of metabolic imaging to localize the primary tumor and other systemic metastases, thereby obviating the need for additional tests.

Regardless of whether a patient has a diagnosis of cancer or not, a broad differential should be entertained. Box 17.1 includes the most common alternative diagnoses including primary brain tumor, abscess, herpetic infection, granuloma, and demyelination.

★ TIPS AND TRICKS

Radiation necrosis in a previously treated patient is frequently mistaken for tumor recurrence. To differentiate the two, a number of different imaging modalities including fluorodeoxyglucose positron emission tomography (FDG PET), magnetic resonance spectroscopy, as well as perfusion and diffusion-weighted MRI have been employed. Unfortunately, none has been shown to be entirely accurate.

Box 17.1. Differential diagnosis.

- Primary brain tumors
- Vascular lesions: hemorrhage, vascular anomaly, infarct
- Infections: abscess, viral infection
- Side effects of therapy: radionecrosis, leukoencephalopathy
- Other: multiple sclerosis

Prognosis

Though the median prognosis for a patient with brain metastases is on the order of months, early diagnosis and vigorous treatment can often reverse neurologic deficits and restore significant quality of life. This is of particular importance for long-term survivors.

While the outcome of individual patients cannot be predicted, several prognostic factors have been identified. These include control of extracranial disease, baseline performance status, age, the sensitivity of the tumor to treatment, and clinical response to steroids. The number, size, and location of brain metastases also impacts survival as patients with fewer than three surgically accessible lesions tend to do better.

Table 17.4. Radiation Therapy Oncology Group (RTOG) recursive partitioning analysis classes.

Prognostic class	Karnofsky performance status (KPS)*	Age	Systemic disease status	Median survival (months)
Class I	≥70	<65	Controlled primary and no extracranial metastasis	7.1
Class II	≥70	Not specified	Not specified	4.2
Class III	<70	>65	Not specified	2.3

*KPS of 70 identifies a patient who can care for himself, but who is unable to carry on normal activity or perform active work.

EVIDENCE AT A GLANCE

The Radiation Therapy Oncology Group (RTOG) performed recursive partitioning analysis (RPA) to predict prognosis following WBRT. Table 17.4 outlines the three classes of patients they identified and the median survivals associated with each.

Box 17.2. Overview of treatment for brain metastases.

Symptomatic treatment
- Corticosteroids
- Anticonvulsants

Definitive treatment
- Whole-brain radiotherapy (WBRT)
- Focal
  - Surgery
  - Stereotactic radiosurgery (SRS)
- Combination
  - Surgery + SRS
  - Surgery + WBRT
  - SRS + WBRT
- Systemic treatment
  - Traditional chemotherapy

Treatment

As outlined in Box 17.2, treatment for patients with brain metastases may be categorized as either symptomatic or definitive. The former seeks to alleviate symptoms engendered by brain metastases or their treatment while the latter takes aim directly at intracranial disease in an effort to control or eliminate it entirely.

Symptomatic treatment

The effective management of the patient's symptoms is an essential component of any comprehensive treatment plan and the judicious and tailored use of symptomatic treatments can significantly impact quality of life. Stimulants may alleviate fatigue associated with radiation; antidepressants often improve mood; and physical therapy can maintain functional status among patients left debilitated by weakness. While it is beyond the scope of this chapter to address all of these in turn, two symptomatic treatments – corticosteroids and anticonvulsants – merit further discussion given the frequency with which they are both used and misused by neurologists and oncologists alike.

Corticosteroids

By reducing vasogenic edema, corticosteroids rapidly ameliorate the neurologic dysfunction produced by brain metastases and should therefore be deployed in all symptomatic patients. Moreover, in addition to their impact on tumor-related edema, steroids have a number of additional salutary effects, particularly for the patient with terminal or pre-terminal cancer. They function as antiemetics, improve appetite, reduce fatigue, and may also have analgesic properties. However, steroids should not be initiated reflexively in the asymptomatic patient. Doing so risks subjecting him or her to unwanted side effects and may, as in the case of metastatic lymphoma, obscure the diagnosis.

Though the optimal dose and timing has not been established, dexamethasone is usually the preparation of choice because of the absence of mineralocorticoid effect. A good rule of thumb is to start with a bolus of 10–24 mg followed by a similar daily dose divided into a morning dose taken on waking and a second one in the early evening. Bedtime dosing should generally be avoided to reduce the likelihood of insomnia. Ideally, steroids should be tapered upon completion of more definitive therapy with either surgery or radiation. At the risk of producing side effects ranging from mild tremulousness to life-threatening gastric perforation, the lowest possible dose needed to control a patient's neurologic symptoms should be used. In cases where patients require prolonged steroid use – typically over 4 weeks – prophylactic antibiotics against *Pneumocystis jirovecii* pneumonia should also be prescribed. Bactrim given three times per week or atovaquone once daily for those with sulfa allergies are the most commonly employed agents.

Anticonvulsants

Anticonvulsants are frequently prescribed reflexively in patients with brain metastases, regardless of seizure history. Yet, there is no evidence to support such indiscriminate use beyond the 1- to 2-week perioperative period, particularly as patients with brain metastases may be more vulnerable to side effects such as neurocognitive dysfunction and sedation. By contrast, patients who experience seizures do merit long-term treatment. In such cases, a non-cytochrome P450-inducing agent is preferred to reduce potential interactions with other agents including dexamethasone. Though not approved for monotherapy in the United States, levetiracetam has rapidly become the agent of choice among neuro-oncologists for this reason as well as its overall tolerability.

EVIDENCE AT A GLANCE

A meta-analysis of 12 studies – four with Class I data – was performed by the Quality Standards Subcommittee of the AAN to address the question of whether patients with brain tumors should be treated prophylactically with anticonvulsants. Based on the available data, they concluded that prophylactic use not only lacked efficacy in preventing seizures, but could even harm patients with untoward side effects.

Definitive treatment

Historically, WBRT has been the modality of choice in the treatment of brain metastases and it remains a key weapon in the neuro-oncologist's arsenal. Over the past two decades, however, refinements in surgical techniques and the development of stereotactic radiotherapy have led practitioners towards more individualized approaches. As outlined in Figure 17.1, important considerations involved in developing a treatment plan include: systemic disease status, overall lesion burden, location of the metastases, as well as the tumor's radiosensitivity. Age, functional status, and patient preference are also key factors involved in generating treatment options. In general, for patients with three or fewer lesions, a focal approach is preferred, while for those with four or more metastases, WBRT remains the best choice.

Whole-brain radiotherapy

Although it is one of the oldest treatments for brain metastases, WBRT remains unsurpassed as a simple noninvasive means of controlling metastatic deposits throughout the brain. Numerous trials have confirmed that WBRT not only effectively palliates neurologic symptoms, but even provides a modest 3–6 month survival advantage. Younger patients with better performance status, fewer lesions, and radiosensitive tumors such as lung and breast cancer tend to do better. Conversely, older patients with poor baseline functioning, more than three metastases, and radioresistant tumors such as melanoma and renal carcinoma are less likely to benefit.

Despite its advantages, WBRT is not without drawbacks – the major one being that normal brain is exposed to the untoward effects of ionizing radiation. Short-term toxicities include headache, hair loss, desquamation, otitis media, and lethargy. Acute encephalopathy, though rare,

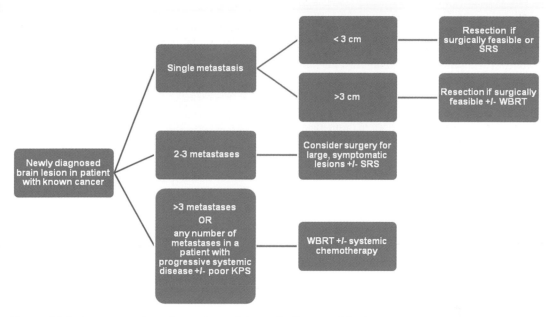

Figure 17.1. An approach to the patient with newly diagnosed brain metastases.

has also been described in patients – particularly those with large tumor burden and evidence of increased intracranial pressure.

Demyelination resulting from damage to oligodendroglia and subsequent breakdown of myelin sheaths is thought to produce many of the early delayed side effects of radiation. These usually make their appearance in a variety of ways within 2 weeks to 4 months of radiotherapy and often resolve over the same time frame. Most commonly, patients or their families report generalized cognitive slowing. Fortunately, this tends to be transient and clinicians ought not to misinterpret such early dysfunction as predictive of radiation-induced dementia, a more disabling sequela of treatment. In addition to vague cognitive changes, patients may also present 2–3 months after radiotherapy with the reappearance or worsening of their original neurologic symptoms. In such cases, one should not automatically presume progression has occurred. Rather, the affected patient should be supported with corticosteroids and monitored closely with frequent clinical and radiographic follow-up.

> **⚓ CAUTION!**
>
> Brain edema acutely worsens in the setting of WBRT. Patients should be protected with dexamethasone initiated at least 48–72 hours before initiating radiotherapy, particularly if intracranial pressure is symptomatic. The authors typically use a dose of 8–16 mg every 24 hours.

Paradoxically, as treatment for systemic disease improves, neurologists are increasingly likely to encounter some of the long-term sequelae of radiation including atrophy, leukoencephalopathy, neurocognitive deficits, and even dementia. Necrosis, one of the most feared consequences of radiation, usually begins 1–2 years after radiotherapy is completed, but may present within 3 months. When present, symptoms tend to mimic those of the brain tumor and may easily be mistaken for recurrence.

WBRT at a dose of 30 Gy delivered in 10 fractions (3 Gy per fraction) has been widely accepted as an effective means of providing safe rapid palliation. Radiation oncologists may diverge from this standard, tailoring their regimens based on a given patient's overall clinical picture. Whatever the schedule, median survival ranges from 2.3 to 13.5 months depending on recursive partitioning analysis (RPA) class and the tumor's radiosensitivity. Ultimately, most patients succumb to systemic as opposed to brain disease.

Focal treatment – surgery

First reported in 1926 by Grant, surgical resection has only recently gained widespread acceptance as an important and viable treatment option for patients with brain metastases. While numerous retrospective and uncontrolled trials have demonstrated a benefit to surgery, all are flawed by selection bias as only the most functional patients are taken to the operating room. Nonetheless, these data do suggest that among select patients, including those with a single brain metastasis, limited systemic disease, a favorable Karnofsky Performance Status (KPS), or extensive edema, surgery can be an important adjunct to radiation with the ability to extend survival by as much as 16 months. By contrast, patients with widely metastatic cancer or with deep inaccessible lesions are less likely to benefit. In addition to its potential therapeutic effects surgery also provides histologic verification of metastatic disease. This is especially important for patients without active systemic disease or among those who are extensively immunosuppressed (Table 17.5).

Focal treatment – stereotactic radiosurgery

Stereotactic radiotherapy or radiosurgery (SRS) delivers a highly focused dose of ionizing radiation (usually 14–20 Gy) in either a single fraction or several fractions to a precise target within a three-dimensional coordinate system. In contrast to treating the whole brain, SRS has the advantage of limiting toxicity to viable surrounding brain tissue while simultaneously allowing for dose escalation within the confines of a specific field. Because they tend to be spherical and relatively well delineated, brain metastases are, in many respects, the ideal targets for such volumetric conformal radiation delivery. Though first used over 50 years ago to treat nonmalignant brain lesions such as vascular malformations, the technique has now been widely adopted in the treatment of cancer patients, particularly those whose lesions are not readily accessible to surgery.

★ TIPS AND TRICKS

There are several stereotactic radiosurgery systems in existence and while each have their proponents, all work on the same principle of high dose, focused radiation. Gamma Knife® delivers gamma rays from multiple cobalt-60 sources and is capable of submillimeter targeting. In order to achieve this precision, it requires a head frame to be

---

Table 17.5. Randomized trials of whole-brain radiotherapy (WBRT) with and without surgery for single brain metastases.

Study and year	Number of patients	Therapy	Median survival time (weeks)	1-Year survival (%)	Median time of functional independence
Patchell *et al.* (1990)	23	WBRT	15	5	8
	25	WBRT + surgery	40	45	38
Vecht *et al.* (1993)	31	WBRT	26	23	14
	32	WBRT + surgery	43	41	30
Mintz *et al.* (1996)	43	WBRT	27.3	30.2	–
	41	WBRT + surgery	24.3	12.2	–

bolted on to the skull of the patient. Linear particle accelerators (LINACs), which deliver X-rays, were developed by modification of standard linear accelerators. CyberKnife® relies on robotics and real-time imaging capability to delineate the target. Novalis®, a fourth option, is produced by BrainLAB and uses infrared fiducial markers attached to the patient to allow for precise tracking of patient position and subsequent adjustment of radiation vectors. Finally, charged particle radiation therapy uses proton or carbon ion beams produced by a cyclotron. Though touted as more precise than conventional photon radiotherapy, there are limited data to suggest any advantage to its use in brain disease. Moreover, its availability is limited by expense and significant infrastructure needs.

The advantages of radiosurgery are well established: it is minimally invasive, has few immediate risks, and may be performed on an outpatient basis. Moreover, radiosurgery is ideally suited to patients whose systemic disease limits their surgical candidacy or whose lesions are simply not amenable to resection by dint of their location. Importantly, radiosurgery does not provide histologic verification – no small disadvantage when one considers that 5–11% of patients with known systemic disease and a brain lesion have nonmetastatic disease. In comparison with surgery, which rapidly alleviates symptoms, the treatment effects of SRS are relatively delayed. In fact, patients may experience transient worsening after SRS as a result of edema from the provoked inflammatory response and may ultimately require higher doses of steroids for longer periods of time. SRS also carries an increased risk of radiation necrosis, especially when performed after a patient has received WBRT. Radiotherapy necrosis can look radiographically and clinically just like tumor growth, so the diagnosis must be considered in these patients.

⚠ CAUTION!

Although some brain metastases decrease in size after SRS, most remain the same or even transiently increase. Therefore it is important not to prematurely categorize every enlarging tumor as treatment failure. Unless a patient becomes symptomatic, lesions should be followed.

The number and size of lesions are important considerations in determining whether a patient is likely to benefit from SRS. In general, SRS is best used to treat patients with brain metastases that are less than or equal to 3 cm in maximal diameter, as larger volumes increase the risk of neurotoxicity. If such a small lesion is deep within the brain, SRS may be the only available focal treatment. However, which modality is superior for small, surgically accessible lesions is less evident and remains an area of ongoing debate. At present, a rational approach takes into consideration tumor size, location, clinical presentation, and systemic disease status. In general, among patients with lesions amenable to either surgery or SRS (1.5–3 cm diameter maximum), those who are symptomatic should be considered for the former while those who are neurologically intact can be treated with the latter.

Combined modalities

The objective of both SRS and resection is to achieve improved survival and quality of life by targeting focal deposits of metastatic disease while limiting toxicity to the brain. WBRT, however, also has its advantages. By treating the brain in its entirety, it may eliminate microscopic disease and prevent distant recurrence. To date, the appropriate means of combining focal and whole brain therapies remains an area of extensive debate. Questions linger as to when and how to deploy each treatment.

Though surgical resection has largely been established as the preferred approach in patients with a single large symptomatic lesion, the question of whether any radiotherapy is beneficial as an adjunct is still uncertain.

Patchell *et al.* investigated patients who underwent resection and compared those who received postoperative WBRT with those who did not. CNS recurrence was lower in the radiated group, but the study did not demonstrate a survival advantage. Similar results were achieved when WBRT was added to SRS. More recently, a large randomized phase III trial was performed comparing patients who received a focal therapy (either surgery or SRS) and WBRT to those treated wtih focal therapy alone. Again, no significant difference in overall survival was observed.

These studies have not answered the important question of when to radiate. Proponents argue that radiotherapy reduces local recurrence and may preserve neurologic function, and therefore should be used early. Opponents advocate for deferral of radiation until recurrence as a means to prevent neurocognitive toxicity, especially in patients of a good RPA class who have a better chance at long-term survival and thus are more likely to experience the long-term effects of radiotherapy.

An alternative approach might be to combine surgery with focal radiation. In an effort to avoid or delay the toxicities of WBRT while simultaneously eradicating residual tumor deposits, some institutions have practiced a strategy of cavity-directed SRS or hypofractionated radiotherapy following resection of brain metastasis. Additional nonresectable lesions, detected either before surgery or immediately thereafter, are typically radiated at the same time. In this manner, while some patients will ultimately require WBRT for treatment failure, a proportion may avoid it altogether. To be effective, close follow-up monitoring with serial MRI is of the essence to provide timely salvage therapy to those who need it.

Chemotherapy

Unfortunately – due, in part, to oncologists' reluctance to include patients with brain metastases on clinical trials – there is a paucity of data supporting the use of systemic agents for intracranial metastases. Previously, chemotherapy was applied in only two situations: as salvage treatment after all radiation and surgical options were exhausted and in small asymptomatic lesions discovered at time of diagnosis before patients had initiated any treatment. However, increasing evidence suggests that there may be a broader role for both classic cytotoxic drugs as well as more novel agents, particularly the so-called "smart drugs" – small molecules aimed at specific aberrant proteins found only in cancer cells. Chemotherapy will likely be the most important treatment modality of the future, as further advances in surgery or radiotherapy are unlikely to improve treatment of brain metastases dramatically in the future, and thus the future lies heavily on neuro-oncologists and medical oncologists.

Two major factors determine responsiveness of a brain metastasis to systemic agents: the permeability of the blood–brain barrier (BBB) and the chemosensitivity of the tumor. Theories as to the role of the BBB in the development and recalcitrance of intracranial metastases have evolved. Previously, the thinking was that the BBB simply blocked access of chemotherapeutic agents to tumor cells, thereby limiting their cytotoxic effect. However, the very fact that these lesions enhance on MRI challenges this concept, as the BBB must be breached in order for gadolinium uptake to occur. Newer theories suggest that the BBB may provide sanctuary for microscopic cancer deposits. While the rest of the body is treated – sometimes successfully – with any number of cytotoxic agents, these metastatic cells lie dormant, sequestered within the CNS from whence they emerge only later as full-blown enhancing tumors. In such cases, one might argue that patients with quiescent systemic disease and a new enhancing intracranial metastasis merit a re-challenge with agents that had worked in the past. Alternatively, one could postulate that if an intracranial metastasis has developed after many rounds of chemotherapy, then it is very likely to have developed resistance.

The sensitivity of any given tumor to chemotherapy is perhaps the most important factor in determining treatment response. Brain metastases secondary to melanoma and renal cell carcinoma remain the most resistant.

While chemotherapy agents with better BBB penetration, such as temozolomide, may prove beneficial, an immense amount of research and work has been carried out recently investigating newer, molecularly targeted therapies which attempt to disrupt biologic pathways aberrant in specific cancers. For example, EGFR inhibitors, such as erlotinib, may have value in treating brain metastases from non-SCLC (NSCLC) harboring specific genetic mutations. Bevacizumab, a monoclonal antibody that blocks angiogenesis, is another targeted therapy that may have therapeutic benefit in brain metastases. It is currently approved for the treatment of NSCLC, breast cancer, and colon cancer, as well as recurrent glioblastoma. Previously, concerns about the risk of intracranial hemorrhage precluded its use in patients with brain metastases, but more recent data and experience suggest that it may be safe, especially given its safety in glioblastoma. As scientists' evolving understanding of cancer biology continues to drive the development of such targeted therapies, it is likely that the role of systemic therapy for the treatment of brain metastases will only expand in the years to come.

Selected bibliography

Aoyama H, Shirato H, Tago M, Nakagawa K, Toyoda T, Hatano K, *et al.* (2006) Stereotactic radiosurgery plus whole-brain radiation therapy vs stereotactic radiosurgery alone for treatment of brain metastases: a randomized controlled trial. *JAMA* **295**, 2483–91.

Bernstein M, Berger M (eds) (2008) *Neuro-oncology: The Essentials*, 2nd edn. Thieme, New York.

Borgelt B, Gelber R, Kramer S, Brady LW, Chang CH, Davis LW, *et al.* (1980) The palliation of brain metastases: final results of the first two studies by the Radiation Therapy Oncology Group. *Int J Radiat Oncol Biol Phys* **6**, 1–9.

Cairncross JG, Kim JH, Posner JB.(1980) Radiation therapy for brain metastases. *Ann Neurol* **7**, 529–41.

DeAngelis LM, Posner JB. (2009) *Neurological Complications of Cancer*, 2nd edn. Oxford University Press, New York.

Gaspar L, Scott C, Rotman M, Asbell S, Phillips T, Wasserman T, *et al.* (1997) Recursive partitioning analysis (RPA) of prognostic factors in three Radiation Therapy Oncology Group (RTOG) brain metastases trials. *Int J Radiat Oncol Biol Phys.* **37**, 745–51.

Gaspar LE, Scott C, Murray K, Curran W. (2000) Validation of the RTOG recursive partitioning analysis (RPA) classification for brain metastases. *Int J Radiat Oncol Biol Phys* **47**, 1001–6.

Glantz MJ, Cole BF, Forsyth PA, Recht LD, Wen PY, Chamberlain MC, *et al.* (2000) Practice parameter: anticonvulsant prophylaxis in patients with newly diagnosed brain tumors. Report of the Quality Standards Subcommittee of the American Academy of Neurology. *Neurology* **23**, 1886–93.

Kocher M, Soffietti R, Abacioglu U, Villà S, Fauchon F, Baumert BG, *et al.* (2011) Adjuvant whole-brain radiotherapy versus observation after radiosurgery or surgical resection of one to three cerebral metastases: results of the EORTC 22952-26001 study. *J Clin Oncol* **29**, 134–41.

Lassman AB, DeAngelis LM. (2003) Brain metastases. *Neurol Clin* **21**, 1–23, vii.

Leyland-Jones B. (2009) Human epidermal growth factor receptor 2-positive breast cancer and central nervous system metastases. *J Clin Oncol* **27**, 5278–86.

Louis DN, Ohgaki H, Wiestler OD, Cavenee WK. (eds) (2007) *WHO Classification of Tumours of the Central Nervous System*, 4th edn. International Agency for Research on Cancer, Lyon.

Mintz AH, Kestle J, Rathbone MP, Gaspar L, Hugenholtz H, Fisher B, *et al.* (1996) A randomized trial to assess the efficacy of surgery in addition to radiotherapy in patients with a single cerebral metastasis. *Cancer* **78** (7), 1470–6.

Nussbaum ES, Djalilian HR, Cho KH, Hall WA. (1996) Brain metastases: histology, multiplicity, surgery, and survival. *Cancer* **78**, 1781–8.

Paget S. (1989) The distribution of secondary growths in cancer of the breast. *Cancer Metastasis Rev* **8**, 98–101.

Patchell RATP, Walsh JW. (1990) A randomized trial of surgery in the treatment of single metastases to the brain. *N Engl J Med* **322**, 494–500.

Posner JB. (1978) Intracranial metastases from systemic cancer. *Adv Neurol* **19**, 579–92.

Vecht CJ, Haaxma-Reiche H, Noordijk EM, Padberg GW, Voormolen JH, Hoekstra FH, *et al.* (1993) Treatment of single brain metastasis: radiotherapy alone or combined with neurosurgery? *Ann Neurol* **33** (6), 583–90.

18

Spinal Cord Compression

Melike Mut

Department of Neurosurgery, Hacettepe University, Ankara, Turkey

Spinal cord compression

Neurologic dysfunction related to spinal cord involvement is a common complication of systemic cancer. Compression of spinal cord, cauda equina, or roots from tumor growth in the spinal epidural space in cancer patients is commonly referred to as spinal epidural metastasis (SEM).

Epidemiology

SEM occurs in 5–10% of all patients with cancer. Median age at the time of the first episode of SEM is 62 years (64 years for men and 58 years for women), with a slight male predominance (57%); the cumulative incidence decreases each decade after 40 years. Prostate, breast, and lung cancer are the most common offenders, and each constitutes 15–20% of SEM, representing more than 50% of SEM cases. Non-Hodgkin lymphoma, multiple myeloma, and kidney cancer typically each account for an additional 5–10%. Colorectal cancer, tumors of unknown primary (most of which emanate from unrecognized lung or gastrointestinal tumors), and sarcomas are other common causes. Autopsy series indicate that SEM are far more common than are clinically detected; 90% of autopsied patients with prostate cancer have vertebral metastases, as do 74% with breast cancer, 45% with lung cancer, 29% with lymphoma or kidney cancer, and 25% with gastrointestinal cancers. In the pediatric population, sarcomas (especially Ewing), neuroblastomas, renal tumors, germ cell tumors, and Hodgkin disease are the most common causes of SEM.

Metachronous presentation (SEM developing in patients who are known to have cancer) is most common, especially for breast and prostate cancers. Synchronous presentation (presentation of SEM at the time of cancer diagnosis) of SEM occurs in 0.23% of all cancer patients. It is disease-specific, ranging from <0.01% in head and neck cancer to 1.95% in myeloma.

The median survival duration in patients with SEM varies from 3 to 11 months after diagnosis. Pretreatment neurologic status and tumor type are the most important predictors of outcome.

Pathophysiology

Dissemination of cancer cells through the vasculature is the presumed mechanism leading to spinal cord compression. The most popular theory for explaining the development of SEM is the access of cancer through the valveless venous system known as Batson plexus, which drains both the vertebrae and skull, and anastomoses

Neuro-oncology, First Edition. Edited by Roger J. Packer, David Schiff.
© 2012 John Wiley & Sons, Ltd. Published 2012 by John Wiley & Sons, Ltd.

with veins draining the breasts, thoracic, abdominal, and pelvic organs. Experimental models have also emphasized the role of arterial seeding of the vertebrae with tumors analogous to brain metastases. The vertebral body is more commonly involved than the posterior elements, presumably because highly vascular red marrow of the vertebral body promotes metastatic growth and the mass of the body is large compared to the posterior elements. The entrance point of vertebral vessels is the posterior part of the vertebral body; the tumor grows and invades the epidural space. Tumor growth through the vertebral neural foramina from the paraspinal region into the spinal canal accounts for 10% of cases.

The pathophysiology of neurologic deterioration associated with SEM is vascular insufficiency and impingement of the epidural venous plexus resulting in venous hypertension and vasogenic edema in the spinal cord rather than direct compression. Direct pressure from the tumor on the spinal cord may also contribute. Without successful treatment, spinal cord infarction will eventually occur.

Clinical features

The thoracic cord is the most common site of metastases where 60% of SEM are located; the next common site is the lumbosacral region (30%). Spinal metastasis is found to reside in the vertebral body and at least one of the pedicles in 68% of cases at the time of diagnosis of spinal metastasis on a recent magnetic resonance imaging (MRI) based study. Isolated anterior compression with metastatic disease restricted to vertebral body occurs in only 3% of episodes. Circumferential soft tissue compression of the spinal cord occurs in 22% of cases.

Although neurologic dysfunction is related to the localization of the tumor, pain is the most frequent symptom (in 83–95% of patients) by the time of diagnosis and has usually been present for several weeks as a result of involvement of bone with tumor. Pain is localized to the involved vertebral segment initially but increases in intensity and expands as weeks pass. Notably, acute neurologic deterioration suggests acute spinal cord compression due to pathologic fracture or dislocation. A characteristic feature of SEM

attributed to distention of the epidural venous plexus is pain during recumbency.

Chronologically, back pain usually precedes motor weakness, which in turn tends to precede sensory changes and sphincter dysfunction. Considering the importance of ambulatory status for neurologic prognosis, it is crucial to recognize the early symptoms of SEM: back pain, weakness, and sphincter dysfunction.

Weakness is present in 60–85% of patients at the time of diagnosis. Two-thirds of patients with SEM are nonambulatory when diagnosed. Involvement of muscle groups is usually asymmetrical and the iliopsoas muscles are often preferentially affected. Weakness is most severe with thoracic SEM given the anatomic features of thoracic spine (i.e. kyphosis, relatively narrow spinal canal, and vascular supply of spinal cord – the zone located between the fourth and ninth thoracic vertebrae has the least blood supply and these levels corresponds to the narrowest region of the spinal canal). Sensory deficits are less common; however, bowel and bladder disturbances are seen in about half of patients with advanced SEM.

> ☆ TIPS AND TRICKS
>
> A characteristic feature of SEM attributed to distention of the epidural venous plexus is pain during recumbency.

Diagnosis

Diagnosis of SEM begins with clinical suspicion. A multivariate analysis of diagnostic tools showed that the main predictors of SEM in a patient with a known systemic malignancy were night pain and low Karnofsky Performance Score. A thorough neurologic examination focused on motor, sensory deficits, and incontinence and radiologic studies must be performed; an MRI of the entire spine is recommended when SEM is suspected. The situation becomes more complicated with SEM as the initial presentation of cancer; because there may be a tendency to avoid or delay costly radiographic studies as most back pain in the general population has a benign etiology.

The predictive value of plain radiographs is very low. Classic radiographic abnormalities such as pedicle thinning, widening of the neural foramina, compression fractures, altered osseous density, and paravertebral soft tissue masses are relatively late findings on plain radiographs during the course of disease. Furthermore, plain radiography can only show bony changes and cannot address the question of soft tissue impingement on the thecal sac or spinal cord. Most metastases are osteolytic, although breast and prostate can cause osteoblastic or sclerotic lesions. Erosion of fine cortical margins of the spinal canal may be the earliest valuable finding on the plain radiographs. The most common finding on plain radiograph is known to be thoracic and lumbar spine pedicle erosion.

Plain radiographs have certain uses but major limitations. Plain films are falsely negative in 10–17% of cases. Reasons include the need for >50% of bone to be destroyed before plain radiography turns positive, the failure of some paraspinal masses invading the neural foramen to produce radiographic changes, and the fact that the multiplicity of bony metastases as seen in some common tumors such as breast and prostate may confuse the picture.

Bone scanning of the entire body with Tc-99m MDP is more sensitive than plain radiography although less sensitive than MRI for demonstrating bone metastases. Positron emission tomography using fluorodeoxyglucose (FDG PET) has been shown to be superior to scintigraphy in the detection of metastases because it detects the presence of tumor directly by metabolic activity, rather than indirectly by showing tumor involvement by increased bone mineral turnover. This allows the detection of metastatic foci earlier with PET than with bone scintigraphy.

Computed tomography (CT) is highly sensitive to alterations in bone density and the extent of bony involvement; a high quality CT sometimes reveals soft tissue compression. CT myelography is still an alternative when MRI is unavailable or cannot be used because of patient size, presence of implanted metallic objects, severe claustrophobia, inability to lie flat for the duration of the test, or uncontrolled pain. CT is still preferred in the guidance of percutaneous needle biopsies. CT with bone windows is also important for surgical planning.

MRI is the most sensitive technique; it is the first and often the only technique used in cases of cord compression, MRI also demonstrates bone lesions without epidural components, intramedullary metastases, and sometimes leptomeningeal tumor deposits. Knowledge of the presence of multiple metastases is clinically important for planning of radiation ports and surgery. Consequently, many authorities recommend either imaging the entire spine or at least the thoracic and lumbar spine in addition to the symptomatic region; asymptomatic epidural deposits are rarely found in the cervical spine.

★ TIPS AND TRICKS

Magnetic resonance imaging is the most sensitive technique in detecting SEM.

Treatment

Surgery

Advances in surgical technique have made surgery an indispensable part of the management of spinal metastases. Surgery is useful to make a definitive diagnosis in some cases, effectively palliate pain, improve neurologic function, reconstruct the stability of the spine, and increase response to adjuvant therapies. Complete paraplegia, which almost never improves with surgery, is a relative contraindication to surgery.

Several preoperative scoring systems have been proposed to help surgical planning and discuss surgical outcomes. General medical condition, number of extraspinal metastases, number of vertebral metastases, visceral metastases, primary tumor type, and presence of neurologic deficit are assessed to decide whether excisional or palliative procedures are preferred.

Another prognostic factor that has an influential effect in determining the differential neurologic outcome after surgery is the type of primary tumor. Patients with lung or prostate cancer are significantly older than patients with other types of primary cancers. Patients with prostate cancer have the highest prevalence of preoperative motor deficits and the shortest average duration of preoperative symptoms prior to surgical intervention. Additionally, patients with breast cancer have the highest incidence of vertebral compression fractures that are associated with poor ambulatory outcomes. Perioperatively, patients with gastrointestinal cancer have the highest rate of incidence of wound dehiscence requiring operative intervention. Patients with primary lung cancer have the highest rate of incidence of cerebrospinal fluid (CSF) leakage requiring operative intervention. The rate of recovery of ambulatory function is highest in patients with lung cancer, and these patients may therefore benefit most from decompressive surgery rather than major surgeries to maintain and/or regain ambulation because they usually have more extensive spinal involvement and a short expected duration of survival.

Generally, the results of surgical decompression in patients with spinal cord compression are superior to the results of radiation series and this is particularly applicable to radioresistant tumors. In surgical series, 74–100% of patients are ambulatory after decompression with 57–82% of nonambulatory patients recovering the ability to ambulate. Postoperative morbidity and mortality rates are in the range of 7–31%. Surgery also improves the quality of life; preoperative pain and paralysis are found to be relieved in 53% and 88%, respectively.

Patchell et al. conducted a prospective randomized multi-institutional trial comparing external beam radiation (30 Gy in 10 fractions) with decompressive surgery and instrumentation followed by external beam radiation therapy in symptomatic patients with spinal cord compression. Patients undergoing surgery and radiation therapy had statistically significant improvement compared with radiation alone in terms of the ambulation, bowel and bladder continence, narcotic requirement, and survival. An evidence-based systematic review concluded that patients with high grade epidural spinal cord compression resulting in myelopathy from solid metastasis should undergo decompressive surgery and instrumentation. A subgroup analysis suggested that patient age is an important factor; the beneficial effect of surgery was found to be diminished and not superior to radiation therapy alone in patients aged 65 years and older.

A recent study by Rades et al. has called into question whether Patchell's study could be reiterated with similar results. They conducted a matched pair analysis comparing surgery followed by radiotherapy with radiotherapy alone for metastatic spinal cord compression. In contrast to Patchell et al.'s study, surgery followed by radiotherapy did not show any significant advantage over radiotherapy alone. Improvement in motor function occurred in 27% of patients after surgery plus radiotherapy and 26% after radiotherapy alone. Post-treatment ambulatory rates were 69% after surgery plus radiotherapy and 68% after radiotherapy alone. Of the nonambulatory patients, 30% and 26%, respectively, regained ambulatory status after treatment. One-year local control rates were 90% after surgery plus radiotherapy and 91% after radiotherapy alone. One-year overall survival rates were 47% and 40%, respectively. They concluded that a new randomized trial comparing both treatments was justified. However, it seems unlikely if this will ever take place.

Different surgical approaches are used for spinal metastatic disease. In a multicenter prospective study, patients harboring spinal metastases underwent surgery ranging from palliative procedures or debulking to en bloc resection. Postoperatively, 71% of the entire group had improved pain control, 53% regained or maintained their independent mobility, and 39% regained urinary sphincter function. The median survival was 18.8 months for the en bloc group, 13.4 months for the debulking group, and 3.7 months for the palliative group. Those who underwent excision had improved quality of life, as this approach provided better pain control, enabling patients to regain or maintain mobility and offering improved sphincter control.

Laminectomy is a less extensive procedure and generally a palliative procedure for patients harboring spinal metastases; however, it is still the procedure of choice in patients in whom the bulk of epidural tumor is posteriorly located, in a subgroup of pediatric spinal sarcoma metastases, and in patients who have short survival expectancy for palliative purposes. Laminectomy generally allows the partial resection of spinal metastases considering the preferential localization of these tumors in the vertebral body; nevertheless, it usually results in amelioration of motor function, pain, and continence and therefore improves patient quality of life. Laminectomy alone may contribute to further spinal instability (up to 52%) and lead to clinical deterioration (25%). Because most deposits are located in the vertebral body and spare the lamina, the collapse of vertebral structures should be prevented with spinal stabilization techniques while radical removal of tumor is performed.

More extensive procedures, such as anterior or anterolateral approaches, allow surgical decompression of pathologic fracture of a vertebral body with extension of tumor and retropulsed bone fragments into the epidural spinal canal with simultaneous stabilization of the spinal column. If tumor involves lateral and/or posterior columns in addition to the anterior column, more extensive approaches with both anterior and posterior decompression and stabilization are necessary.

The role of *de novo* surgery was established in a prospective study in which the initial therapy for epidural spinal cord compression was surgical decompression. Forty-four percent of patients were nonambulatory before the surgery, and all regained the ability to ambulate postoperatively; approximately two-thirds received radiation treatment postoperatively. These results are superior to those reported after external radiation therapy and steroids alone. Additionally, prior radiation increases the risk of wound infection by three times compared with patients who undergo *de novo* surgery. Considering the timing of surgery, patients undergoing emergency surgery were more likely than those undergoing elective surgery to experience functional improvement such as recovered ambulation (61.5% vs. 25%). Thus, *de novo* surgery, including emergency surgery when necessary, seems to be the optimal surgical approach to SEM.

Radiation therapy

Radiation therapy has been the preferred treatment for most patients with SEM. The optimum fractionation schedule for radiotherapy is not known. To minimize the harmful effects of radiation on normal tissues, radiation is usually fractionated into small doses administered over a few days to weeks. Total doses of 2500–3600 cGy in 10–15 fractions are standard. An increased number of fractions is associated with improved pain control. The schedule of 30 Gy in 10 fractions is commonly utilized for patients with a markedly reduced life expectancy. Additionally, the delivery of two fractions of 800 cGy 1 week apart in SEM patients with poor neurologic prognosis is safe and apparently as efficacious as more conventional schedules. Once the anatomic limits of the epidural tumor have been identified, radiation oncologists specify treatment fields that extend one to two vertebral bodies above and below these limits and encompass the lateral dimensions of the SEM.

In most cases, radiation therapy is efficacious in terms of preventing further tumor growth and neurologic damage. The most important prognostic factor is pretreatment neurologic status. The time to develop motor deficits before radiation therapy is a significant prognostic indicator. A slower development of motor deficits predicts a better functional outcome. Current literature suggests that survival outcome after conventional radiotherapy is around 4.3 months (range 2–20 months). Patients with radiosensitive tumors and a single spinal metastasis do best, while patients with lung cancer, multiple vertebral metastases, or visceral or brain metastases have shorter survival. Survival rates are higher in patients who are ambulatory either before or after radiation. Level 1 evidence shows that 60–74% of patients remain ambulatory after conventional radiation in the setting of cord compression, whereas 19–33% of nonambulatory patients are able to walk after radiation. Fifty to 70% (range 57–100%) of patients were found to have improvement in pain after radiation therapy and approximately 70% of patients recovered sphincter function. The local control rate was 77% (range 61–89%).

An important prognostic factor is the primary cancer site. Median survival in patients undergoing radiotherapy for SEM varies between 3 and 6 months. The more radiosensitive tumors – breast, prostate and small cell lung cancer, lymphoma, and myeloma – are the most likely to shrink with radiotherapy. Melanoma and renal cell carcinoma are among the most radioresistant cancers; although such patients may still obtain significant palliation with radiation for SEM, the chances of major functional recovery or a long-lasting response to radiotherapy are much smaller than with the radiosensitive tumors. Radiosurgery can be used for more radioresistant tumors when feasible. The extent of subarachnoid impingement from an epidural metastasis has some prognostic value; as expected, patients with large masses have poorer outcome.

Recently, a new scoring system has been proposed by Rades *et al.*. Six prognostic factors determine the score: type of primary tumor (breast cancer vs. prostate cancer vs. myeloma/lymphoma vs. lung cancer vs. other tumors); interval between tumor diagnosis and metastatic spinal cord compression (less than 15 months vs. more than 15 months); presence of other bone metastases at the time of radiotherapy; presence of visceral metastases at the time of radiotherapy; pretreatment ambulatory status (ambulatory vs. non-ambulatory); and time of developing motor deficits before radiotherapy (1–7 days vs. 8–14 days vs. more than 14 days). The total scores range between 20 and 45 points. The 6-month survival rates are 14% (for those with 20–30 points), 56% (for those with 31–35 points), and 80% (for those with 36–45 points), respectively. This scoring system has been developed and validated in patients treated with radiotherapy alone, and its value in patients undergoing decompressive surgery is unknown.

Conventional radiation for spine metastases confers short-term reversible toxicity such as fatigue, mucositis, or myelosuppression, depending on the spinal segment irradiated. The most feared complication is radiation myelopathy, which typically takes 1–2 years to manifest, beyond the expected survival of most patients undergoing conventional radiation therapy. Although the actual tolerance of the spinal cord is unknown, a commonly accepted spinal cord dose to give a 5% or less risk of radiation myelopathy at 5 years is 50 Gy to less than 5 cm of cord, given in standard fractions. Dose fractionation schedules used for conventional radiation of SEM fall below this dose limit.

Spinal radiosurgery refers to the use of precisely targeted radiation to a small spinal tumor with the goals of achieving a tumoricidal radiation dose while not injuring sensitive structures such as the spinal cord. Current indications for the use of radiosurgery as a treatment modality for metastatic spine disease include pain (palliative benefit) related to a specific involved vertebral body, radiographic tumor progression, as a primary treatment modality, for progressive neurologic deficit, or after open surgical intervention.

Spinal radiosurgery appears to offer improved local control rates compared with external beam radiotherapy. Use of this modality is restricted to cases where the spinal cord dose can be kept lower than the tumor dose and below the threshold associated with radiation myelopathy. Spinal radiosurgery is frequently used to treat radiographic tumor progression after conventional irradiation treatment or after prior surgery. When used as a primary treatment modality, radiosurgery provides long-term radiographic tumor control in 90% of cases (breast, lung, and renal cell carcinoma metastases, and 75% of melanoma metastases).

If a tumor is only partially resected during open surgery, radiosurgery may be used to treat the residual tumor at a later date. A range of prescribed doses have been reported and include single-fraction radiosurgery ranging from 8 to 24 Gy or hypofractionated regimens consisting of $4\,Gy \times 5$ fractions, $6\,Gy \times 5$ fractions, $8\,Gy \times 3$ fractions, and $9\,Gy \times 3$ fractions. There is currently no evidence to support one regimen over another. Fifty-seven to 92% of patients experienced improvement of neurologic symptoms after radiosurgery. Despite the low quality of the available evidence, the reported outcomes are remarkably consistent, with 85–100% of reported patients experiencing effective palliation of pain.

Multimodality treatment

Although direct decompressive surgery combined with external beam radiotherapy can improve the ability to walk significantly compared with radiotherapy alone, many patients with SEM have multiple areas of metastases and have a poor overall condition. Consequently, an invasive surgical approach is feasible only in the minority of cases with better prognostic features. Radiosurgery has recently been added as another modality of radiotherapy for SEM in selected cases.

Treatment of SEM with a multimodality approach – surgery followed by radiation therapy – has the advantages of both surgery and radiation treatment. The choice of surgical procedure depends on the patient's general condition and life expectancy. Radiation therapy should follow within 1 month after surgery, generally to a total dose of 30–36 Gy (3 Gy per fraction). Long-lasting remission of pain and the recovery of neurologic deficit are obtained in 80% and 70% of patients, respectively. In selected patients, survival rates are also highly satisfactory, with an overall survival of 44% and 37% at 1 and 2 years, respectively.

Patients with moderately to highly radiosensitive tumors (lymphoma, multiple myeloma, breast, and prostate carcinoma) may undergo surgery first and then postoperative conventional radiation treatment or may undergo radiotherapy first in the absence of spinal instability. Radiosurgery may be an initial or postoperative option for radioresistant tumors (melanoma, renal cell, thyroid, non-small cell lung, and colon carcinoma). Although there are limited data available, high dose single fraction radiation may provide better local tumor control than conventional radiation treatment for radioresistant tumors when used as a postoperative adjuvant. Thus, the need for reoperation may be reduced. Should reoperation be required for neurologic salvage or local tumor control, image-guided intensity modulated radiotherapy may be offered either as high dose, single fraction or hypofractionated radiation to facilitate local tumor control. The ability to perform additional radiation therapy potentially will augment the success of operations for local disease control.

★ TIPS AND TRICKS

Treatment of SEM with a multimodality approach, surgery followed by radiation therapy, has the advantages of both surgery and radiation treatment. However, most SEM patients receive radiation treatment alone because of poor clinical condition and the presence of extensive disease.

Recurrent SEM

Even after treatment, recurrence of SEM is common and multiple recurrences in the same patient are not rare, placing patients at risk for paralysis. About half of patients surviving 2 years, and nearly all patients surviving 3 years or longer, develop recurrent SEM. Recurrence of spinal metastasis leads to neurologic deterioration in 69% of patients within 1 year of surgery who underwent surgery within 1 year and in 96% of surgical patients within 4 years. Patients with breast carcinoma develop recurrent SEM more frequently than those with lung carcinoma because of their longer survival. Thus, these patients are more likely to present with a recurrence due to ultimate failure of standard radiation therapy.

The recurrence of SEM occurs about as often at the initial level (55%) as at a different level (45%). Surgery may be the only way to prevent impending neurologic deficit by high grade epidural spinal cord compression because patients with previous extensive radiation therapy to the region cannot receive additional radiation. In one series, highly selected patients with adequate systemic cancer control and general state of health underwent 1–4 reoperations at the same level. The median time between the initial operation and the first reoperation at the same spinal level due to tumor recurrence was 8.3 months. A median survival time of 12.4 months was noted after the first reoperation, and a median survival time of 9.1 months was noted after the last reoperation. At their last follow-up 65% of patients were ambulatory, and the median time between loss of ambulation and death was 1 month. Repeat surgeries improved both the survival and functional status of the patients with acceptable surgical complication rates. These findings indicate that surgery should be considered as a first line option in recurrent SEM depending on the patient's performance status and extent of disease. When recurrent SEM is at a different spinal level, or when the previous radiation dose was low or the geometry favorable, radiosurgery may be a good option. In selected cases, radiosurgery control rates are reportedly >90% for recurrent SEM.

General supportive measures

The most debilitating symptoms of SEM are pain and weakness. Severe pain can be managed with narcotics. Corticosteroids have favorable effects on pain related to bone metastases, spinal cord compression, and vasogenic edema in the spinal cord. Consequently, their use is recommended in patients with neurologic dysfunction or severe pain until definitive therapies are undertaken. Dexamethasone is the most commonly used agent; the optimal dexamethasone regimen has not been established, but general practice is to administer a bolus of 10–100 mg IV, followed by 4–24 mg IV every 6 hours.

Opiates, inactivity related to pain or neurologic deficit, and autonomic spinal dysfunction may all contribute to constipation, and Valsalva maneuvers frequently exacerbate pain, so an aggressive bowel regimen should be instituted when diagnosis is suspected. Bisphosphonates may prevent pathologic fractures and can palliate bone pain caused by a variety of solid tumors.

Chemotherapy

Chemotherapy is a reasonable treatment option for SEM when the underlying tumor is likely to be chemosensitive. Chemotherapy has been successfully used for both Hodgkin and non-Hodgkin lymphoma, as well as breast cancer, germ cell tumors, and neuroblastoma.

Rehabilitation

Patients with SEM usually have neurologic deficits and pain; constipation, decubitus ulcers, and incontinence may accompany motor deficits. Patients with anticipated longer survival are appropriate for rehabilitation programs targeting longer term goals, while patients with shorter survival are more suitable for short, directed rehabilitation programs. Patients who can walk after treatment have a longer median survival (7.9 months) than do patients who cannot walk (1.2 months). Patients who walked after treatment lived longer, were ambulatory for most of their remaining life, had less pain, and had a lower incidence of depression. Patients with short expected survival may achieve functional improvements in mobility and self-care, and be discharged home.

Conclusions

Almost all patients with SEM will benefit from some form of radiation, and some will benefit from surgery as well. Surgeons and radiation oncologists should both be consulted promptly in cases of SEM. Local control of SEM can be achieved with surgery and subsequent radiation therapy with tolerable treatment-related morbidity and mortality in selected cases. Radiosurgery is increasingly used in the management of SEM, while chemotherapy has a smaller role limited to chemosensitive tumors. Overall survival and prognosis depend mainly on the extent of neurologic dysfunction at diagnosis of SEM, and the type and stage of the primary malignancy.

Selected bibliography

Bach F, Larsen BH, Rohde K, Borgesen SE, Gjerris F, Boge-Rasmussen T, et al. (1990) Metastatic spinal cord compression: occurrence, symptoms, clinical presentations and prognosis in 398 patients with spinal cord compression. *Acta Neurochir (Wien)* **107**, 37–43.

Bilsky MH, Laufer I, Burch S. (2009) Shifting paradigms in the treatment of metastatic spine disease. *Spine* **34** (22 Suppl), 101–7.

Chaichana KL, Pendleton C, Sciubb DM, Wolinsky JP, Gokaslan Z. (2009) Outcome following decompressive surgery for different histological types of metastatic tumors causing epidural spinal cord compression. *J Neurosurg Spine* **11**, 56–63. [Clinical article]

Chi JH, Gokaslan Z, McCormick P, Tibbs PA, Kryscio RJ, Patchell RA. (2009) Selecting treatment for patients with malignant epidural spinal cord compression: does age matter? Results from a randomized clinical trial. *Spine* **34** (5), 431–5.

Choi D, Crockard A, Bunger C, Harms J, Kawahara N, Mazel C, et al. (2010) Review of metastatic spine tumour classification and indications for surgery: the consensus statement of the Global Spine Tumour Study Group. *Eur Spine J* **19**, 215–22.

Gerszten PC, Mendel E, Yamada Y. (2009) Radiotherapy and radiosurgery for metastatic spine disease: what are the options, indications, and outcomes? *Spine* **34** (22 Suppl), 78–92.

Helweg-Larsen S, Sorensen PS. (1994) Symptoms and signs in metastatic spinal cord compression: a study of progression from first symptom until diagnosis in 153 patients. *Eur J Cancer* **30A**, 396–8.

Helweg-Larsen S, Sørensen PS, Kreiner S. (2000) Prognostic factors in metastatic spinal cord compression: a prospective study using multivariate analysis of variables influencing survival and gait function in 153 patients. *Int J Radiat Oncol Biol Phys* **46** (5), 1163–9.

Ibrahim A, Crockard A, Antonietti P, Boriani S, Bünger C, Gasbarrini A, *et al.* (2008) Does spinal surgery improve the quality of life for those with extradural (spinal) osseous metastases? An international multicenter prospective observational study of 223 patients. Invited submission from the Joint Section Meeting on Disorders of the Spine and Peripheral Nerves, March 2007. *J Neurosurg Spine* **8** (3), 271–8.

Kienstra GE, Terwee CB, Dekker FW, Canta LR, Borstlap AC, Tijssen CC, *et al.* (2000) Prediction of spinal epidural metastases. *Arch Neurol* **57**, 690–5.

Laufer I, Hanover A, Lis E, Yamada Y, Bilsky M. (2010) Repeat decompression surgery for recurrent spinal metastases. *J Neurosurg Spine* **13** (1), 109–15.

Maranzano E, Latini P. (1995) Effectiveness of radiation therapy without surgery in metastatic spinal cord compression: final results from a prospective trial. *Int J Radiat Oncol Biol Phys* **32** (4), 959–67.

Mut M, Schiff D, Shaffrey ME. (2005) Metastasis to nervous system: spinal epidural and intramedullary metastases. *J Neurooncol* **75** (1), 43–56.

Patchell RA, Tibbs PA, Regine WF, Payne R, Saris S, Kryscio RJ, *et al.* (2005) Direct decompressive surgical resection in the treatment of spinal cord compression caused by metastatic cancer: a randomised trial. *Lancet* **366**, 643–8.

Rades D, Douglas S, Veninga T, Stalpers LJ, Hoskin PJ, Bajrovic A, *et al.* (2010) Validation and simplification of a score predicting survival in patients irradiated for metastatic spinal cord compression. *Cancer* **116** (15), 3670–3.

Rades D, Huttenlocher S, Dunst J, Bajrovic A, Karstens JH, Rudat V, *et al.* (2010) Matched pair analysis comparing surgery followed by radiotherapy and radiotherapy alone for metastatic spinal cord compression. *J Clin Oncol* **28** (22), 3597–604.

Rades D, Karstens JH, Alberti W. (2002) Role of radiotherapy in the treatment of motor dysfunction due to metastatic spinal cord compression: comparison of three different fractionation schedules. *Int J Radiat Oncol Biol Phys* **54**, 1160–4.

Schiff D. (2003) Spinal cord compression. *Neurol Clin North Am* **21**, 67–87.

Sundaresan N, Steinberger AA, Moore F, Sachdev VP, Krol G, Hough L, *et al.* (1996) Indications and results of combined anterior–posterior approaches for spine tumor surgery. *Neurosurg* **85**, 438–46.

Tan M, New P. (2011) Survival after rehabilitation for spinal cord injury due to tumor: a 12-year retrospective study. *J Neurooncol* **104**, 233–8.

Tanaka M, Nakahara S, Ito Y, Kunisada T, Misawa H, Koshimune K, *et al.* (2009) Surgical treatment of metastatic vertebral tumors. *Acta Med Okayama* **63** (3), 145–50.

Taylor JW, Schiff D. (2010) Metastatic epidural spinal cord compression. *Semin Neurol* **30** (3), 245–53.

Tokuhashi Y, Matsuzaki H, Toriyama S, Kawano H, Ohsaka S. (1990) Scoring system for the preoperative evaluation of metastatic spine tumor prognosis. *Spine* **15**, 1110–3.

Tomita K, Kawahara N, Kobayashi T, Yoshida A, Murakami H, Akamaru T. (2001) Surgical strategy for spinal metastases. *Spine* **26**, 298–306.

19

Leptomeningeal Metastases

Sean Grimm[1] and Marc Chamberlain[2]

[1]Northwestern University, Chicago, IL, USA
[2]Department of Neurology and Neurological Surgery, Fred Hutchinson Cancer
Research Center, University of Washington *and* Division of Neuro-Oncology
Seattle Cancer Care Alliance, Seattle, WA, USA

Introduction

Cancer cells that spread to the subarachnoid (cerebrospinal fluid [CSF]) space are referred to as leptomeningeal metastases (LM). Other commonly used terms used include leukemic meningitis (a consequence of leukemia), lymphomatous meningitis (a result of lymphoma), carcinomatous meningitis (due to solid cancer), and neoplastic meningitis (all tumor types). LM usually occurs as a late manifestation of cancer (>75% of all instances of LM), at a time when widespread systemic metastases are present. Rarely, LM may be the first or only manifestation of cancer (<10%). Although LM is a rare complication of cancer (affecting 1–3% of all patients with cancer), it results in significant neurologic morbidity and mortality.

CSF is produced in the choroid plexus of the lateral, third, and fourth ventricles. CSF is a filtrate of blood plasma produced by both passive and active transport of blood substances. A normal adult produces approximately 21 mL/hour (500 mL/day). CSF circulates throughout the neuraxis and initially is actively ejected from the ventricles by arterial pulsations of the choroid plexus. CSF is primarily produced in the choroid plexus of the lateral ventricles and flows caudally and sequentially through the following structures: third ventricle (via the paired interventricular foramina of Monro), cerebral aqueduct, fourth ventricle, cisterna magna (via the foramina of Magendie and Luschka). Once in the cistern magna, CSF fluid may travel superiorly toward the cerebellar hemispheres to the basal cisterns, or inferiorly toward the spinal subarachnoid space. CSF in the spinal subarachnoid space posterior (dorsal) to the spinal cord is directed in the caudal direction towards the lumbar thecal sac (lumbar cistern) before CSF circulates anterior (ventral) to the spinal subarachnoid space. The direction of CSF ventral to the spinal cord is in the cephalad direction, returning CSF to the basilar cisterns and upward over the lateral and superior surfaces of the cerebral hemispheres where it is reabsorbed at the arachnoid granulations, emptying into the superior sagittal sinus. Obstruction or increased resistance at any point along this pathway by tumor adhesions may lead to elevated intracranial pressure (ICP) and a communicating hydrocephalus. CSF circulates 3–4 times each day and with each circulation the entire CSF volume re-enters the venous circulation by way of the superior sagittal sinus. A physiologic blood–CSF barrier (analogous to the blood–brain barrier) excludes water-soluble sub-

Neuro-oncology, First Edition. Edited by Roger J. Packer, David Schiff.

stances, such as chemotherapy, from entering the CSF.

Cancer cells metastasize to the CSF compartment by several mechanisms including hematogenous spread, direct extension from brain parenchymal disease, and retrograde spread along peripheral nerves. Once cancer enters the subarachnoid space, it spreads by way of CSF circulation, eventually emigrating to invade brain, spinal cord, and exiting nerves. The most common sites of subarachnoid bulk disease include the ventricles, basal cisterns, and cauda equina. Any cancer may spread to the subarachnoid space, but certain cancers have an increased propensity (see discussion below). Hematologic tumors (leukemia and lymphoma) have the highest risk for spread into the CSF, although the incidence of leukemic meningitis is low because of the infrequency of the disease and CNS prophylaxis at time of initial diagnosis and treatment. Among solid tumors the incidence is highest (in order of frequency) in breast, lung, melanoma, and gastrointestinal cancers. As systemic cancer therapy becomes more effective, it is likely that there will be an increased incidence of CNS metastasis including LM as the CNS provides a pharmacologic sanctuary from the majority of cancer therapy.

Clinical features

Because the signs and symptoms of LM are poorly recognized by oncologists and neurologists, their presence is under-recognized and, consequently, LM is often underdiagnosed. In an autopsy series of patients with cancer, LM were noted in 25%, while only 7% were diagnosed during life.

The hallmark of LM is multifocal neurologic dysfunction of subacute onset, reflecting the presence of tumor deposits at multiple sites throughout the neuraxis. The anatomic regions affected by LM can be separated into three domains: the cerebral hemispheres (15% of all instances of LM), cranial nerves (35%) and spinal cord and nerve roots (60%). Specific clinical presentations (i.e. cauda equina syndrome, communicating hydrocephalus, cranial neuropathy) should prompt a careful search for LM in a patient with known cancer:

- New onset seizures
- Unexplained encephalopathy
- Headache
- Gait unsteadiness (apraxic or "magnetic" gait)
- Blurred vision (optic neuropathy)
- Diplopia
- Face numbness ("numb chin")
- Face weakness – Bell's palsy (unilateral or bilateral)
- Vertigo
- Hearing loss
- Radicular pain
- Back pain
- Foot drop
- Leg weakness
- Bowel or bladder incontinence.

★ TIPS AND TRICKS

LM should be suspected when a cancer patient presents with multifocal neurologic dysfunction affecting the cerebral hemispheres, cranial nerves, or spinal cord and nerve roots.

Cerebral hemisphere dysfunction

LM cause hemispheric dysfunction via several mechanisms: increased ICP, superficial invasion and neuronal injury, mass effect, and ischemia by small vessel occlusion.

Increased intracranial pressure

LM may cause impaired flow and cause outflow obstruction of CSF at any site within the CSF compartment (most commonly at the level of the ventricles, basal cisterns, spinal subarachnoid space, and superior sagittal sinus), resulting in hydrocephalus and increased ICP. It is important to recognize that CSF flow disruption and associated ICP may be present, even in patients without evidence of hydrocephalus on neuroimaging.

Patients with LM may have compensated hydrocephalus and chronically elevated ICP. As a consequence, they often experience intermittent episodes of neurologic dysfunction that result from sudden elevations of intracranial pressure, termed plateau waves. Plateau waves are thought to arise from an increase in cerebral blood volume, following a sudden decrease in cerebral vascular resistance. Plateau waves can occur spontaneously or be precipitated by sneezing, coughing, Valsalva maneuver, and particularly when rising from a lying or sitting position. Symptoms can be quite variable, but the most common include headache, transient altered consciousness ("staring spells"), and sudden weakness of both lower extremities with collapse but preservation of consciousness. The episodes are often misdiagnosed as focal seizures and many patients are unnecessarily treated with anticonvulsants. Symptoms from plateau waves and increased ICP may be improved with placement of a ventriculoperitoneal (VP) shunt. Notably, seizures are relatively uncommon in patients with LM (<15%).

Metabolic competition and ischemia

LM directly competes with neurons for essential metabolites such as glucose. The tumor may grow along the Virchow–Robin spaces and thereby penetrate brain at some distance from the arachnoid space. LM may involve small blood vessels of exiting nerves (vasa nervorum), resulting in thrombosis and nerve ischemia.

Cerebral hemisphere clinical symptoms

Headache

Headache is the most common complaint in patients with LM. It is usually nonspecific and diffuse and may be associated with nausea, vomiting, or lightheadedness. Severe headache that is episodic suggests the presence of plateau waves (see above).

Gait dysfunction

Patients with LM often have a gait disturbance, which may reflect either hemispheric disturbance or spinal cord dysfunction. Some patients may develop an apraxic or "magnetic" gait that is seen in a patient with normal pressure hydrocephalus; urinary incontinence is an associated feature.

Episodic altered consciousness

Episodic loss of consciousness in patients with LM is usually caused by seizures. Plateau waves, causing staring spells and brief alterations of consciousness, should also be considered and are often misdiagnosed as seizures. Differentiating between these two possibilities is important as treatment differs.

Encephalopathy

Patients may experience diffuse cognitive dysfunction that resembles delirium or a confusional state. LM must be considered in cancer patients with altered mental status, particularly if no other cause is demonstrable (i.e. brain metastasis, electrolyte disturbance, medication effect).

Cranial nerve dysfunction

The cranial nerves travel through (*pari passu*) the subarachnoid space so as to exit the CNS and innervate peripheral targets. LM may infiltrate or cause ischemia in an exiting cranial nerve, causing symptoms.

LM may affect any cranial nerve. Common complaints include blurred vision (CN II), binocular diplopia (CN III, IV, or VI), facial numbness (CN V), facial weakness (CN VII), vertigo or hearing loss (CN VIII), and tongue weakness (CN XII).

Spinal nerve root dysfunction

Although LM may affect any spinal nerve root, involvement of the cauda equina is most common. Patients with cauda equina involvement usually present with asymmetric lower extremity weakness and dermatomal sensory disturbance which ultimately evolves into paraparesis, sensory loss, and urinary incontinence. Subtle lower extremity weakness is often the only evidence of LM affecting the spine. LM may also infiltrate exiting nerve roots causing radicular pain and radiculopathy. Nuchal rigidity is rarely present (15%) despite disease of the spinal cord.

Diagnosis

Neurologic examination

The hallmark of LM is dysfunction of the nervous system separated in time and space; patients suspected of harboring LM should be examined carefully for neurologic abnormalities that may not be associated with symptoms. A classic example is the finding of a lower extremity monoparesis (early cauda equina syndrome) in a patient complaining of diplopia and manifesting abducens palsy.

Neurologic examination findings suggestive of LM include extraocular muscle dysfunction (VI > III > IV), facial sensory loss, facial weakness, hearing loss, alteration of gag reflex, tongue deviation, extremity weakness (in a lower motor neuron nerve pattern), confusion, and gait disorder.

> ## ✭ TIPS AND TRICKS
>
> The finding of multifocal neuraxis disease in a patient with known malignancy is highly suggestive of LM. In patients with LM, signs on examination frequently exceed patient-reported symptoms.
>
> Cranial mononeuropathy and cauda equina syndrome represent two very characteristic clinical presentations of LM.

Imaging

Patients suspected of harboring LM should undergo magnetic resonance imaging (MRI) of the brain and complete spinal axis (cervical, tho-racic, and lumbar). In the appropriate clinical setting, abnormal leptomeningeal enhancement is consistent with a diagnosis of LM. Classic brain MRI findings include cortical leptomeningeal enhancement (often focal), cerebellar folia enhancement (Figure 19.1), ventricular enhancement, enhancement of the brainstem surface, and nodular enhancement of cranial nerves. Coexistent parenchymal brain metastasis is common and seen in 30–40% of all patients with LM. Hydrocephalus may be present (<10%), although subtle, and may be appreciated only if a prior study is available for comparison. Brain CT may show similar findings but is less sensitive than cranial MRI.

The classic finding on spine MRI is nodular contrast enhancement of the cauda equina nerve roots (Figure 19.1b). Patients may also have clumping of nerve roots or enhancement of the spinal cord surface. A computed tomography (CT) myelogram can be performed in patients unable to undergo MRI.

Approximately 30% of patients with LM have impaired CSF flow (i.e. a disturbance of CSF circulation caused by adhesive tumor deposits in the CSF space). Physicians should consider obtaining radionuclide (either [111]indium-diethylenetriamine pentaacetic acid or [99]Tc

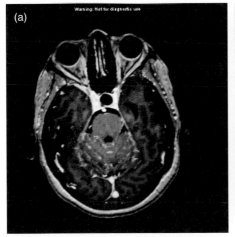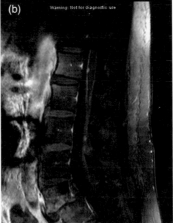

Figure 19.1. Magnetic resonance T1-weighted, post-contrast imaging of (a) brain demonstrating contrast enhancement of the cerebellar folia and (b) lumbar spine region demonstrating enhancement of the conus medullaris and lumbar nerve roots.

macroaggregated albumin) ventriculography in all patients with LM from solid tumors to evaluate CSF flow dynamics because results influence treatment and are prognostically important. This is particularly important if intra-CSF therapy is under consideration.

> ☆ TIPS AND TRICKS
>
> Many patients (30%) with LM have impaired or obstructed CSF flow. Radionuclide ventriculography to evaluate the CSF circulation should be considered in all patients with LM from solid tumors so that an appropriate treatment strategy can be determined.

CSF analysis

CSF examination should be performed in all patients suspected of having LM. CSF assessment should include opening pressure, cytology (to determine if pathologically malignant cells are present in instances of solid cancers) or flow cytometry (most sensitive for hematologic malignancies), cell count, protein, and glucose.

Opening pressure

All patients undergoing CSF sampling to assess for LM should have an opening pressure measured. The measurement should be obtained with the patient in the lateral decubitus position. Measurements obtained in the sitting or prone (e.g. procedures under fluoroscopic guidance) position may under- or overestimate ICP. Elevated CSF pressure measured by lumbar puncture is defined as >20 cm H$_2$O (normal is approximately 12 cm H$_2$O). Occasional patients (particularly with breast cancer) may have strikingly elevated opening pressure even when hydrocephalus is not obvious on imaging.

Protein

Elevated protein is the most common CSF abnormality found in patients with LM. The finding is nonspecific and not required for diagnosis. Normal CSF protein in the lumbar space and ventricle is <45 mg/dL and <25 mg/dL, respectively.

Pleocytosis

Patients with LM often have an increased CSF white count, usually with lymphocyte predominance. CSF leukocytosis is defined as >4 cells/mm^3. The number of CSF white blood cells in patients with LM is most often <50 cells/mm^3 and higher number of leukocytes or neutrophil predominance in the CSF should raise the possibility of chemical or infectious meningitis.

Glucose

Low CSF glucose (hypoglycorrhachia) is a common finding (30%) in patients with LM. Hypoglycorrhachia is defined as CSF glucose less than two-thirds of serum glucose. Because patients may have rapidly fluctuating serum glucose and it takes several hours for serum glucose to equilibrate with CSF glucose, an absolute value of less than 40 mg/dL is considered low in patients without diabetes mellitus.

Cytology

The demonstration of malignant cells in the CSF is pathologically diagnostic of LM. However, a negative cytology does not rule out the diagnosis because of a high false negative rate (>40%). The poor sensitivity results from a combination of sampling error and difficulty with specimen processing. Sampling error occurs because of a small number of cancer cells circulating in CSF and the random event of capturing suspended tumor cells in a comparatively large fluid volume. LM cells adhere at various locations in the CSF compartment, diminishing the number of suspended cells available for analysis. The yield of cytology is improved by sending a large volume of CSF for analysis, ideally >10 mL. The entire CSF cytology sample is centrifuged to concentrate the available cells for analysis. The CSF collected should be processed immediately or mixed with a preservative (CytoLyt® in a ratio of 1:1) to prevent cell lysis. In some cases, a cervical puncture may improve yield (especially in patients where the LM are predominantly located along the brainstem). In a patient with an intraventricular access device (e.g. an Ommaya reservoir), a sample can also be obtained from the lateral ventricle. Even with correct specimen processing, the false negative rate is still high; up to 50% of patients with eventual positive CSF cytology have a negative initial examination. With a second CSF examination the yield is increased to 80%. Minimal benefit is obtained from a third CSF specimen if the first two CSF samples are negative for malignant cells. Importantly, nearly half of all patients with LM have persistently negative CSF cytology, suggesting that positive CSF cytology is not the only parameter that defines LM. Neuroimaging (nearly 50% of all studies are negative for LM) and clinical examination often provide the only evidence for LM.

★ **TIPS AND TRICKS**

CSF cytology is diagnostic of LM but has low sensitivity. The false negative rate can be minimized by sending at least 10 mL of CSF for cytology, obtaining CSF near the site of disease on imaging, delivering the CSF to the laboratory for immediate processing, and performing a repeat lumbar puncture. In most cases, a third lumbar puncture is not helpful in making the diagnosis.

Flow cytometry

Flow cytometry is the analysis of cell surface markers by fluorescent probes to identify a monoclonal population of tumor cells. This laboratory technique is most useful and is more sensitive than CSF cytology in patients with lymphoma or leukemia. The identification of a monoclonal population of lymphocytes in a CSF sample (predominantly B cells) distinguishes neoplastic from reactive cells (overwhelmingly T cells).

Biochemical markers

Biochemical markers can be evaluated in the CSF, but their use in most cases is limited by poor sensitivity and specificity; they are less useful than CSF cytology or flow cytometry. Tumor markers such as carcinoembryonic antigen (CEA) from adenocarcinoma, carbohydrate antigen (CA) 15-3 in breast, melanin in melanoma, CA 125 in ovarian cancer, oncofetoproteins in germ cell tumors, and immunoglobulin M (IgM) in multiple myeloma can be tested in the CSF. If

the level is elevated in the absence of markedly elevated serum levels, it implies CSF production of the biochemical marker. Caution must be exercised when interpreting results as the biomarker may exude through an intact blood–CSF barrier when serum levels are significantly elevated or show up in the CSF specimen sent from a "traumatic tap." To avoid this confusion, simultaneous specimens from the serum and CSF should be sent for analysis. In addition to occasional diagnostic utility, CSF biomarkers may be useful for monitoring therapeutic response.

Treatment

The medical literature provides little guidance on the optimal treatment of LM. Jayson and Howell summarized the problems inherent in interpreting the available literature:

1 Most series include patients with LM that have arisen from different primary malignancies, which are likely associated with differing median survival.
2 There have been few prospective randomized investigations of treatment modalities in patients with LM from a particular tumor type.
3 The definition of response varies from one report to another so that some response rates refer to cytologic changes in the CSF while other consider clinical, cytologic, and biochemical parameters.
4 Reports include patients with and without parenchymal metastases or bulky subarachnoid disease, and the natural history of LM in the two situations may differ.

It is believed that treatment can palliate symptoms and in some cases improve neurologic disease-related survival; however, there has never been a properly powered trial determining the benefit of intra-CSF chemotherapy in the treatment of LM. Determining which patients to treat with LM is challenging, and one such guideline is provided in Figure 19.2. Treatment options for LM include surgery, radiation therapy, intra-CSF chemotherapy, and systemic chemotherapy. In most instances, a combination of treatment modalities is utilized.

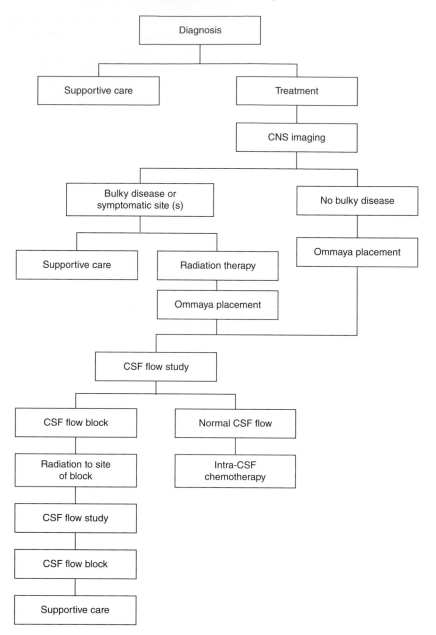

Figure 19.2. Decision and treatment algorithm of neoplastic meningitis. CNS, central nervous system; CSF, cerebrospinal fluid.

Surgery

Patients with symptoms from increased ICP or plateau waves may achieve symptomatic improvement following the placement of a VP shunt. Complications of VP shunt placement include bleeding, subdural fluid collection, infection, and shunt malfunction requiring revisions. Clinicians are often concerned that peritoneal shunting of LM will lead to peritoneal carcinomatosis. Although this is of theoretical concern, it is rarely seen in clinical practice. Rarely, and in patients without known cancer, a meningeal biopsy directed at radiographic abnormalities may be required to obtain a diagnosis. The most common surgical procedure is placement of a ventricular access device (i.e. an Ommaya or Rickham reservoir) to facilitate intra-CSF chemotherapy administration.

Radiotherapy

Radiotherapy is the most effective treatment for the resolution of symptoms associated with LM, although it is only a palliative measure. Because the entire neuraxis is involved in LM, the brain and spinal CSF compartments must be treated. Without so-called craniospinal irradiation, tumor present in untreated CSF regions will reseed regions that were treated with radiotherapy. Radiating the entire neuraxis is often associated with significant myelosuppression (particularly in adults with prior exposure to systemic chemotherapy and radiotherapy overlapping the spine) and acute gastrointestinal toxicity. To reduce treatment toxicity, local or involved-field radiotherapy is usually preferable. The strategy is to treat symptomatic areas such as whole brain, base of skull, segmental spinal cord, or cauda equina. Patients treated with local radiotherapy may experience improvement of cranial neuropathies or pain whereas focal neurologic deficits such as gait, bowel/bladder dysfunction and weakness rarely improve. Focal radiotherapy is also useful for asymptomatic patients in treating areas of bulky subarachnoid or parenchymal disease and in order to improve CSF flow dynamics when CSF flow is compromised, allowing the subsequent use of intra-CSF chemotherapy.

Intra-CSF chemotherapy

Chemotherapy can be administered directly into the CSF space. The three agents most commonly used are methotrexate, cytarabine (including liposomal cytarabine), and thiotepa. The doses and schedules of these drugs are shown in Table 19.1.

EVIDENCE AT A GLANCE

Table 19.2 summarizes the randomized clinical trials of intra-CSF agents used for LM.

Table 19.1. Intra-cerebrospinal fluid (intra-CSF) chemotherapy options for leptomeningeal metastases (LM).

Drug	Dose	Schedule
Methotrexate	10–15 mg	Twice weekly for 4 weeks, then every other week for 4 weeks, then monthly
Cytarabine	30–100 mg	Twice weekly for 4 weeks, then every other week for 4 weeks, then monthly
DepoCyt (liposomal cytarabine)	50 mg	Every 2 weeks for four treatments, then monthly for six treatments
Thiotepa	10 mg	Three times weekly for 4 weeks, then every other week for 4 weeks, then monthly

The advantage of intra-CSF treatment is that cytotoxic CSF drug concentrations can be achieved at doses that do not usually cause systemic toxicity. The predominant toxicity of intra-CSF chemotherapy is the induction of transient chemical aseptic meningitis manifested by headache, nausea, vomiting, CSF pleocytosis, and occasionally confusion. As the symptoms of aseptic meningitis occur within hours after injection, bacterial infection is not often a consideration. Rare side effects of intra-CSF chemotherapy include acute encephalopathy (confusion or seizure) and myelopathy (treatment-related cauda equina). Prolonged survivors of LM may be at risk for developing a delayed late leukoencephalopathy (dementia, urinary incontinence, and gait apraxia), especially likely if previous

Table 19.2. Randomized clinical trials of intra-cerebrospinal fluid (intra-CSF) chemotherapy agents.

Study	Design	Response	Toxicity
Shapiro et al. (2006)	Solid tumors (n = 103), DepoCyt vs. MTX; lymphoma (n = 25), DepoCyt vs. ara-C	DepoCyt vs. MTX/ara-C: PFS,* 35 vs. 43 days DepoCyt vs. MTX: PFS, 35 vs. 37.5 days DepoCyt vs. ara-C: CR,* 33.3% vs. 16.7% PFS, 34 vs. 50 days	DepoCyt vs. MTX/ara-C: drug-related AEs, 48% vs. 60% serious AEs, 86% vs. 77%
Boogerd et al. (2004)	n = 35, breast cancer; i.t. vs. no i.t. treatment†	i.t. vs. no i.t.: improvement or stabilization, 59% vs. 67% TTP, 23 vs. 24 weeks median survival, 18.3 vs. 30.3 weeks	i.t. versus no i.t.: neurologic complications, 47% vs. 6%
Glantz et al. (1999b)	n = 28, lymphoma; DepoCyt vs. ara-C	DepoCyt vs. ara-C: TTP,* 78.5 vs. 42 days OS,* 99.5 vs. 63 days RR, 71% vs. 15%	DepoCyt vs. ara-C: headache, 27% vs. 2% nausea, 9% vs. 2% fever, 8% vs. 4% pain, 5% vs. 4% confusion, 7% vs. 0% somnolence, 8% vs. 4%
Glantz et al. (1999a)	n = 61, solid tumors; DepoCyt vs. MTX	DepoCyt vs. MTX: RR,* 26% vs. 20% OS,* 105 vs. 78 days TTP, 58 vs. 30 days	DepoCyt vs. MTX: sensory/motor, 4% vs. 10% altered mental status, 5% vs. 2% headache, 4% vs. 2%
Grossman et al. (1993)	n = 59, solid tumors and lymphoma (in 90%); i.t. MTX vs. thiotepa	i.t. MTX vs. thiotepa: neurologic improvements, none median survival, 15.9 vs. 14.1 weeks	i.t. MTX vs. thiotepa: serious toxicities similar between groups; mucositis and neurologic complications more common in MTX group

AE, adverse event; CR, complete response; i.t., intra-CSF; MTX, methotrexate; N/V, nausea/vomiting; OS, overall survival; PFS, progression-free survival; RR, response rate; TTP, time to progression.

*No significant differences between groups.

†Appropriate systemic chemotherapy and/or radiotherapy given in both arms.

treatment utilized methotrexate and whole-brain radiotherapy. Aseptic meningitis, the most common side effect of intra-CSF chemotherapy, usually resolves within 1–5 days following treatment and can be symptomatically treated with oral antipyretics, antiemetics, and corticosteroids.

Although intra-CSF chemotherapy is the mainstay of treatment for LM, there are several limitations. First, intra-CSF chemotherapy should not be administered to patients with CSF obstruction or impaired flow dynamics as demonstrated by a radionucleotide ventriculography study. Impairment of the normal CSF circulation leads to stasis of fluid in the ventricles and other regions depending upon the site of CSF obstruction. Chemotherapy injected into a noncommunicating CSF compartment does not circulate and consequently fails to treat the entire CSF space. In addition, the administered intra-CSF drug is effectively concentrated in the blocked compartment resulting in increased drug exposure and potential chemotherapy-related neurotoxicity. Involved field radiotherapy to the site of CSF flow obstruction may alleviate obstruction and permit safe intra-CSF drug administration. Second, with few exceptions (e.g. breast cancer), the available intra-CSF chemotherapy drugs have poor efficacy against solid tumors. Third, administration of intra-CSF chemotherapy is sometimes technically challenging. Intra-CSF chemotherapy can be administered into the lumbar space by repeated lumbar punctures (intrathecal therapy) or into the ventricle via an Ommaya or Rickham reservoir (an intraventricular catheter attached to a subgaleal reservoir). Both routes of intra-CSF drug delivery have limitations. Chemotherapy delivered via lumbar puncture is limited by patient discomfort, thrombocytopenia (platelets >50,000 are required to reduce the risk of epidural hematoma), and coagulopathy. In addition, the drug is not infrequently (approximately 12% of all injections) injected into a subdural or epidural space such that intrathecal therapy is not administered. Notwithstanding intrathecal injection, therapeutic drug concentrations in the ventricular space may not be reliably achieved in nearly one-third of patients and as a consequence compromise efficacy.

Because a ventricular access device avoids these issues, it is recommended in the majority of patients who are treated with intra-CSF chemotherapy. However, treatment with a ventricular access device is not without complication. The device is subject to infection (in nearly 10% of all patients with a ventricular device) and may occasionally be misplaced at time of surgical implantation. Importantly, any ventricular access device requires that patients undergo a surgical procedure.

✋ CAUTION!

Patients with LM frequently have impaired CSF flow dynamics as demonstrated by radionucleotide ventriculography studies. When CSF flow is impaired, diffusion from the CSF into the periventricular brain white matter often results in neurotoxicity when intra-CSF chemotherapy is administered. Patients with obstruction of CSF outflow should not receive intra-CSF chemotherapy unless the block is restored to normal by treatment with involved field radiotherapy.

Systemic chemotherapy

The use of systemic chemotherapy for LM is limited because the physiologic blood–CSF barrier prohibits most chemotherapy agents from entering the CSF. This physiologic barrier is analogous to the blood–brain barrier which is well recognized as a limitation for systemic chemotherapy for brain metastases. The use of specific systemic chemotherapy agents is discussed in the appropriate sections below.

🔬 SCIENCE REVISITED

The blood–CSF barrier is composed of tight junctions between the choroid cells (in contrast to the blood–brain barrier where the tight junctions are between epithelial cells) which limit the passage of water-soluble agents. In addition, choroid plexus cells possess enzymes that can metabolize several drugs in a manner similar to liver detoxification. Most lipid-soluble substances enter the CSF freely by crossing the blood–CSF barrier.

Prognosis

The prognosis for solid tumor patients with LM is poor, reflecting the fact that LM is usually diagnosed late in the cancer disease course, underlying tumors are often refractory to systemic treatment, and the particular difficulty of treating tumor in the subarachnoid space. Median survival is 4–6 weeks without treatment and 2–3 months with treatment. Patients with radiotherapy and chemotherapy "sensitive" tumors such as breast cancer and hematologic malignancies may fare better; however, 1-year survival is only 15%.

For solid tumor patients with widespread metastatic disease, the goal of therapy is to improve or stabilize neurologic function and improve quality of life, as most patients will expire from their systemic disease. To prevent the development and progression of disabling neurologic symptoms and signs (rarely reversed with treatment), early diagnosis followed by treatment of LM in appropriate patients is optimal.

Treatment of specific tumors

Leukemia

The leukemias are among the malignancies at highest risk for the development of LM. In the 1970s the incidence of LM from acute lymphoblastic leukemia was 30–66%. With current treatment regimens that include prophylactic intra-CSF chemotherapy, the incidence has decreased to <5%. Prophylactic CNS chemotherapy is effective in preventing CSF relapse, but only marginally effective in treating established disease. Two issues arise with prophylactic CNS treatment of leukemia. First, there is risk of leukemic seeding of the CSF during the lumbar puncture. As such, the first lumbar puncture is usually performed after reducing the peripheral blast count with induction chemotherapy and the first dose of intra-CSF chemotherapy is administered at the time of diagnostic lumbar puncture. The second issue is differentiating between a "traumatic" tap and leukemic meningitis. For acute lymphoblastic leukemia, guidelines have been established. A CSF flow study is not usually necessary in leukemic patients treated with CNS prophylaxis as without LM, CSF compartmentalization rarely occurs.

Lymphoma

The CSF space is the most common site of central nervous system (CNS) metastasis in systemic lymphoma (in contrast to primary CNS lymphoma in which parenchymal brain involvement is more common). The diagnosis is made by a combination of flow cytometry, clinical examination, and neuroradiography. Liposomal cytarabine has, in a small randomized trial, been shown to be more effective than free cytarabine in lymphomatous meningitis. There are limited data to suggest intra-CSF rituximab (a monoclonal antibody directed at malignant CD20-expressing B lymphocytes) may be effective for lymphomatous meningitis.

Breast cancer

Breast cancer is the solid tumor with the highest incidence of LM; approximately 5% of patients will develop LM. Whether there is increased risk of LM in breast cancers that overexpress human epidermal growth factor receptor-2 (HER2) is controversial. Unlike other solid tumors, breast LM may respond to treatment and occasional long-term survivals have been reported. The percentage of patients alive with breast LM at 1 year is 11–25%. Aggressive treatment is usually indicated in the majority of patients with breast cancer-associated LM.

Patients with normal CSF flow dynamics (as documented by radionucleotide ventriculography), limited systemic and CNS disease burden can be treated with intra-CSF chemotherapy. Methotrexate, thiotepa, and cytarabine appear to have similar efficacy, although one study favored DepoCyt over methotrexate for quality of life and cause of death (neurologic vs. systemic), suggesting that liposomal cytarabine be considered the intra-CSF chemotherapy agent of choice. Intra-CSF trastuzumab (a monoclonal IgG1 antibody to HER2) is being investigated in clinical trials for breast cancer with HER2 overexpression and LM.

Several systemic treatment options are available for breast LM. Therapeutic CSF concentrations have been demonstrated with high dose methotrexate ($3.5–8\,g/m^2$) administration. Capecitabine has demonstrated efficacy for both LM and brain metastases in small studies. Lapatinib is not an option for breast-related LM as it has demonstrated minimal response in brain metastases, likely because of limited CNS penetration.

Lung cancer

Lung is the solid tumor with second highest incidence of LM. Lung cancer is separable into two histologic categories: small cell lung cancer (SCLC) and non-small cell lung cancer (NSCLC) with differing neurotropism and response to treatment.

SCLC is a solid tumor that frequently metastasizes to the CSF; LM occurs in 9–25% of patients and 2-year cumulative incidence is 10%. The overall incidence is decreasing as smoking rates decline. It is one of the most chemosensitive and radiation-sensitive solid tumors. However, there are no studies that have examined the response to treatment of SCLC and LM.

NSCLC is poorly responsive to standard intra-CSF chemotherapy (i.e. methotrexate and cytarabine) though the use of topotecan may be more promising.

Melanoma

Melanoma is uncommon, but has the third highest incidence of LM, reflecting the strong neurotropism of melanoma. LM melanoma is highly resistant to treatment and intra-CSF chemotherapy is usually ineffective. Not well tested is whether intra-CSF alpha interferon or thiotepa may provide a more rational tumor-specific therapy for melanoma and LM.

Colorectal cancer

Colon cancer rarely metastasizes to the leptomeninges although LM may occur following resection of cerebellar metastasis. Colon and other gastrointestinal cancers have a predilection to metastasize to the cerebellum. Standard intra-CSF chemotherapy treatments have limited effectiveness but there are no prospective trials using a pre-specified LM therapy in these cancers and consequently treatment guidelines are lacking.

Summary

Despite the fact that the prognosis is poor for the majority of patients with LM, treatment is often administered in patients with limited systemic and CNS disease, good performance, and reasonable life expectancy. Treatment goals of LM are palliative, attempting to slow or stabilize neurologic disease so as to delay or prevent disabling neurologic symptoms which negatively impact quality of life. Patients with radiographic, clinical, or pathologic defined LM should be treated with focal radiotherapy to the anatomic site causing symptoms, sites of CSF flow disruption (if intra-CSF chemotherapy is to be administered), and to sites of bulky CNS disease (Figure 19.2). Following radiotherapy, patients with chemoresponsive tumors should be considered for treatment with an intra-CSF chemotherapy agent appropriate and with activity against the primary cancer (Figure 19.2). Patients with encephalopathy, bulky CNS disease, or abnormal CSF flow study refractory to radiotherapy should be considered for supportive hospice care. Figure 19.2 outlines a general treatment algorithm for LM.

Selected bibliography

Boogerd W, van den Bent MJ, Koehler PJ, Heimans JJ, van der Sande JJ, Aaronson NK, et al. (2004) The relevance of intraventricular chemotherapy for leptomeningeal metastasis in breast cancer: a randomised study. Eur J Cancer 40 (18), 2726–33.

Bromberg JE, Breems DA, Kraan J, Bikker G, van der Holt B, Smitt PS, et al. (2007) CSF flow cytometry greatly improves diagnostic accuracy in CNS hematologic malignancies. Neurology 68 (20), 1674–9.

Chamberlain MC. (1998) Radioisotope CSF flow studies in leptomeningeal metastases. J Neurooncol 38 (2–3), 135–40.

Chamberlain MC. (2008) Neoplastic meningitis. Oncologist 13 (9), 967–77.

Chamberlain MC, Kormanik PA, Barba D. (1997) Complications associated with intraventricular chemotherapy in patients with leptomeningeal metastases. J Neurosurg 87 (5), 694–9.

Chamberlain MC, Kormanik PA, Glantz MJ. (2001) A comparison between ventricular and lumbar cerebrospinal fluid cytology in adult patients with leptomeningeal metastases. Neuro Oncol 3 (1), 42–5.

DeAngelis LM, Posner JB. (2009) Neurologic Complications of Cancer, 2nd edn. Oxford University Press, Oxford; New York.

Glantz MJ, Cole BF, Glantz LK, Cobb J, Mills P, Lekos A, *et al.* (1998) Cerebrospinal fluid cytology in patients with cancer: minimizing false-negative results. *Cancer* **82** (4), 733–9.

Glantz MJ, Jaeckle KA, Chamberlain MC, Phuphanich S, Recht L, Swinnen LJ, *et al.* (1999a) A randomized controlled trial comparing intrathecal sustained-release cytarabine (DepoCyt) to intrathecal methotrexate in patients with neoplastic meningitis from solid tumors. *Clin Cancer Res* **5** (11), 3394–402.

Glantz MJ, LaFollette S, Jaeckle KA, Shapiro W, Swinnen L, Rozental JR, *et al.* (1999b) Randomized trial of a slow-release versus a standard formulation of cytarabine for the intrathecal treatment of lymphomatous meningitis. *J Clin Oncol* **17** (10), 3110–6.

Grossman SA, Finkelstein DM, Ruckdeschel JC, Trump DL, Moynihan T, Ettinger DS; Eastern Cooperative Oncology Group. (1993) Rand-omized prospective comparison of intraventricular methotrexate and thiotepa in patients with previously untreated neoplastic meningitis. *J Clin Oncol* **11** (3), 561–9.

Hitchins RN, Bell DR, Woods RL, Levi JA. (1987) A prospective randomized trial of single-agent versus combination chemotherapy in meningeal carcinomatosis. *J Clin Oncol* **5** (10), 1655–62.

Jayson GC, Howell A. (1996) Carcinomatous meningitis in solid tumours. *Ann Oncol* **7** (8), 773–86.

Seute T, Leffers P, ten Velde GP, Twijnstra A. (2005) Leptomeningeal metastases from small cell lung carcinoma. *Cancer* **104** (8), 1700–5.

Shapiro WR, Schmid R, Glantz M, *et al.* (2006) A randomized phase III/IV study to determine benefit and safety of cytarabine liposome injection for treatment of neoplastic meningitis. *J Clin Oncol* **24** (Suppl 6), 1528.

20

Immune-Mediated Paraneoplastic Neurologic Disorders: An Overview

Myrna R. Rosenfeld and Josep Dalmau

Department of Neurology, Hospital Clinic/Institute of Biomedical Investigation (IDIBAPS), University of Barcelona, Barcelona, Spain

Introduction

Paraneoplastic neurologic disorders (PND) are cancer-associated neurologic disorders that result from a variety of pathogenic mechanisms. This chapter focuses on some of the more common PND that are known or strongly suspected to be immune-mediated. The autoimmune etiology of these PND is supported by the detection in the serum and cerebrospinal fluid (CSF) of antibodies that react with antigens expressed by the nervous system, the frequent presence of inflammatory cells in the CSF, the clinical response to immunomodulatory therapies, and experimental work demonstrating a direct pathogenic effect of some antibodies.

Pathogenesis and incidence

The exact pathogenesis of immune-mediated PND remains unclear. It is generally accepted that expression of neuronal proteins by a systemic cancer breaks immune tolerance to proteins normally expressed in the nervous system. In response patients develop antineuronal antibodies that may be found in serum and CSF and serve as markers of the paraneoplastic origin of the neurologic symptoms. When directed against cell surface or synaptic antigens, the antibodies are pathogenic and produce neurologic dysfunction by interfering with neuronal cell signaling or synaptic transmission. When the associated antibodies are directed against intracellular antigens, the pathogenic mechanisms appear to be mediated by cytotoxic T cells.

The incidence of immune-mediated PND varies with tumor type. PND occur more commonly in association with tumors that express neuroendocrine proteins such as small cell lung cancer (SCLC) or neuroblastoma, tumors that contain nervous tissue such as teratomas, and tumors that affect organs with immunoregulatory functions (thymoma). Less common but often associated with highly typical neurologic syndromes are neoplasms of the ovary, breast, and germ cell tumors of the testis. There are also the immune-mediated PND associated with plasma cell malignancies or B-cell lymphomas. In these disorders, the immunoglobulins synthesized by the neoplastic cells likely cause neurologic dysfunction by direct antibody activity against peripheral nerve antigens or nonspecific deposition of immunoglobulin fragments in peripheral nerves. These disorders are not further discussed here.

Neuro-oncology, First Edition. Edited by Roger J. Packer, David Schiff.

Diagnosis of the neurologic syndrome and cancer

The diagnosis of PND is based on recognition of the neurologic syndrome, demonstration of the associated cancer, and detection of serum and CSF neuronal antibodies. As early tumor treatment and immunotherapy are associated with increased likelihood of stabilization or improvement of the PND, it is vital that diagnosis not be delayed. Some neurologic syndromes, such as Lambert–Eaton myasthenic syndrome (LEMS) or an acute onset cerebellar syndrome in an older patient are so strongly associated with cancer (called classic PND) that their recognition should prompt a search for the commonly associated cancer type. While many PND develop and progress rapidly exceptions do occur, and some patients develop insidious forms of PND that can be misdiagnosed as chronic degenerative disorders. The PND that affect the central nervous system (CNS), dorsal root ganglia, or proximal nerve roots are often associated with CSF abnormalities. CSF findings that are consistent but not specific of PND include pleocytosis with lymphocyte predominance, normal or elevated protein levels, intrathecal synthesis of immunoglobulins, and oligoclonal bands. Evaluation of the CSF is also important to rule out other cancer complications, such as infectious or neoplastic meningitis.

Neuroimaging, best performed with magnetic resonance imaging (MRI), can be helpful to rule out metastatic lesions or other cancer-related complications. In most PND of the CNS the blood–brain barrier is intact and the affected brain regions rarely enhance with contrast. There have been a few reports of paraneoplastic cerebellar degeneration with contrast enhancement of the cerebellar folia which initially suggested leptomeningeal disease. In limbic encephalitis, T2 and fluid attenuated inversion recovery (FLAIR) abnormalities on MRI often are seen at early stages of the disorder. In the early stages of PND, [18]fluorodeoxyglucose positron-emission tomography (FDG PET) may reveal increased metabolic activity, likely representing inflammatory changes, in areas where the MRI is normal.

In more than half of cases, symptoms of PND develop before the cancer diagnosis has been made and at a time when the cancer may be quite small and difficult to demonstrate. In addition to a review of cancer risk factors and serologic cancer markers, a comprehensive radiologic assessment including computed tomography (CT) scan of the chest, abdomen, and pelvis is a reasonable start. Studies have demonstrated that combined CT and FDG PET scanning is useful in identifying occult tumors although there are reports in which the detection of antineuronal antibodies led to the discovery of an occult cancer that was not detected by CT or PET. The use of specific tests will vary with the neurologic syndrome, patient's gender and age, and, if present, the specific antineuronal antibody.

Patients with a previously characterized antineuronal antibody and neurologic dysfunction in whom a cancer is not initially found should have close tumor surveillance. Ideally, these patients should have evaluations every 6–9 months as most PND-associated cancers manifest within the first year of neurologic symptom presentation. Less commonly, several years will elapse before the cancer is detected. Patients in cancer remission who develop a PND should be assessed for tumor recurrence.

Detection and significance of paraneoplastic antineuronal antibodies

The detection of specific and well-characterized antineuronal antibodies in serum or CSF can rapidly confirm the diagnosis of a PND. While low titers of antineuronal antibodies may be identified in the serum of some patients with cancer but without PND, detection of high titers of antibodies in serum or of any titer of antibodies in the CNS is strongly supportive of PND. In contrast, the absence of an antineuronal antibody does not rule out that a syndrome could be paraneoplastic. In this case it is possible that the antibody has not yet been identified, or that other immune (or nonimmune) mechanisms are involved. When antibodies are found it is important to remember that not all antineuronal antibodies have the same significance; some antibodies associate with one or a limited number of PND and histologic types of cancer while others are less syndrome and tumor-specific.

Table 20.1. Antibodies to intracellular antigens, syndromes, and associated cancers.

Antibody	Associated neurologic syndrome(s)	Tumors
Anti-Hu	Encephalomyelitis, subacute sensory neuronopathy	SCLC
Anti-Yo	Cerebellar degeneration	Ovary, breast
Anti-Ri	Cerebellar degeneration, opsoclonus	Breast, gynecologic, SCLC
Anti-Tr	Cerebellar degeneration	Hodgkin lymphoma
Anti-CRMP5	Encephalomyelitis, chorea, optic neuritis, uveitis, peripheral neuropathy	SCLC, thymoma, several
Anti-Ma proteins	Limbic, hypothalamic, brainstem encephalitis	Testicular (Ma2), several (Ma)
Anti-amphiphysin	Stiff person syndrome, encephalomyelitis	Breast, SCLC
Anti-GAD65	Stiff person, cerebellar syndrome, refractory epilepsy	Infrequent tumor association (thymoma)

CRMP, collapsing response-mediator protein; GAD, glutamic acid decarboxylase 65; SCLC, small cell lung cancer.

Antibodies that target intracellular antigens

There are two groups of antibodies that target intracellular antigens. In one group are those antibodies that are strongly associated with characteristic neurologic syndromes and histologic types of cancers; they serve as markers of PND. This group includes anti-Hu, Yo, Ma2, Ri, CV2/CRMP5, and amphiphysin antibodies (Table 20.1). Detection of one of these antibodies strongly supports the diagnosis of PND even if no tumor is found at evaluation. Some antibodies are more syndrome-specific than others; for example, anti-Yo antibodies almost always associate with predominant cerebellar degeneration, and anti-Ma2 with limbic or upper brainstem dysfunction, while anti-Hu or anti-CV2/CRMP5 antibodies associate with a much wider spectrum of symptoms.

In the second group are those antibodies that are markers for the presence of a cancer but not of the neurologic syndrome. This group includes antibodies that target the SOX and Zic families of proteins. The utility of these antibodies is therefore confined to clinical settings where their detection suggests that the patient has an underlying tumor. For example, LEMS can occur with or without a cancer association, almost always an SCLC. However, the presence of SOX antibodies in a patients with LEMS is significantly associated with the presence of an SCLC.

Antibodies that target cell surface or synaptic proteins

These antibodies are directed against neuronal cell surface or synaptic proteins that have important roles in synaptic function such as synaptogenesis, synaptic transmission and plasticity, hemisynaptic organization and synaptic assembly, and regulation of membrane excitability (Table 20.2). Detection of antibodies against any of these antigens usually associates with a characteristic syndrome that may occur with or without a cancer association. Thus, these antibodies are markers of the neurologic syndrome but not of paraneoplasia. A common property of these disorders is that, despite the severity of the related syndromes, most patients respond to immunotherapy. This group includes antibodies to the excitatory glutamate N-methyl-D-aspartate receptor (NMDAR), alpha-amino-3-hydroxy-5-methyl-4-isoxazolepropionic acid receptor (AMPAR), inhibitory gamma-aminobutyric acid (GABA$_B$) receptor, leucine-rich glioma-inactivated 1 (LGI1), contactin associated protein-like 2

Table 20.2. Antibodies to cell surface or synaptic antigens, syndromes, and associated tumors.

Antibody	Neurologic syndrome	Tumor type when associated
Anti-NMDAR	Anti-NMDAR encephalitis	Teratoma (frequency depends on gender and age)
Anti-AMPAR	Limbic encephalitis with relapses; psychiatric symptoms	Thymoma, breast, SCLC
Anti-GABA$_B$R	Limbic encephalitis, seizures	SCLC, neuroendocrine
Glycine receptor	Encephalomyelitis with rigidity, stiff person syndrome	Infrequent tumor association
Anti-LGI1	Limbic encephalitis	Infrequent tumor association (thymoma, SCLC)
Anti-Caspr2	Morvan syndrome, neuromyotonia, encephalitis	Limited experience to assess tumor frequency (thymoma may occur)
Anti-mGluR1	Cerebellar degeneration	May occur with Hodgkin lymphoma or without tumor
Anti-VGCC	Cerebellar degeneration, LEMS	SCLC
Anti-ganglionic AChR*	Autonomic ganglionopathy (pandysautonomia)	Infrequent tumor association

AChR, acetylcholine receptor; AMPAR, α-amino-3-hydroxy-5-methyl-4-isoxaolepropionic acid receptor; Caspr2, contactin associated protein-like 2; GABA$_B$R, gamma-amino-butyric acid B receptor; LEMS, Lambert–Eaton myasthenic syndrome; LGI1, leucine-rich glioma inactivated 1; mGluR1, metabotropic glutamate receptor 1; NMDAR, N-methyl-D-aspartate receptor; SCLC, small cell lung cancer; VGCC, voltage-gated calcium channel.
*Not discussed in this chapter.

(CASPR2) and the alpha 1 subunit of the glycine receptor.

Frequently encountered paraneoplastic neurologic disorders associated with immune responses

When a patient with cancer develops neurologic symptoms, a thorough clinical history, knowledge of the temporal association with cancer therapies, and results of ancillary tests usually reveal the cause. When no etiology is identified, the diagnosis considered is often that of a PND. There are several PND that are encountered frequently enough or for which the clinical syndrome is highly suggestive of PND, that it is reasonable to consider this diagnosis at the initial encounter. If correct, this offers the possibility for early intervention and improved outcome. These PND include paraneoplastic cerebellar degeneration (PCD), sensory neuronopathy, encephalomyelitis (PEM), limbic encephalitis, and the encephalitides with antibodies to cell surface or synaptic proteins. Opsoclonus-myoclonus is less common but so distinctive clinically that when seen, the diagnosis of PND should be strongly considered. LEMS and myasthenia gravis are two other common syndromes that may occur with or without a cancer association. As these disorders have been well studied and detailed descriptions are available they are not further discussed here.

Cerebellar degeneration

In adults, there are only a few causes for an acute to subacute onset of diffuse cerebellar dysfunction. In patients with a known cancer, the differential diagnosis includes metastatic complications and side effects of cancer treatment, including cerebellar toxicity of 5-fluorouracil and cytosine arabinoside.

Neuroimaging and CSF studies are useful to rule out metastatic disease. In PCD, the CSF may show inflammatory cells or mild increase in proteins while MRI of the brain is often normal at symptom presentation or may rarely show cerebellar cortical enhancement with gadolinium. As the disease evolves cerebellar atrophy develops. Almost all antineuronal antibodies that target intracellular antigens have been reported in PCD although 30–40% of patients with PCD do not have antineuronal antibodies and the diagnosis is by exclusion of other causes. Antibodies to voltage-gated calcium channels (VGCC) can occur with or without LEMS in a subgroup of patients with PCD and SCLC.

Paraneoplastic encephalomyelitis

Patients with PEM develop symptoms of multifocal involvement of the CNS, often in association with sensory and autonomic deficits. The symptoms of PEM develop rapidly and progress over weeks or months until stabilization or death. The CSF is almost always abnormal with mild to moderate lymphocytic pleocytosis, increased protein concentration, and oligoclonal bands or increased immunoglobulin G (IgG) index. Brain MRI is often abnormal, showing FLAIR or T2 sequence hyperintensities in involved areas and sometimes clinically silent regions. Contrast enhancement is more likely to occur in some forms of encephalitis (e.g. limbic-diencephalic encephalitis associated with anti-Ma2 antibodies) than others (e.g. limbic encephalitis associated with anti-Hu antibodies). The antibodies more frequently encountered in PEM are Hu, CRMP5, Ma2, and amphiphysin.

Paraneoplastic myelitis usually occurs in the context of a more widespread involvement of the nervous system, such as encephalomyelitis, and has the same antibody associations. Nonetheless, there are cases of pure or predominant myelopathy as a paraneoplastic manifestation of several types of cancers, predominantly of the lung and breast. In this disorder the MRI findings along with CSF inflammatory abnormalities,

with negative cytology, may lead to the diagnosis. In about one-third of patients the MRI is normal, but close to 50% of cases show a characteristic pattern that consists of symmetric longitudinally extensive T2 signal abnormality in a tract or gray matter distribution that often shows symmetric enhancement. The differential diagnosis includes neuromyelitis optica (predilection for central gray matter, but the enhancement is usually patchy), amyotrophic lateral sclerosis, and vitamin B_{12} deficiency (tract-specific T2 signal changes, but no contrast enhancement). While metastases of the spinal cord and leptomeninges are accompanied by MRI findings of nodular areas of enhancement or pial enhancement, the MRI of paraneoplastic myelopathy does not show nodular or pial areas of enhancement.

Paraneoplastic sensory neuronopathy

Paraneoplastic sensory neuronopathy (PSN) may occur in isolation, but often occurs in association with PEM. In more than 80% of patients with PSN the associated tumor is SCLC, and frequently the neurologic symptoms develop before the cancer diagnosis has been made. Patients develop pain, numbness, and sensory deficits that can affect limbs, trunk, and cranial nerves. Proprioception is often most affected, leading to sensory ataxia and pseudoathetoid movements. The deficits are often asymmetric and may initially suggest radiculopathy or mononeuritis multiplex. Nerve conduction studies show decreased or absent sensory nerve action potentials with normal or near-normal motor conduction velocities. The most commonly associated antibody is anti-Hu, with some patients having additional antibodies to CV2/CRMP5 or others; up to 18% of patients with PSN have no detectable antibodies.

Paraneoplastic opsoclonus-myoclonus

Opsoclonus consists of involuntary, arrhythmic, chaotic, multidirectional saccades without intersaccadic intervals. When paraneoplastic it generally occurs in association with myoclonus and ataxia. MRI studies are usually normal, and the CSF is normal or shows lymphocytic pleocytosis, increased protein concentration, or oligoclonal bands. In adults, the tumors more frequently involved are SCLC, gynecologic, and breast cancers; in children, there is a strong association with neuroblastoma. Other than anti-Ri antibodies found in some women with breast or gynecologic cancers and less frequently SCLC, most patients with paraneoplastic opsoclonus-myoclonus do not have well-characterized antineuronal antibodies.

Treatment of pediatric opsoclonus-myoclonus involves resection of the neuroblastoma, if present, and immunotherapy, including corticosteroids, adenocorticotropic hormone (ACTH), intravenous immunoglobulin (IVIg), plasmapheresis, rituximab, or cyclophosphamide. Children frequently respond well to the initial treatment, but they are often left with behavioral, speech, and sleep problems. Relapses are frequent, usually during intercurrent illnesses or attempts to reduce immunotherapy. In adults, corticosteroids or IVIg can accelerate improvement in patients with idiopathic disease, but those with paraneoplastic opsoclonus-myoclonus only benefit from immunotherapy when the tumor is controlled.

Stiff person syndrome

This disorder associates with muscle stiffness, rigidity, and spasms that are triggered by sensory, auditory, or emotional stimuli. Symptoms improve with sleep and diazepam and have a characteristic electrophysiologic pattern of continuous motor neuron activity simultaneously involving agonist and antagonist muscles. The disorder can occur with or without tumor association and the antibody association varies accordingly.

In 85% of cases with stiff person syndrome the etiology is not paraneoplastic and these patients usually have antibodies against glutamic acid decarboxylase 65 (GAD65). GAD65 antibodies can also occur in some patients with cerebellar ataxia and refractory epilepsy, and these symptoms can overlap with stiff person syndrome. GAD65 antibodies have been reported in a few patients with stiff person syndrome in association with thymoma and other tumors. Although GAD65 antibodies can be detected in non-neurologic disorders (such as type 1 diabetes), the presence of antibodies in the CSF is specific for neurologic disease.

The paraneoplastic form of the disorder often associates with amphiphysin antibodies; the tumors more frequently involved are SCLC and breast cancer. Patients with paraneoplastic stiff person syndrome are more likely to be older, have asymmetric and distal distribution of symptoms, frequent cervical involvement, and may have spinal myoclonus and pruritus.

In addition to treating the tumor and immunotherapy, symptomatic treatment with diazepam, baclofen, sodium valproate, vigabatrin, or tiagabin is often effective.

Encephalomyelitis with rigidity is associated with stiff person syndrome. Patients with this disorder usually have brainstem dysfunction and there is recent evidence that a subgroup of these patients have glycine receptor (GlyR) antibodies (discussed below). Most patients with GlyR antibodies do not appear to have cancer. As occur with other antibodies against neuronal cell surface antigens, the identification of patients with GlyR antibodies is important because symptoms usually respond to immunotherapy.

Syndromes with antibodies against cell surface antigens

Unlike most of the syndromes described above, which almost always occur as manifestations of an underlying cancer, the disorders associated with antibodies to cell surface antigens can occur with or without cancer; the frequency of an underlying tumor varying among age, gender, and type of antibody. Although recently described these disorders are at least five times more frequent than all classic paraneoplastic disorders with antibodies to intracellular antigens.

Anti-NMDAR encephalitis

This disorder usually affects young woman or children of either sex, although adult male patients can also be affected. Symptoms of anti-NMDA receptor encephalitis develop and resolve as a multistage process. Most patients experience a viral-like prodrome followed by psychosis, memory, behavioral and cognitive deficits, seizures, and dyskinesias (orofacial, limb, and trunk). There is frequent autonomic and breathing instability that result in the need for intensive care monitoring and mechanical ventilation. The majority of children are brought to medical attention as a result of changes in mood, behavior, personality, insomnia, and language disintegration, at times associated with seizures. The symptom presentation in children may initially suggest late onset autism, early onset schizophrenia, or childhood disintegrative disorder.

The CSF often shows lymphocytic pleocytosis; about 60% have oligoclonal bands and one-third have increased proteins. Early in the course, MRI abnormalities occur in about half of cases, most commonly increased signal on FLAIR or T2 sequences in the cerebral or cerebellar cortex, medial temporal lobes, subcortical regions, basal ganglia, or brainstem. In most patients, the EEG shows generalized slow, delta, or theta activity without epileptic discharges although these findings may overlap with electrographic seizures.

Just over half of patients have an associated tumor, most commonly an ovarian teratoma that can be mistaken for a benign cyst. Women older than 18 years are more likely to have a tumor than those who are younger. In males, the detection of a tumor is rare. Isolated cases associated with other tumor types include teratoma of the mediastinum, SCLC, Hodgkin lymphoma, neuroblastoma, breast cancer, and germ cell tumor of the testes.

✋ CAUTION!

Patients with anti-NMDAR encephalitis (and some cases of encephalitis associated with antibodies against other cell surface antigens) are often given incorrect initial diagnoses. The adults are often young women thought to have acute psychosis, catatonia, schizophrenia, viral encephalitis, drug abuse, or neuroleptic malignant syndrome among others. A history of a viral-like prodrome and the development of prominent psychiatric manifestations, seizures, and dyskinesias (in particular orofacial) along with autonomic and breathing instability strongly support the diagnosis of anti-NMDAR encephalitis that can be confirmed by the presence of NMDAR antibodies. Almost 40% of cases are children and teenagers who develop changes in mood, behavior, personality, insomnia, and language disintegration, at times associated with seizures. Some of these symptoms can be mistaken for late onset autism, early onset

schizophrenia, or childhood disintegrative disorder. Early diagnosis and institution of therapy shortens recovery time and increases the likelihood of full recovery.

Anti-AMPAR encephalitis

The disorder most commonly affects middle-aged women, who acutely develop limbic dysfunction, at times with prominent psychiatric symptoms and sometimes seizures. About 70% of patients have an underlying tumor in the lung, breast, or thymus. Patients may have other autoimmune disorders.

CSF findings are similar to that of anti-NMDA receptor encephalitis with predominant lymphocytic pleocytosis. Brain MRI usually shows abnormal FLAIR signal involving the medial temporal lobes, rarely with transient signal changes in other areas.

Anti-GABA$_B$ receptor encephalitis

The encephalitis associated with antibodies to the GABA$_B$ receptor has been described in both men and women (median age 62 years). Patients present with limbic encephalitis and seizures and about half of the patients have an associated tumor, either SCLC or a neuroendocrine tumor of the lung. As in anti-AMPA encephalitis, these patients frequently have additional autoantibodies (thyroid peroxidase, SOX, ANA, or N-type voltage-gated calcium channels) suggesting a susceptibility to autoimmunity. Imaging and CSF findings are similar to other types of limbic encephalitis. Patients with paraneoplastic limbic encephalitis and GAD antibodies often have GABA$_B$ receptor antibodies, which likely drive the neurologic syndrome.

Anti-LGI1 limbic encephalitis

This disorder was previously attributed to antibodies targeting the voltage-gated potassium channels (VGKC). Patients with antibodies to LGI1 develop memory disturbances, confusion, and seizures, sometimes preceded by short tonic seizures that can be mistaken for myoclonus or startle disorders. The MRI findings are usually typical of limbic encephalitis but the CSF is often normal or with mild changes. Only 20% of cases are associated with a neoplasm, most commonly thymoma or SCLC.

Anti-CASPR2 associated syndromes (neuromyotonia, Morvan syndrome, encephalitis)

This group of disorders had been previously attributed to VGKC, but the target antigen is CASPR2. Patients usually develop peripheral nerve hyperexcitability (neuromyotonia), cognitive impairment, memory loss, hallucinations, seizures, autonomic dysfunction, or a combination of neuromyotonia and CNS dysfunction (Morvan syndrome). Some patients have, in addition, other immune-mediated disorders such as myasthenia gravis with anti-acetylcholine or MuSK antibodies. The peripheral signs and symptoms may lead to the diagnosis of atypical motor neuron disease in some patients. The diagnosis of anti-CASPR2 associated symptoms is important to establish because the disorder responds to immunotherapy. Anti-CASPR2 associated syndromes may occur with or without an associated tumor, usually thymoma.

Anti-GlyR associated symptoms

Antibodies to the alpha1 subunit of the GlyR occur in some patients with progressive encephalomyelitis with rigidity and myoclonus (PERM), acquired hyperekplexia, and atypical stiff person or stiff limb syndrome without GAD65 antibodies. In a report of three patients, atypical symptoms included alterations of behavior and sleep, seizures, trismus, and neurogenic pruritus. None of the patients had cancer, and only one had substantial neurologic recovery.

General treatment strategies

The first therapeutic strategy for PND is the identification and treatment of the tumor as this appears to offers the best chance of neurologic stabilization or improvement. As noted above, in many PND of the CNS associated with antibodies to intracellular antigens, cytotoxic T-cell mechanisms are likely important in mediating neuronal destruction and therefore these PND tend to be poorly responsive to treatment. In addition to treatment of the tumor, initiation of immunomodulatory therapies while the PND is still progressing may be useful as the neuronal damage may not be complete. Initial therapies include corticosteroids, IVIg, or rituximab. If there is no initial response to these therapies and the patient is still losing neurologic functions, more aggressive immunosuppression can be attempted with cyclophosphamide, tacrolimus, or cyclosporine.

Concerns that the use of immunosuppression in cancer patients will favor tumor growth or result in increased toxicity if combined with ongoing cancer therapies appear unfounded. Experience with PND and other disorders such as lymphoma demonstrates that immunosuppressive therapies are well tolerated by most patients who are also receiving chemotherapy and do not worsen tumor outcomes.

The disorders associated with antibodies to cell surface or synaptic antigens are often quite responsive to antibody depleting and immunosuppressive therapies as the antibodies are directly responsible for the neurologic dysfunction. This is particularly true for disorders of the peripheral nervous system such as LEMS, myasthenia gravis, and neuromyotonia. For those disorders of the CNS (e.g. anti-NMDAR encephalitis and others), IVIg or plasma exchange are often useful at early stages of the disease. However, later in the course, when there is high intrathecal synthesis of antibodies, these treatments are often insufficient and additional therapy with rituximab and cyclophosphamide is frequently required. While in the syndromes related to intracellular autoantigens patients almost never improve unless the tumor is treated, those associated with cell surface autoantigens may respond to immunotherapy before the tumor is treated. However, treatment of the tumor along with immunotherapy are both necessary to reduce relapses and accelerate the neurologic recovery.

☆ TIPS & TRICKS

Symptoms of PND develop before there is a known cancer diagnosis in almost half of patients, and if a tumor is found this is usually small and localized. If suspicion is high for a PND based on clinical presentation, syndrome, presence of inflammatory cells in the CSF and/or antineuronal antibodies, a thorough search for cancer should be performed. Detection of antineuronal antibodies focuses the search to the tumor type more commonly associated with those antibodies. If the tumor does not express the target antigen, a search for a second neoplasm should be undertaken. Patients with classic antineuronal antibodies without a detectable tumor should have repeat cancer screening within 3–6 months, and then every 6 months for 4 years. Keep in mind that there are reports of tumors being found several years after PND onset. Patients in cancer remission who develop a PND should be assessed for tumor recurrence.

☆ TIPS AND TRICKS

The PND associated with antibodies to intracellular antigens often do not improve with therapy. The best chance for stabilization or improvement is when treatment is instituted when there is ongoing evidence of active inflammation in the CSF or when the patient is still actively deteriorating. Those disorders associated with antibodies to cell surface antigens are highly responsive to treatment, with better outcomes observed in those who are treated early with immunotherapy and tumor removal, if appropriate. Even when critically ill these patients should be aggressively treated. Experience demonstrates that these procedures are tolerated and shorten time to recovery and increase the likelihood of full recovery.

Selected bibliography

Alexopoulos H, Dalakas MC. (2010) A critical update on the immunopathogenesis of stiff person syndrome. *Eur J Clin Invest* **40**, 1018–25.

Bataller L, Graus F, Saiz A, Vilchez JJ. (2001) Clinical outcome in adult onset idiopathic or para-neoplastic opsoclonus-myoclonus. *Brain* **124**, 437–43.

Dalmau J, Lancaster E, Martinez-Hernandez E, Rosenfeld MR, Balice-Gordon R. (2011) Clinical experience and laboratory investigations in patients with anti-NMDAR encephalitis. *Lancet Neurol* **10**, 63–74.

Gorman MP. (2010) Update on diagnosis, treatment, and prognosis in opsoclonus-myoclonus-ataxia syndrome. *Curr Opin Pediatr* **22** (6), 745–50.

Graus F, Delattre JY, Antoine JC, Dalmau J, Giometto B, Grisold W, *et al.* (2004) Recommended diagnostic criteria for paraneoplastic neurological syndromes. *J Neurol Neurosurg Psychiatry* **75**, 1135–40.

Hughes EG, Peng X, Gleichman AJ, Lai M, Zhou L, Tsou R, *et al.* (2010) Cellular and synaptic mechanisms of anti-NMDA receptor encephalitis. *J Neurosci* **30**, 5866–75.

Hutchinson M, Waters P, McHugh J, Gorman G, O'Riordan S, Connolly S, *et al.* (2008) Progressive encephalomyelitis, rigidity, and myoclonus: a novel glycine receptor antibody. *Neurology* **71**, 1291–2.

Lai M, Hughes EG, Peng X, Zhou L, Gleichman AJ, Shu H, *et al.* (2009) AMPA receptor antibodies in limbic encephalitis alter synaptic receptor location. *Ann Neurol* **65**, 424–34.

Lancaster E, Huijbers MGM, Bar V, Boronat A, Wong A, Martinez-Hernandez E, *et al.* (2011) Investigations of caspr2, an autoantigen of encephalitis and neuromyotonia. *Ann Neurol* **69** (2), 303–11.

Lancaster E, Lai M, Peng X, Hughes E, Constantinescu R, Raizer J, *et al.* (2010) Antibodies to the GABA(B) receptor in limbic encephalitis with seizures: case series and characterisation of the antigen. *Lancet Neurol* **9**, 67–76.

Lancaster E, Martinex-Hernandez E, Dalmau J. (2011) Encephalitis and antibodies to synaptic and neuronal cell surface proteins. *Neurology* **77** (2), 179–89.

Mas N, Saiz A, Leite MI, Waters P, Baron M, Castaño D, *et al.* (2011) Antiglycine-receptor encephalomyelitis with rigidity. *J Neurol Neurosurg Psychiatry* **82**, 1399–401.

Murinson BB, Guarnaccia JB. (2008) Stiff-person syndrome with amphiphysin antibodies:

distinctive features of a rare disease. *Neurology* **71**, 1955–8.

Psimaras D, Carpentier AF, Rossi C. (2010) Cerebrospinal fluid study in paraneoplastic syndromes. *J Neurol Neurosurg Psychiatry* **81**, 42–5.

Rosenfeld MR, Dalmau J. (2011) Anti-NMDA-receptor encephalitis and other synaptic autoimmune disorders. *Curr Treat Options Neurol* **13** (3), 324–32.

Tanaka K, Tanaka M, Inuzuka T, Nakano R, Tsuji S. (1999) Cytotoxic T lymphocyte-mediated cell death in paraneoplastic sensory neuronopathy with anti-Hu antibody. *J Neurol Sci* **163**, 159–62.

Titulaer MJ, Klooster R, Potman M, Sabater L, Graus F, Hegeman IM, *et al.* (2009) SOX antibodies in small-cell lung cancer and Lambert–Eaton myasthenic syndrome: frequency and relation with survival. *J Clin Oncol* **27**, 4260–7.

21

Neurotoxicity of Radiation Therapy and Chemotherapy

Eudocia Quant Lee

Center for Neuro-Oncology, Dana-Farber/Brigham and Women's Cancer Center, Boston, MA, USA

Introduction

Neurotoxicity resulting from cancer therapies is an important source of morbidity in oncology. Cytotoxic chemotherapy, radiation, and novel targeted therapies can adversely impact the central and/or peripheral nervous systems. The severity of these manifestations ranges from reversible self-limited conditions to severe life-threatening disorders. Some neurologic complications may occur during treatment, while others may not be detectable for months or years after completion of therapy. Neurotoxicity may also lead to reduction of dosages or cessation of therapy, thus limiting potential therapies. Treatment regimens must be optimized to eradicate disease without excessive injury of normal neural structures. Because neural tissue repair is limited, prevention and early recognition are key to avoiding permanent neurologic damage. As a neurologist, it is also important to differentiate therapy-related neurotoxicity from other etiologies such as compression or infiltration by tumor, metabolic factors, nutritional deficiencies, infections, and paraneoplastic disorders. For the purpose of this chapter, "chemotherapy" will refer to all systemic antineoplastic agents including cytotoxic chemotherapy as well as novel targeted agents.

CNS toxicity from antineoplastic agents

Neurotoxicity from chemotherapy can affect the central nervous system (CNS) diffusely (e.g. encephalopathy, delirium, or dementia) or focally (e.g. cerebellar ataxia). Several chemotherapy-induced CNS disorders are well characterized. An acute cerebellar syndrome with ataxia and somnolence may occur with high dose cytarabine (Figure 21.1). Symptoms are usually noted 3–8 days after initiating treatment and usually resolve a few days after discontinuing cytarabine. Intrathecal methotrexate or liposomal cytarabine produces aseptic meningitis, which can be ameliorated with prophylactic dexamethasone. Acute high dose methotrexate neurotoxicity is characterized by somnolence, confusion, and seizures within 24 hours of treatment. Symptoms usually resolve spontaneously without sequelae. Chronic leukoencephalopathy occurs commonly with high dose methotrexate, but has also been described with vincristine, fluorouracil, and ifosfamide. Specific agents (e.g. thymidine for fluorouracil, methylene blue for ifosfamide,

Neuro-oncology, First Edition. Edited by Roger J. Packer, David Schiff.

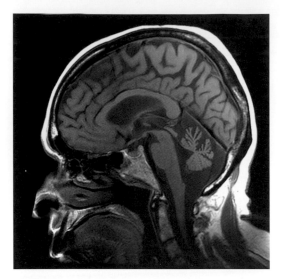

Figure 21.1. This patient received high dose cytarabine for acute promyelocytic leukemia. Her leukemia went into remission, but she developed dysarthria and gait instability following a few cycles of treatment. A sagittal T1-weighted MRI obtained almost 20 years after treatment demonstrates cerebellar atrophy.

and folinic acid for methotrexate) may minimize the encephalopathy caused by these chemotherapies.

✋ CAUTION!

The major delayed complication of methotrexate therapy is a leukoencephalopathy. Although this syndrome may be produced by methotrexate alone, it is exacerbated by radiotherapy, especially if radiotherapy is administered before or during methotrexate therapy. This neurotoxicity usually occurs following repeated administration of intrathecal or high dose intravenous methotrexate, but has been described after standard dose intravenous doses.

Posterior reversible encephalopathy syndrome (PRES) is typically associated with uncontrolled hypertension or immunosuppressants such as cyclosporine and tacrolimus, but has also been described in relationship to a variety of combination and single anticancer agents such as gemcitabine, cisplatin, cyclophosphamide, bevacizumab, and sunitinib. Symptoms may include headache, confusion, visual disturbances, and seizures. Typical magnetic resonance imaging (MRI) findings in PRES include symmetric white matter edema in the posterior cerebral hemispheres. Symptoms usually resolve spontaneously with conservative management, including removal of the offending agent, blood pressure regulation, seizure control, and management of any co-morbid conditions (e.g. electrolyte imbalances, infections).

⚖ SCIENCE REVISITED

Posterior reversible leukoencephalopathy (PRES), also known as reversible posterior leukoencephalopathy, is attributed to disordered cerebral autoregulation and endothelial dysfunction. Although commonly considered reversible with conservative management, PRES can rarely result in permanent damage such as cerebral infarctions caused by compression of microcirculation from the mass effect of vasogenic edema.

An increasingly recognized neurotoxicity occurring during or after chemotherapy is cognitive impairment known as "chemo brain." Chemo brain most often refers to problems with memory, multitasking, and/or concentration. Even though many patients improve after completing chemotherapy, subsets of patients continue to experience cognitive impairments. Symptoms may be subtle but can adversely affect quality of life. Neuropsychologic profiles suggest disruption of frontal–subcortical networks including problems with short-term memory, executive function, working memory, and sustained attention. Epidemiologic studies of chemo brain have demonstrated conflicting results regarding its frequency and severity, and may be difficult to interpret for a variety of reasons including the lack of cognitive evaluation prior to chemotherapy and inconsistency in defining what constitutes cognitive dysfunction. Unfortunately, data regarding prevention or treatment of chemotherapy-induced cognitive impairment are limited.

Even though many chemotherapeutic agents are associated with neurotoxicity, many other factors conspire to cause mental status changes in cancer patients. A thorough evaluation is warranted in such patients to rule out other causes. The differential diagnosis includes electrolyte imbalances, dehydration, organ failure, intracranial disease (such as brain or leptomeningeal metastases), paraneoplastic syndromes, endocrine dysfunction, infections (such as urinary tract infections), seizures, other medications (such as opioids) and nutritional deficiencies.

Chemotherapy-induced peripheral neuropathy

Peripheral neuropathy is the most common neurologic complication of chemotherapy, with vinca alkaloids, platinum compounds, taxanes, thalidomide, and bortezomib as the most neurotoxic. Chemotherapy-induced peripheral neuropathy (CIPN) may lead to dose reduction, treatment delay, or treatment discontinuation. The cumulative toxic dose associated with clinical manifestations varies according to chemotherapy (e.g. greater than 30–50 mg for vinca alkaloids and greater than 300–400 mg/m^2 for platinum analogues). CIPN is often characterized by a painful sensory neuropathy, initially presenting as paresthesias and dysesthesias in the fingers and toes. The symptoms may spread proximally to affect upper and lower extremities in a stocking–glove distribution. Pathophysiology also varies according to chemotherapy; mechanisms include disruption of microtubule assembly and axonal transport. Nerve conduction studies may demonstrate a length-dependent axonal pattern or a sensory neuronopathy depending on the chemotherapeutic agent. Other patterns of peripheral nervous system involvement include autonomic neuropathy with vincristine, ataxic neuropathy with cisplatin, cranial neuropathies with vinca alkaloids, proximal motor neuropathy with taxanes, and transient neuromyotonia with oxaliplatin. CIPN can be exacerbated by co-morbid conditions associated with peripheral neuropathy, such as diabetes, alcoholism, nutritional deficiencies (e.g. thiamine, vitamin B$_{12}$), metabolic disorders (e.g. hypothyroidism), compressive injuries, and vascular damage. Therefore, diagnostic work-up should exclude these disorders. Symptoms from CIPN often improve with drug discontinuation or dose reduction, but recovery may take months and may be incomplete. Symptoms may occasionally progress even after discontinuation, as seen with cisplatin. Several agents have been investigated for the prevention or treatment of CIPN, but data are insufficient to warrant routine use in clinical practice.

Bortezomib, a proteosome inhibitor used in the treatment of multiple myeloma, causes a small fiber, axonal sensory neuropathy that is one of its main dose-limiting toxicities. The incidence is in the range of 30–40%, and the prevalence increases through the first five treatment cycles. Neuropathic pain is more prominent than sensory loss or paresthesias. Examination typically reveals loss of pain and temperature distally with preservation of vibration sense, muscle strength, and ankle reflexes. As with other small fiber neuropathies, nerve conduction studies may be unremarkable. Most patients experience resolution or improvement of their neuropathy symptoms with dose reduction or drug discontinuation. The cause of bortezomib-related neuropathy is unknown.

Oxaliplatin is another chemotherapy commonly associated with peripheral neuropathy. This is a third generation platinum compound used for metastatic colorectal cancer. Two distinct syndromes are described:

1 An acute reversible neurotoxicity characterized by paresthesias, cold hypersensitivity, jaw and eye pain, ptosis, leg cramps, and visual and voice changes occurring during or shortly after an infusion; and
2 A chronic sensory distal axonal neuropathy occurring with cumulative doses of oxaliplatin.

Strategies for minimizing the latter syndrome include interspersing oxaliplatin with a nonoxaliplatin-containing regimen and lengthening the duration of infusion. Calcium and magnesium infusions may also reduce the severity of oxaliplatin-induced chronic peripheral neuropathy without reducing response rates, but further studies are needed to determine their true role in preventing oxaliplatin peripheral neuropathy (Table 21.1).

★ TIPS AND TRICKS

Chemotherapy-induced peripheral neuropathy (CIPN) is characterized by a painful, sensory neuropathy in a stocking–glove distribution and can be a significant source of morbidity for patients. Recovery from CIPN is variable depending on the offending agent. Gradual improvement may occur over months with oxaliplatin and bortezomib.

Radiation toxicity

The effectiveness of radiotherapy is frequently limited by the tolerance of the nervous system. Although radiation is carefully planned to minimize damage to normal neural structures, radiation toxicity can still affect any part of the neuroaxis resulting in encephalopathies, myelopathies, brachial and lumbosacral plexopathies, malignant peripheral nerve sheath tumors, brain tumors, and a variety of other neurologic disorders. Certain neural tissues are particularly vulnerable to radiation damage including the hypothalamus, resulting in endocrine dysfunction, and optic nerves, resulting in vision loss or blindness. The cerebrovascular system is also susceptible to delayed effects from radiation, resulting in vascular malformations, aneurysms, accelerated atherosclerosis, and strokes. Risk factors associated with radiation-induced nervous system complications include fraction doses >200 cGy, cumulative radiation doses >5000 cGy, volume of brain irradiated, concomitant or subsequent chemotherapy, age <7 or >60 years, pre-existing CNS damage, and vascular risk factors.

Cranial irradiation is an important component of primary and metastatic brain tumor management, but can cause acute, subacute, and chronic complications. During or shortly following radiation, patients may experience progressive fatigue and signs of intracranial pressure attributed to disruption of the blood–brain barrier and cerebral edema. Fatigue generally resolves following completion of radiation. Corticosteroids can improve mild symptoms, but increased intracranial pressure sometimes requires more aggressive management. Subacute, or early delayed, effects occur approximately 6–12 weeks following radiation. Symptoms include generalized weakness, fatigue, and somnolence caused, in part, by transient demyelination and disruption of the blood–brain barrier.

The most severe complications of radiation neurotoxicity are delayed or chronic. Delayed cerebral radionecrosis occurs months to years after radiation to brain parenchyma. This can affect a diffuse area of the brain, as seen following whole-brain radiation, or can be localized, as seen following focal radiation. Although best characterized following external beam radiation, focal cerebral radionecrosis may be relatively more common after stereotactic radiosurgery or interstitial brachytherapy. In patients with glioblastoma, the combination of temozolomide with fractionated radiotherapy increases the risk of radiation necrosis and can produce changes on imaging that mimic tumor progression. Presenting signs and symptoms of delayed cerebral radionecrosis are nonspecific and include headaches, confusion, seizures, cognitive dysfunction (discussed further below), and focal neurologic deficits. Both vascular and glial damage have been implicated in the pathophysiology. Cerebral radionecrosis may be difficult to distinguish from tumor recurrence. Occasionally, biopsy is needed for definitive diagnosis. Clinical improvement has been reported in small series following treatment with corticosteroids, anticoagulation, hyperbaric oxygen therapy, or bevacizumab but further studies are needed to clarify the role of these agents in radiation necrosis.

One dreaded manifestation of delayed radiation injury is cognitive dysfunction, although the existing data characterizing this complication in adults are limited. Varying degrees of cognitive impairment have been reported, although as many as 12% of patients may develop frank dementia. Radiation-induced cognitive dysfunction must be distinguished from other causes of cognitive decline such as disease progression, chemotherapy, medications (including corticosteroids and anticonvulsants), paraneoplastic dis-

Table 21.1. Common neurologic complications associated with chemotherapy.

Agent	Common uses	Neurologic complications
Platinum compounds		
Cisplatin	Sarcoma, small cell lung cancer, ovarian cancer, lymphoma, germ cell tumors	Sensory large fiber neuropathy Ototoxicity
Oxaliplatin	Colorectal cancer	Acute neurotoxicity characterized by paresthesias Chronic sensory neuropathy
Vinca alkaloids		
Vincristine	Non-Hodgkin lymphoma, Hodgkin disease, leukemia, nephroblastoma	Sensory > motor neuropathy Autonomic neuropathy
Taxanes		
Paclitaxel	Ovarian, breast, lung, head and neck cancers	Sensory neuropathy Motor neuropathy causing proximal muscle weakness Acute pain syndrome with myalgias and arthralgias (within days of administration)
Nab-Paclitaxel (protein-bound paclitaxel)	Breast cancer	Sensory neuropathy
Docetaxel	Breast, ovarian, non-small cell lung cancer	Sensory neuropathy (less frequent than paclitaxel) Motor neuropathy (less frequent than paclitaxel)
Antimetabolites		
Methotrexate	Lymphoma, leukemia	Aseptic meningitis and transverse myelopathy (less common) with IT administration Acute encephalopathy (high doses and IT) Delayed leukoencephalopathy
Cytarabine	Leukemia, lymphoma	Aseptic meningitis with IT administration Acute cerebellar dysfunction (high doses)
Nelarabine	Leukemia	Encephalopathy Headache Seizures Peripheral neuropathy (leg weakness and paresthesias)

(Continued)

Table 21.1. (*Continued*)

Agent	Common uses	Neurologic complications
5-fluorouracil (5-FU)	Colorectal cancer	Acute encephalopathy Acute cerebellar dysfunction (rare) Subacute multifocal leukoencephalopathy
Ifosfamide	Testicular, breast, lung, cervical, ovarian, bone cancers; lymphomas; sarcomas	Acute encephalopathy (high doses)
Epothilones		
Ixabepilone	Breast cancer	Sensory neuropathy
Others chemotherapies		
Thalidomide	Multiple myeloma	Sensory neuropathy Somnolence
Bortezomib	Multiple myeloma, mantle cell lymphoma	Sensory neuropathy
Sunitinib	Renal cell carcinoma, gastrointestinal stromal tumor	Muscle cramps and myalgias
Interferon-alpha	Leukemia, lymphoma	Depression Headaches, encephalopathy, seizures (high doses)
L-asparaginase	Leukemia	Venous sinus thrombosis

IT, intrathecal.

orders, and toxic metabolic disorders. In addition, cognitive dysfunction may not become apparent for several years. In a longitudinal study of low grade gliomas comparing irradiated patients with nonirradiated patients, no differences in cognitive function were detected at a mean of 6 years after diagnosis. Yet, re-evaluation of the same cohort at a mean of 12 years after diagnosis did reveal cognitive disabilities in 53% of the patients who had radiation compared to 4% of the patients who were radiotherapy-naïve. Typically, in patients with radiation-induced cognitive dysfunction, neuropsychologic testing reveals deficits in memory, visual motor processing, quantitative skills, and attention. Brain MRI may demonstrate leukoencephalopathy, progressive brain atrophy, or radiation necrosis, but patients with mild to moderate cognitive dys-

function often have normal-appearing neuroimaging. The underlying pathology may be related to inflammation, metabolic derangements, and long-term damage of various neural cell types including stem and progenitor cells. In addition, cranial irradiation can profoundly inhibit neurogenesis in the hippocampus, an area of the brain essential to learning and memory. Both methylphenidate and donepezil improve cognition in brain tumor patients. Ventriculoperitoneal shunting may benefit patients with radiation-induced hydrocephalus.

Loss of hormonal functions of the hypothalamic–pituitary axis is a common adverse event following cranial irradiation. Patients in pediatric as well as adult populations who receive radiation involving the parasellar or hypothalamic regions may be at greater risk for endocrine deficits and may require neuroendocrine surveillance. The onset may be insidious over months to years, and hypothalamic–pituitary axis radiation can result in deficiencies involving growth hormone (GH), adrenocorticotrophic hormone (ACTH), and/or thyroid-stimulating hormone (TSH). The manifestations depend upon which hormones are lacking. Hormone deficiencies are correctable with hormone replacement.

Another well-described toxicity affecting the nervous system is radiation-induced plexopathy. This can affect the brachial plexus following radiation for lung or breast cancer or the lumbosacral plexus following radiation for pelvic or lower abdominal tumors. A patient may present with progressive weakness and paresthesias in the arms or legs several months following radiation therapy. Pain is uncommon, which may help distinguish radiation plexopathy from tumor infiltration or compression. Diagnosis is often clinical although electromyography may demonstrate mykyomia. Imaging studies can be used to exclude tumor infiltration or compression from the differential diagnosis. Treatment is generally conservative (Table 21.2).

Table 21.2. Common neurologic complications associated with radiation.

Time course	Neurologic complications
Acute	Fatigue
	Increased intracranial pressure (headache, nausea, mental status changes, etc.)
Subacute	Generalized weakness, fatigue, somnolence
Chronic	Focal radionecrosis
	Cognitive dysfunction
	Hydrocephalus
	Brachial/lumbosacral plexopathy
	Endocrine dysfunction
	Vascular malformations, aneurysms, accelerated atherosclerosis, strokes

Conclusions

Neurotoxicity is a common dose-limiting toxicity for chemotherapy and radiation therapy. The neurologist can have an important role in the care of cancer patients through early recognition. Work-up should also include a thorough evaluation for other conditions that can mimic neurotoxicities from anticancer treatments.

Selected bibliography

Albers J, Chaudhry V, Cavaletti G, Donehower R. (2007) Interventions for preventing neuropathy caused by cisplatin and related compounds. *Cochrane Database Syst Rev*, **1**, CD005228.

Antoine JC, Camdessanche JP. (2007) Peripheral nervous system involvement in patients with cancer. *Lancet Neurol* **6**, 75–86.

DeAngelis LM, Posner JB. (eds) (2009) *Neurologic Complications of Cancer*, Oxford University Press, New York, pp. 447–510.

Dietrich J, Monje M, Wefel J, Meyers C. (2008) Clinical patterns and biological correlates of cognitive dysfunction associated with cancer therapy. *Oncologist* **13**, 1285–95.

Douw L, Klein M, Fagel SS, van den Heuvel J, Taphoorn MJ, Aaronson NK, *et al.* (2009) Cognitive and radiological effects of radiotherapy in patients with low-grade glioma: long-term follow-up. *Lancet Neurol* **8**, 810–8.

Khasraw M, Posner JB. (2010) Neurological complications of systemic cancer. *Lancet Neurol* **9**, 1214–27.

Marinella MA, Markert RJ. (2009) Reversible posterior leucoencephalopathy syndrome associated with anticancer drugs. *Intern Med J* **39**, 826–34.

Monje M. (2008) Cranial radiation therapy and damage to hippocampal neurogenesis. *Dev Disabil Res Rev* **14**, 238–42.

Richardson PG, Briemberg H, Jagannath S, Wen PY, Barlogie B, Berenson J, *et al.* (2006) Frequency, characteristics, and reversibility of peripheral neuropathy during treatment of advanced multiple myeloma with bortezomib. *J Clin Oncol* **24**, 3113–20.

Schiff D, Wen PY, van den Bent MJ. (2009) Neurological adverse effects caused by cytotoxic and targeted therapies. *Nat Rev Clin Oncol* **6**, 596–603.

Shih HA, Loeffler JS, Tarbell NJ. (2009) Late effects of CNS radiation therapy. *Cancer Treat Res* **150**, 23–41.

Sioka C, Kyritsis AP. (2009) Central and peripheral nervous system toxicity of common chemotherapeutic agents. *Cancer Chemother Pharmacol* **63**, 761–7.

Vardy J, Rourke S, Tannock IF. (2007) Evaluation of cognitive function associated with chemotherapy: a review of published studies and recommendations for future research. *J Clin Oncol* **25**, 2455–63.

Wefel JS, Wltgert ME, Meyers CA. (2008) Neuropsychological sequelae of non-central nervous system cancer and cancer therapy. *Neuropsychol Rev* **18**, 121–31.

Wolf S, Barton D, Kottschade L, Grothey A, Loprinzi C. (2008) Chemotherapy-induced peripheral neuropathy: prevention and treatment strategies. *Eur J Cancer* **44**, 1507–15.

Yoshii Y. (2008) Pathological review of late cerebral radionecrosis. *Brain Tumor Pathol* **25**, 51–8.

Index

Neuro-oncology, First Edition. Edited by Roger J. Packer, David Schiff.
© 2012 John Wiley & Sons, Ltd. Published 2012 by John Wiley & Sons, Ltd.

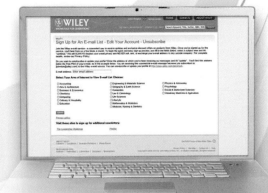
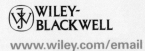